AF754845

Sex Offending Behavior of Persons with an Intellectual Disability:

A Multi-Component Applied Behavior Analytic Approach

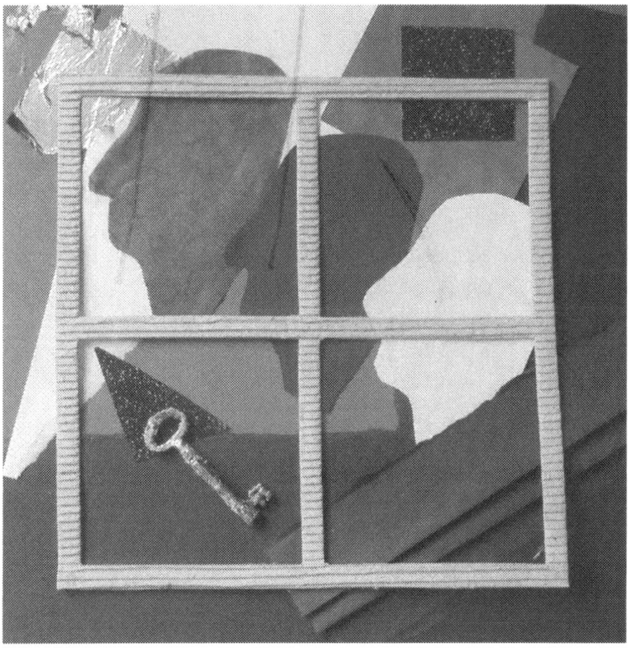

Dorothy M. Griffiths, Kendra Thomson, Stephanie Ioannou, Jordan Hoath and Robin J. Wilson

With contributions from Jan Frijters

Foreword by Peter Sturmey

NADD An association for persons with developmental disabilities and mental health needs.

132 Fair Street
Kingston, New York 12401

ISBN: 978-1-57256-123-6
LCCN: 2018966276

Printed in the United States of America

About our Authors

Jan C. Frijters is an Associate Professor in the Department of Child and Youth Studies at Brock University. His research focuses on learning difficulties, motivation, and intervention. He also has a passion for quantitative research methods, especially for techniques such as multilevel modeling, person-centered, and structural equation modeling approaches that can help sort out how developmental processes unfold over time and within specific learning contexts.

Dorothy Griffiths is a Professor Emerita in the Department of Child and Youth Studies and the Department of Applied Disabilities at Brock University. She has published and presented extensively in the area of challenging behavior and persons with intellectual and developmental disabilities, with special interests in sexually offending behavior and issues regarding human rights and persons with disabilities. She is a member of the Order of Ontario and the Order of Canada.

Jordan Hoath has been supporting individuals with intellectual disabilities in a variety of roles for 15 years. His clinical and research interests include ethics of treating problematic sexual behaviors and the community reintegration of high risk offenders.

Stephanie Ioannou is a Board Certified Behavior Analyst who has provided assessment and treatment to persons with dual diagnosis and sexual offending behavior in community settings. Within a bio-psycho-social framework, she has worked with adults with dual diagnosis and challenging behaviors and provided clinical oversight of the delivery of ABA services to children/youth with autism and their families.

Kendra Thomson is an Associate Professor in the Department of Applied Disability Studies at Brock University and a Doctoral-level Board Certified Behavior Analyst (BCBA-D). Her research is investigating best practices for training others (parents, support staff, etc.) how to provide evidence-based support to individuals with intellectual and developmental disabilities and how that impacts individuals and their families.

Robin J. Wilson is a board certified clinical and consulting psychologist with more than 30 years' experience in sexual violence prevention. His research and practice focus on the assessment, treatment, and risk management of persons with sexual behavior problems, particularly, individuals with intellectual disabilities and persons returning to the community after long-term incarceration or hospitalization.

Acknowledgements

This book is dedicated to the memory of Susan Tough, former Director of York-Simcoe Behavior Management Services (currently renamed as Mackenzie Health Centre for Behaviour Health Sciences). In her memory and in respect for her contribution to the research and practice related to persons with intellectual disabilities who have committed sexually offending behaviors, the proceeds of this book will be donated to the Susan Tough Award that is given to a graduate student in the Applied Disability Department at Brock University in St. Catharines, Ontario.

The authors also wish to express our thanks to the late William Lindsay who inspired us to write this book. Bill was one of the most prolific researchers in the field of treatment for persons with intellectual disability who had sexually offended. We hope this book would be what he had hoped it would become.

Another thank you to Maurice Feldman who encouraged us by suggesting that a book that firmly grounded the principles of Applied Behavior Analysis into the current applied practice in the treatment of persons with intellectual disabilities who have sexually offended was a much needed addition to the field.

TABLE OF CONTENTS

About our Authors iii
Acknowledgements v
Foreword ix
Preface xiii

PART I: FOUNDATIONS

Chapter 1. Introduction 3

Chapter 2. Sex offending behavior and persons with an intellectual disability 23

Chapter 3. Towards a multi-component decision model for assessment and treatment of sexual offending behavior of persons with an intellectual disability 43

PART II: ASSESSMENT

Chapter 4. Exploring antecedents and consequences related to sex offending behaviors of persons with an intellectual disability 57

Chapter 5. Exploring the role of motivating operations of sex offending behavior of persons with an intellectual disability 87

Chapter 6. Exploring the functions of sex offending behavior of persons with an intellectual disability 101

Chapter 7. Combining assessment components into an integrated treatment plan 117

PART III: TREATMENT

Chapter 8. Setting the stage for success in treating sexual offending behavior 143

Chapter 9. Teaching alternative or coping skills for sex offending behavior 173

Chapter 10. Corrective and remedial consequences 201

PART IV: GENERALIZATION AND MAINTENANCE

Chapter 11. Long term management 223

Chapter 12. Pulling it all together 243

PART V: ETHICAL DILEMMAS

Chapter 13. Ethical dilemmas in treating persons with intellectual disabilities who have sexually offended 269

Foreword

Peter Sturmey, Ph.D.

The Graduate Center and Queens College, City University of New York

Some forty years ago I remember interviewing an adult with moderate intellectual disabilities on a locked ward of a British mental handicap hospital. It was a dismal picture. He was highly sexually motivated. He would casually inform anyone who asked that he was interested in "men, women, boys and girls" and spent much of his time looking out of the windows in the direction of a nearby junior school which he was very familiar with. The setting was barren and even hostile. There was nothing to do and staff despised him because of his sexual interest in children. When they talked to him – and it was not often – they were curt and often rude. They could not understand him and had no idea what to do about the problem other than try to stop it happening by locked doors, enhanced supervision, hormonal treatment (which was not particularly helpful, but did cause development of breasts), and threats. Professional staff and administrators were no more effective than direct support staff. There were no treatment programs of any kind for men like this, and outcome for him and his victims was poor. He ended up sexually assaulting other residents in part because there was nothing else to do and no other sexual outlets for him.

Without being complacent, I think we have come a long way in forty years: This book by Dorothy Griffiths, Kendra Thomson, Stephanie Ioannou, Jordan Hoath, Robin Wilson and Jan Frijters beautifully illustrates that.

Over the last 40, years we have seen the elimination and downsizing of institutional services with the concomitant enormous increase in community services involving care by families, more early intervention, education, and adult services of all kinds. This change has happened not only for individuals who are easy to support but also those who are truly challenging. Early work on community services focused on individuals with severe externalizing challenging behavior such as aggression (e.g., Toogood et al., 1988) which took ideas from applied behavior analysis (ABA) and attempted to apply and integrate them into typical services. Only later did research-practitioners begin to attend to society's, service, and individual's needs related to persons with intellectual disabilities who had offender sexually. Beginning with the early work of the York Behavior Management Services in Ontario in the 1970s in collaboration with lead researchers, including Gene Abel and Vernon Quinsey, research-practitioners began to address understanding and treating offending behavior in individuals with intellectual disabilities. This seed sprouted and grew into thirty years of applied research and service development in Ontario, but also in the United Kingdom, Australia, and the United States among other countries.

Early ABA work on modification of problematic sexual behavior in various populations demonstrated that both respondent and operant processes were often important, but such work often used simple positive punishment procedures using arbitrary consequences, were often conducted in analog, clinic or institutional settings, and focused on one narrow part of an individual's life. Such approaches may have been justified in the past when little was known, but individuals and their families need more than reduction in a narrowly defined problem behavior treated only by consequences. Researchers initially developed functional assessment and analysis extensively in relationship to self-injury (Carr, 1977). They subsequently extended this approach and subsequently extended in various ways, such as applications to multiple forms of challenging behavior (Hanley, Iwata, & McCord, 2003), positive behavior support (Carr et al., 1999), and applications to a wide variety of clinical problems (Sturmey, 2007), including logical functional analysis (Wulfert, Dougher, & Greenway, 1996). An important contribution of this volume is to take these notions of and expand and integrate their application to sex offending behavior in individuals with intellectual disabilities in the context of contemporary services while addressing important questions such as person-centered planning, staff training, and working with families, police and courts.

Throughout the book the authors make excellent use of case material which is rich, varied, and authentic. The case material makes good teaching material and good models for practitioners. The case material also usefully illustrates the abstract concepts, application to practice, and ethical issues in this challenging field.

I congratulate Dorothy Griffiths, Kendra Thomson, Stephanie Ioannou, Jordan Hoath, Robin Wilson, and Jan Frijters not only for writing this excellent book, but (in some cases) a lifetime dedicated to ethical, practical, and science-based treatment of individuals with intellectual disabilities and sex offending behavior to reduce their challenging behavior, give them a better life, and make the world a better and safer place for all of us.

REFERENCES

Carr, E. G. (1977). The motivation of self-injurious behavior: A review of some hypotheses. *Psychological Bulletin, 84*(4), 800-816. http://dx.doi.org/10.1037/0033-2909.84.4.800

Carr, E. G., Horner, R. H., Turnbull, A. P., Marquis, J. G., Magito McLaughlin, D., ... Doolabh, A., (1999). *Positive behavior support as an approach for dealing with problem behavior in people with developmental disabilities: A research synthesis.* Monographs of the American Association on Mental Retardation. Washington, D.C.: American Association on Mental Retardation.

Hanley, G. P., Iwata, B. A., & McCord, B. E., (2003). Functional analysis of problem behavior: A review. *Journal of Applied Behavior Analysis, 36,* 146-185.

Sturmey, P. (2007). *Functional analysis in clinical treatment.* New York: Elsevier.

Toogood, A., Emerson, E., Hughes, H., Barret, Cummings S., & McCool, C., (1988). Challenging behavior and community services 3: Planning individualised services. *British Journal of Learning Disabilities, 16,* 70-74.

Wulfert, E., Greenway, D., & Dougher, M. J. (1996). A logical functional analysis of reinforcement-based disorders: Alcoholism and pedophilia. *Journal of Consulting and Clinical Psychology, 64(6),* 1140-1151

Preface

Applied behavior analysis (ABA) has been defined as "the science in which tactics derived from the principles of behavior are applied systematically to improve socially significant behavior and experimentation is used to identify the variables responsible for behavior change" (Cooper, Heron &, Heward, 2007, p. 20). Many effective treatment approaches, based on the principles of ABA, have been applied to a variety of socially significant behaviors (e.g., academic skills and addiction to smoking cessation) and across diverse populations (e.g., autism spectrum disorder and acquired brain injury to stroke patients). Treatment for challenging behavior, when exhibited by persons with intellectual disabilities, is most typically addressed through empirically supported behavioral principles. Willner (2005) noted that staff members are often trained in behavioral methods, which are relatively successful in managing most challenging behaviors. However, when the challenging behavior is sexual or of a sex offending nature, behavior analysts often report being ill prepared to approach this area of intervention even though the same principles apply.

At the International Dual Diagnosis Certificate Program (IDDCP) in 2014, Dr. Timothy Vollmer, then editor of the flagship journal in the field of ABA *Journal of Applied Behavior Analysis*, noted that there is a lack of research in the area of sexual violence prevention. Dr. Vollmer cited some of the challenges associated with conducting research on behaviors that are high-risk and often clandestine and infrequent.

In 2015, again addressing IDDCP, Dr. William Lindsay, one of the sexual violence prevention field's most prolific and noted clinicians and authors, suggested that the empirical research on ABA and sexual offending behavior (SOB) may be lacking because ABA techniques have been researched but failed to produce empirically-significant results (e.g., lack of large sample size or highly controlled experimental designs). While this hypothesis is warranted based on the lack of experimentally validated research, the authors of this book pose a rival hypothesis. Our experience based on years of successful clinical practice in this field employing these ABA principles to treat offenders leads us to suggest that while it is true that published research on SOB and ABA and persons who have sexually offended has been sparse in recent decades, there may be an alternative hypothesis to explain this observation.

One potential rival hypothesis may be that the assessment of SOB, if conducted through a rigid lens where researchers are attempting to prove that a certain type of treatment is appropriate for all offenders, is far too simplistic. Years ago, one of the authors reviewed a research proposal that proposed to research the effectiveness of a certain treatment approach applied randomly to a group of sex offenders compared to a group receiving a different type of treatment. There was an implication in this research design that "one size fits all." This type of research violates the basic understanding of efficacious ABA, which is grounded in comprehensive individualized assessment and treatment. In ABA, the assessment of the variables that lead to and maintain behavior, not the topography of the behavior alone, determines treatment. However, even among the sexual violence prevention literature, a clear trend has emerged to suggest there are different paths to offending (i.e., Ward & Hudson, 1998); understanding the importance of assessment pathways to offending has been applied to offenders who have an intellectual disability (Lindsay, Steptoe, & Beech, 2008). The authors of this text contend that research and practice in the area of SOB and ABA must therefore follow a model-based design that ensures that treatment aligns with a protocol of analysis.

An earlier model was introduced by Griffiths, Quinsey, and Hingsburger in 1989. They proposed that to determine an efficacious therapeutic approach for each suspected offender, individualized assessment required investigation of three main components: patterns of sexual arousal, sexual knowledge, socio-sexual skills, and three subcomponents: relationship skills, coping skills, and moral and legal responsibility. They suggested that these six components formed the basis for development of an integrated treatment model. In their model, they proposed that following an assessment of each component, an individual would be provided targeted intervention in the components deemed related to the offense or identified as lacking and, as such, requiring improvement. Hence, where a lack of coping or anger management may have played a part in the offense, this component would be identified as part of a treatment package and similarly for each component including arousal to deviant imagery. It was not assumed that all offenders would show deficits in all areas, and, as such, the model proposed to identify the areas of vulnerability for each offender and provide habilitation or rehabilitation in the areas deemed to be lacking. This model, which was designed for use in community settings, included an active relapse prevention component that included development of a network of support around the individual to build a life that proactively prevented relapses and provided a safety net for early intervention in lapsing behavior.

Wulfert, Greenway, and Dougher (1996) later suggested that by identifying the functional clusters of behavior for sex offending behavior, a logical functional analysis could be formed that would provide a decision model on which to organize assessment and create a stronger link to targeted treatment. They proposed that by following this approach, clinicians could develop intervention guidelines founded on a functional understanding of sexually offending behavior.

Following from the two examples provided above, the authors of this book propose an integrated model that can serve as a basis for behavior analysts to assess and intervene for persons with intellectual disabilities who have sexually offended. In this book, a six-component decision-based model for the behavioral assessment of sexualized offending behavior of persons with intellectual disabilities will be explored. In contrast to the above model, which was largely based on teaching appropriate and replacement skills using behavioral principles, this book proposes to base its model on the use of the current ABA approaches to assessment and treatment that have emerged as standard practice. As such, this book represents a model that will bridge the gap between ABA and the treatment of SOB.

Let's look at three cases below and see what your first impressions are regarding these behaviors.

CASE I

Jerry is a 21-year-old male, diagnosed with a mild intellectual disability, oppositional defiant disorder, and attention deficit hyperactivity disorder. Jerry has a long history of sexual assaults, the first occurring at 16 when he fondled a five-year-old girl in his neighbourhood. There were no charges laid, as Jerry's family dealt with the situation on their own and resolved this with the neighbors by assuring them he would not be allowed to be in the presence of their child again. Later, when Jerry was 17, he invited a 7-year-old neighborhood boy into his family home to watch movies in the basement. Jerry's parents were upstairs at the time and they felt it was okay for him to invite a boy into the basement because "Jerry was like a child himself." Jerry rubbed on top of the boy with their clothes on. When the boy told his parents, the boy's parents called the police who soon arrived at Jerry's house. Jerry's parents minimized the assault and placed blame on the boy's parents for not keeping track of their son. No charges were laid with the agreement that Jerry would be placed elsewhere and, therefore, would no longer live in the neighborhood.

CASE II

Porter is a 21-year-old man who lives in a large multi-bed setting. The staff reported that he was placed there by his family for sexual reasons. Porter has also been reported to have three known episodes of alleged sexually offensive behavior within this multi-bed setting, the latter of which involved a person who was new to the facility. She and Porter had no relationship prior to the offense. The woman had limited cognitive abilities and would have been deemed incapable of giving informed consent to sexual contact. Her family wanted Porter charged and the staff agreed, given that he has a long history of sexual offense.

CASE III

Scott is a 25-year-old man with high functioning cognitive challenges and, because of his abilities, was hired as a "junior staff" in his day program. One of the individuals at day program indicated to staff that Scott had touched his genitals, however the staff were adamant that these behaviors were an accident and that there was no way Scott knew what he was doing. Scott continued the offenses but was better able to hide the behavior and only assaulted individuals who were non-verbal. Scott assigned vulnerable males special tasks that he would oversee and then took advantage of this situation by isolating the members to sexually assault them. Scott's behavior continued. Finally, the day program staff members became aware of it, but they were reluctant to notify the residence in which Scott lived because they believed Scott would be unfairly restricted. On one occasion after many observed incidents, the staff members did notify the authorities, but the police refused to press charges; the responding officers said they had met people with disabilities before and people like Scott don't know what they're doing.

Each of these cases represents different and unique challenges. There is no treatment program that will fit each individual because the path by which they became a person who sexually offended was different. Each person, however, requires a thorough assessment of their general history and specific history related to the 'index offense,' which refers to the last offense that has brought them to the point where they are being assessed by a behavior analyst. The purpose of the functional behavioral assessment is, as with all behaviors, to determine the antecedents, specific target behaviors, maintaining consequences, and any potential motivating operations, to hopefully determine the function of the behavior. Based on an integration of the behavioral assessment model, an individualized treatment plan will be developed that will focus on prevention through setting the stage for success, teaching alternative and coping skills, determining remedial and corrective consequences, and determining a path for long term risk management. Given the nature of the population, additional assessment information may be needed.

In the *Diagnostic Manual-Intellectual Disability* (DM-ID; Fletcher, Loschen, Stavrakaki & First, 2007), the companion to the *Diagnostic and Statistical Manual of Mental Disorders* (DSM-IV-TR; American Psychiatric Association, 2000), the authors of the Sexual and Gender Identity Disorder chapter (Griffiths et al., 2007) suggested that, in addition to standard risk, cognitive, and phallometric assessments, sociosexual knowledge be evaluated when assessing individuals with intellectual disabilities and sexual related offenses.

As behavior analysts have long known, there is no cookie cutter solution to any behavior problem. An effective treatment approach begins with an individualized assessment of the variables that evoke/elicit and maintain the behavior, including the motivating operations at work for a particular person. In this book, we have elaborated the skills necessary to apply these principles to persons with intellectual disabilities who sexually offend.

The book is divided into five parts. Part I provides a description of the foundations of ABA as it applies to persons with intellectual disabilities who have sexually offended and sets the stage for the logical functional model. Part I includes the first three chapters of the book. Chapter 1 provides historical background and an introduction to existing literature as it relates to sex offending behavior and ABA. Chapter 2 provides background on how sex offending behavior with persons with intellectual disabilities is defined, in addition to special considerations that have been identified for this population. Chapter 3 is a foundational chapter focusing on the logical functional model for the assessment and treatment of sexual offending behavior in persons with intellectual disabilities.

Part II consists of Chapters 4 to 7 and includes discussion regarding application of behavioral principles related to the assessment of persons with intellectual disabilities who have sexually offended: the contingencies (including motivating operations), and function of sex offending behavior as it relates to persons with intellectual disabilities. In Chapter 7, the authors revisit the three case examples described above to demonstrate how to incorporate the key elements of the assessment into an integrated treatment package.

Part III of the book provides a foundation for intervention. Chapter 8 introduces guidelines for setting the stage for success to ensure proactive and preventative environmental conditions. Chapter 9 reviews the approaches needed to teach alternative and coping skills for managing sexually offensive behavior in persons with intellectual disabilities. Chapter 10 discusses the nature of corrective or remedial consequences.

Part IV includes Chapters 11 on long term risk management, which addresses issues of generalization and maintenance of treatment gains in the community, and Chapter 12, which pulls together the treatment discussion by demonstrating the application to our three case examples.

Part V (Chapter 13) explores some of the ethical dilemmas in the treatment of sexual offending behavior of persons with intellectual disabilities including implications for research.

In this book, the authors propose a multi-component decision model, based on Wulfert and colleagues (1996) and the behavior analytic literature on functional behavior assessment, to serve as a basis for behavior analysts to assess and intervene with persons with intellectual disabilities who have sexually offended. These components fall into three areas: assessment (determining contingencies, motivating operations, and function), treatment (teaching alternative or coping skills and providing remedial consequences), and long-term risk management (including generalization and maintenance). The outcomes of the assessment component will serve as a foundation for a decision about a path for intervention.

The proposed model is not a new model. Rather, the consensus in the field in working with persons with intellectual disabilities who sexually offend often suggests a comprehensive multi-component model to assessment and treatment (i.e. Pritchard et al., 2011; 2016). This is because there is currently no single treatment model that can best address the unique characteristics of this population. Typically, best practice approaches are drawn from a variety of principles and theoretical models. Therefore, with the creation of this model, the authors have aimed to amalgamate all the best practice principles and combine them into one multi-component model within an ABA framework to be applied to people with intellectual disabilities.

The suggestions and approaches in this model may take extensive time to teach, make environmental modifications, and monitor. People who engage in inappropriate sexual behavior have likely been doing it a long time with strong histories of reinforcement as sexualized behavior in persons with intellectual disabilities is often ignored, dismissed, minimized, or simply managed. The authors recognize that applying this model to people who often present with complex and complicated histories is not a straightforward task. However, we are suggesting that by taking a systematic approach to assessing problematic sexual behavior using the same principles used with other challenging behaviors, we can provide a clear and comprehensive direction for intervention. The underpinning of many effective techniques and strategies used with people who display sexually offensive behavior are grounded in ABA.

REFERENCES

American Psychiatric Association (2000). *Diagnostic and statistical manual of mental disorders (DSM-TR-IV)*. Washington, DC: author.

Cooper, J. O., Heron, T. E., & Heward, W. L. (2007). *Applied behavior analysis* (2nd ed.). Upper Saddle River, NJ: Pearson Education Inc.

Fletcher, R., Loschen, E., Stavrakaki. C. & First, M. *(Eds.) (2007). Diagnostic manual-Intellectual disability* (DM-ID). Kingston, NY: NADD Press.

Griffiths, D., Fedoroff, P., Richards, D., Cox-Lindenbaum, D., Langevin, R., Linsday, W.D., Hucker, S., & Goldman, M. (2007). Sexual and gender identity disorders. In R. Fletcher, E. Loschen, S. Stavrakaki, & M. First (Eds.). *Diagnostic Manual - Intellectual Disability (DM-ID): A textbook of diagnosis of mental disorders in persons with intellectual disability* (pp.411-457). Kingston, NY: NADD Press.

Griffiths, D. M., Quinsey, V. L., & Hingsburger, D. (1989). *Changing inappropriate sexual behavior: A community-based approach for persons with developmental disabilities.* Baltimore, MD: Paul H. Brookes Publishing.

Lindsay, W. R. (June 2015). *Assessment and treatment of sexual offending behavior in persons with developmental disabilities and autism.* International Dual Diagnosis Certificate Program, Brock University, St. Catharines, Ontario

Lindsay, W.R., Steptoe, L., & Beech, A.T. (2008). The Ward and Hudson pathways model of the sexual offense process applied to offenders with intellectual disability. *Sexual Abuse, 20,* 379-92.

Pritchard, D., Graham, N., Penney, H., Owen, G., Peters, S., & Mace, C.F. (2016). Multi-component behavioral intervention reduces harmful sexual behavior in a 17-year-old male with autism spectrum disorder: a case study. *Journal of Sexual Aggression, 22*(3), 368-378.

Pritchard, D., Graham, N., Ikin, A., Penney, H., Kovacs, L., Mercer, D., ... Jones, D. (2011). Managing sexually harmful behavior in a residential special school. *British Journal of Learning Disabilities, 40,* 302-309.

Vollmer, T. (June 2014). *Assessment and intervention with sex offenders with intellectual disabilities.* International Dual Diagnosis Certificate Program, Brock University, St. Catharines, Ontario

Ward, T., & Hudson, S. M. (1998). The construction and development of theory in the sexual offending area: A meta-theoretical framework. *Sexual Abuse: A Journal of Research and Treatment, 10,* 47-63.

Willner, P. (2005). The effectiveness of psychotherapeutic interventions for people with learning disabilities: a critical overview. *Journal of Intellectual Disability Research, 49*(1), 73-85.

Wulfert, E., Greenway, D., & Dougher, M. J. (1996). A logical functional analysis of reinforcement-based disorders: Alcoholism and pedophilia. *Journal of Consulting and Clinical Psychology, 64*(6), 1140-1151.

PART I:

FOUNDATIONS

Chapter One

Introduction

> *(A)lthough ... scientists have largely avoided investigations of human sexuality, leaving this one of the most poorly explored fields in biology, psychology, or sociology, it should be emphasized that there is no aspect of human behavior about which there has been more thought, more talk, more books written (Kinsey, Pomeroy & Martin, 1948, p. 21).*

The field of ABA has undergone many changes in recent decades. Similarly, the field of sexual offender treatment has undergone significant shifts in the focus of assessment and treatment. In this chapter, the authors will explore these changes and how they intersect when providing assessment and intervention for persons with intellectual disabilities who have sexually offended.

BEHAVIORAL APPROACHES IN THE TREATMENT OF SEX OFFENDING

> *Contemporary approaches to sexual deviance owe little to classical psychoanalytical or psychodynamic theory or practice. Rather they are the result of the confluence of two psychologies: the radical behaviorism of John B. Watson...and the descriptive taxonomic approach of Alfred Kinsey and his associates... (Laws & Marshall, 2003, p.77).*

As cited in Laws and Marshall (2003), the development of the behaviorist view by Watson was influenced by Thorndike's earlier laws of learning and Pavlov's demonstration of classical conditioning. Watson's work, using reinforcement to analyze learning in animals, called for the examination of behavior as an objective science that would allow for the prediction and control of behavior, without examining the unobservable consciousness (Laws & Marshall, 2003).

Although Skinner's (1938) principles of operant conditioning shaped much of what occurred in the field of behaviorism in general, Laws and Marshall (2003) noted that it had very little impact on the treatment of sexual deviance, noting that in American academia, operant conditioning became dominant, but in the treatment of sexual deviance Pavlovian (or classical) conditioning was initially more accepted.

McGuire, Carlisle, and Young (1965) theorized that Pavlovian conditioning was at the etiology of sexual deviance, noting that accidental early sexual experiences involving deviant images were later used in fantasies paired with masturbation to create a sexual preference for deviant behavior and a lesser preference for nondeviant sexuality. The natural evolution of this theory into practice was to develop treatment to eliminate the deviant sexual preference. Application of this theory required a method of measurement. Kurt Freund (1965) introduced a method of measurement of sexual preference to erotic visual stimuli based upon changes in penile physiology (either volume, circumference, or both) in a controlled laboratory setting. [This measure known as the Penile Plethysmegraph (PPG) will be discussed later in this chapter and in Chapter 4.] With the scientific evidence to measure sexual arousal, new research demonstrated that punishment, such as electrical shock applied to the arm or leg could be used to modify sexual arousal. In the 1970s, the introduction of behavior therapy as applied to sexual deviance was initially based on reduction of problem behavior using aversion therapy, such as electric shock. Quinsey Chaplin, and Carrigan (1980) demonstrated early promising results suggesting that the effects of signalled punishment might have reduced response to inappropriate sexual stimuli. Follow-up research, however, has failed to find a strong effect of punishment or aversion on sexual preferences. Although intrusive procedures were applied to treat a variety of sexual behaviors which at the time were considered unconventional or deviant, by the 1980s, renowned scientists (Quinsey & Earls, 1990; Quinsey & Marshall, 1983) noted that aversion therapy, despite some immediate results, did not produce long term changes in inappropriate sexual behavior.

In 1958, Wolpe developed an approach called reciprocal inhibition, later renamed systematic desensitization, which at the time was applied to the treatment of deviant sexual interests (Bond & Hutchinson, 1960; Stevenson & Wolpe, 1960). Their work was followed by Marks and colleagues in developing behavioral approaches for the treatment of sexual deviance (Marks & Gelder, 1967; Marks, Gelder, & Bancroft, 1970; Marks, Rachman, & Gelder, 1965).

Marshall (1979) noted that the work of the lesser known Guthrie (1935) had demonstrated that if attempting to eliminate an undesirable behavior, treatment should evoke an alternative, preferably incompatible, response in the presence of the eliciting stimulus, by presenting the stimulus repeatedly to a point where the stimulus effect was exhausted. Marshall (1979) applied a variation of Guthrie's theory to attempt to eliminate arousal to sexually deviant stimuli, which he called satiation. Using a procedure highly similar to that reported by Marshall (1979), Laws (1995) analyzed a behavior therapy called verbal satiation to condition inhibition.

The 1970s saw a surge of interest in behavioral approaches to the treatment of sexual deviance under the influence of Gene Abel, a psychiatrist from the United States. His work and that of others focused not only on the reduction of deviant arousal but the enhancement of appropriate arousal to age appropriate partners (Abel, Blanchard, Barlow, & Flanagan, 1975). This period showed the introduction of a method in which an offender would masturbate while fantasizing about an appropriate sexual encounter (Marquis, 1970). In 1982, Kelly reported that the majority of programs were still employing behavioral suppression, whereas others had introduced treatment aimed at enhancing appropriate sexual behavior or were using both. As Laws and Marshall (2003) noted, it was at this time in the 1970s that a shift began. Although deviant sexual preferences were still considered an important piece of the puzzle of sexually offending behavior, it was becoming clear that understanding deviant sexual behavior would require a more comprehensive theoretical base that also entailed enhancement of appropriate sexual interests.

The 1970s also saw the recognition and integration of cognitive (covert) influences into conditioning therapy. Cautela studied the use of cognitive self-control procedures including covert sensitization, covert reinforcement, and covert extinction (Cautela, 1967, 1970, 1971). Practitioners in the 1970s began to respond to the growing influence of the work of Donald Meichenbaum (1974) regarding the role of perception and thought as cognitive mediating variables in behavior, which led to the emergence of cognitive behavior therapy. This shift was logical in the offender treatment world since altering deviant fantasies had been recognized as an important element in treating sex offenders (Abel & Blanchard, 1974). This recognition of the role of cognition also led Abel, Becker, and Cunningham-Rathner (1984) to identify the concept of cognitive distortion as an important element in sexual offending behavior. Cognitive distortions are biased beliefs regarding sexually deviant interests that do not match those held by society at large (e.g., women who wear short skirts are asking to be raped, some children can consent to sexual activities, etc.). These beliefs can also lead to justification for sexually deviant interests or behaviors (Abel, Gore, Holland, & Camp, 1989).

In their thoughtful review of the early phases of behavioral intervention as applied to those who were considered sexually deviant, Laws and Marshall (2003) concluded that:

> *[T]his early theory (i.e., the sexual preference hypothesis) underpinning behavioral approaches to deviant sexuality failed to account for the complexity of such behaviors, it is important to keep in mind the valuable role such theorizing played in the gradual development of today's more comprehensive approach. It is the nature of good science, and good clinical practice, to begin with the simplest account of a problem and only proceed to more complex conceptualizations as the data dictate. In the philosophy of science, this is called the principle of parsimony (Klee, 1997), and it is a dictum that is well illustrated by the history of behavior therapy in general and the cognitive behavioral treatment of sexual offenders in particular. In clinical practice and behavioral science, theories are to be admired because they have practical relevance to both research and treatment, not because they are eventually shown to be true or false (p. 87).*

The 1970s also saw the introduction of skill-based interventions, aimed at developing prosocial skills that were deemed lacking in offenders and which if enhanced could reduce recidivism, including empathy and perception of others (Marshall, 1971), and the development of social skills (Marshall, 1989). By the 1980s a comprehensive approach to offender treatment began to emerge (Murphy, Abel & Becker, 1980). Programs began to expand their interventions to include an educational focus aimed at enhancing social and relationship skills and sexual knowledge (Marshall & Williams, 1975), as well as assertiveness training and gender role behavior (Abel, Blanchard, & Becker, 1978).

Marshall and Barbaree (1990) proposed an Integrated Theory of Sexual Offending suggesting that offenses are propagated because of a number of interacting distal and proximal factors. They theorized that adverse childhood experiences, which may include abuse, poor parenting, or punitive discipline, could create distortions in the person's functioning regarding relationships, especially those involving sex or aggression. These distortions and a lack of developed social and self-regulation skills merge during adolescence and, together with the surge of hormones during adolescence, can result in a fusion of sexual interests, attitudes, and preferences that are offense-related. They suggested that this path continues into adulthood where failed or rejected relationships may create anger, negative attitudes towards women, and low self-esteem, thereby further fueling negative emotions and the development of deviant sexual fantasies. Masturbatory rehearsal can strengthen the deviant sexual interests which Marshall and Barbaree suggested might include positive reinforcement by enhancing a feeling of control, self-esteem, and/or negative reinforcement by reducing stress or tension. They further noted that behavior can also be maintained by automatic reinforcement and the development of cognitive distortions that allow the behavior to be justified. They also suggested that the model also allows for integration of the influence of risk factors such as alcohol/drug use and stress among other factors.

Ward and Beech (2006) further refined the three systems comprising trait features of Marshall and Barbaree's (1990) Integrated Theory of Sexual Offending. They proposed a model in which:

> *(a) The motivation/emotional system can incorporate the sexual attachment, intimacy, emotional, and needs constructs of the Marshall and Barbaree theory;*
>
> *(b) The action selection and control aspect of our theory can absorb the impulsivity, social skills, and self-regulation components of the Integrated Theory;*
>
> *(c) The perception and memory system are able to integrate the entrenched beliefs, strategies, identity, and values referred to in the Integrated Theory. (p. 60).*

This theory began to move the treatment for sexual offending to examination of the person as a whole, mirroring developments that had occurred in working with other mental health related challenges. From this discourse, a new model developed proposing that there were different pathways to offending or "relapse" (Hudson, Ward, & McCormack, 1999) and a new a self-regulation model to prevent relapse (Ward & Hudson, 1998, 2000).

The focus of the sexual offender research began to take another shift. In the 1980s there emerged a strong emphasis on relapse prevention as a key focus of intervention (Pithers, Kashima, Cumming, Beal, & Buell, 1988). However, by the 1990s, the relapse prevention model came under criticism (Ward & Hudson, 1996; Ward, Hudson, & Siegert, 1995). From that criticism emerged a new approach. Building on their earlier work, Ward and Beech (2006) proposed that there are four pathways to sexual offending. The Pathways Model (Ward & Beech, 2006, p. 60) identified four distinct but "interacting psychological mechanisms: intimacy and social skill deficits, distorted sexual scripts, emotional dysregulation, and cognitive distortions. Each mechanism depicts a specific offence pathway with different psychological and behavioral profiles, and separate aetiologies and underlying deficits." The four pathways are *Avoidant-Passive* (under-regulation and a resistance to offending with a lack of coping abilities), *Avoidant-Active* (resistance to offending that is thwarted by unregulated attempts to control or counterproductive strategies), *Approach-Automatic* (behaviors that are impulsive or poorly planned, marked by under developed self-regulation), or *Approach-Explicit* (active desire to offend using planned self-regulated behavior). Following from their work there emerged a renewed emphasis on the role of self-regulation.

Another key area that developed was determining a scientifically based method to evaluate risk related to recidivism. Actuarial risk assessment instruments emerged in the literature (e.g., *Sexual Offender Risk Appraisal Guide*-SORAG; Quinsey, Harris, Rice & Cormier, 1995). However, some actuarial risk assessment instruments included only static factors (e.g., *Static-99R*; Hanson & Thornton, 2000), which did not allow for evaluation of changes in risk as a result of intervention or other changeable factors. Dynamic factors, sometimes referred to as criminogenic needs (see Andrews & Bonta, 2010), represent potentially changeable factors that have been linked to the offending behavior, such as lack of self-management or self-regulation strategies (see Hanson, Harris, Scott & Helmus, 2007). Accordingly, further prediction scales soon followed focusing on these dynamic factors.

In more recent years there has been an emphasis placed on assessing risk for recidivism as a means to determine the nature of supports, environmental setting, and intensity of intervention a person might need to live safely in the community (Keeling, Rose, & Beech, 2009; Willis & Grace, 2008; 2009). As noted above, this assessment has been based on aggregate ratings of risk based on a combination of static and dynamic risk factors. Commonly used static tools are the aforementioned *Static-99R*, in addition to the VRAG-R (Harris, Rice, Quinsey, & Cormier, 2015) and *Risk Matrix-2000* (Thornton et al., 2003). Most risk assessment scales were designed originally for populations with typical cognitive development; however, Camilleri and Quinsey (2011) suggested that the VRAG-R has produced "promising results" (p. 66) for use with persons with intellectual disabilities. Additionally, Hanson and associates (2013) demonstrated that the *Static-99R* possesses moderate predictive validity in regard to assessing sexual re-offense potential in person with intellectual disabilities. McGrath, Livingston, Falk, and Erickson Warfield (2007) noted that actuarial risk assessment instruments, such as the *Static-99R* have predictive validity for persons with intellectual disabilities in some studies (see Harris & Tough, 2004; Tough, 2001). The range of these static factors may be helpful in determining the level of support and supervision that may be required in keeping with the Risk Principle outlined by Andrews and Bonta (2010) in their seminal Risk-Need-Responsivity model. However, for the purpose of therapeutic outcomes, dynamic risk factors represent contributing conditions that provide critical factors for intervention.

Since static indicators are unchangeable some researchers have challenged the value of these assessments in determining treatment for persons with intellectual disabilities (Harris & Tough, 2004; Wilson, Prescott, & Burns, 2014). The assessment of dynamic risk factors has therefore gained prominence as a method of determining factors that may be addressed in treatment and addressed for long term generalization and maintenance. Sometimes referred to as psychologically meaningful risk factors (see Mann, Hanson, & Thornton, 2010), dynamic factors are the changeable factors, that have been found through assessment, that contribute to a person's recidivism. Dynamic variables may include inappropriate cognitions or attitudes about sexual behavior or styles of general and sexual self-regulation (Lindsay, 2009). To assess for these dynamic factors in persons with intellectual disabilities, Steptoe, Lindsay, Murphy and Young (2008) developed the *Dynamic Risk Assessment and Management System* (DRAMS). Although still being field tested, preliminary results indicated that the items of the scale are predictive of events that preceded an offense for a person and consequently could be used to predict reoffending or establish a program for prevention of relapse.

More recently, a scale has been produced specifically for use with people with intellectual disabilities and sexual behavior problems. The *Assessment of Manageability of Individuals with Developmental and Intellectual Limitations Who Offend-Sexually* (ARMIDILO-S; Boer et al., 2013). This scale, which will be described more fully in Chapter 4, uses a format very similar to the *Stable-2007* (Hanson et al., 2007), but includes a reframing of all factors as potentially protective, as well as including consideration of environmental factors.

In 2010, Andrews and Bonta put forward the Risk, Need, Responsivity (RNR) model, which proposed that interventions are more likely to be successful when the intensity of intervention matches the level of risk posed, and where interventions specifically target known criminogenic needs in a manner that considers client characteristics (e.g., motivation, intellectual ability, learning styles). This model was criticized for a lack of attention to the entire picture of treatment needs, specifically related to issues of responsivity (Ward, Melser, & Yates, 2007). Alternatively, the Good Lives Model (GLM; Ward & Gannon, 2006) for sex offenders in the typically developing population proposed a more holistic approach that includes building a goal-oriented life focused on achieving common human goals that will improve well-being. A third perspective was suggested by Wilson and Yates (2009) who opined that the seeming divide between the two approaches of Risk/Need/Responsibility and the Good Lives Model is a red herring. In examining the two models, Wilson and Yates (2009) suggested that RNR is the overarching framework in which successful interventions are likely to succeed and that GLM is one curriculum that could possibly ensure appropriate attention to need and responsivity in that overarching framework. This would ultimately lead to the development of "an integrated strategy [that] would further assist in reducing offender recidivism, while increasing offender self-efficacy, re-integration potential, and community safety" (p 60).

EVOLUTION OF APPLIED BEHAVIOR ANALYSIS IN DEVELOPMENTAL DISABILITIES

Applied behavior analysis (ABA) includes empirically based approaches to investigate the origins of challenging behavior and to develop targeted strategies based on individualized assessment in people with intellectual disabilities. Jacobson and Holburn (2004, p.1) noted that ABA has played a long, distinguished, and central role in the provision of clinical services to persons with intellectual disabilities since the 1960s, although earlier applications were evident in the literature (e.g., Fuller, 1949). Earlier applications were based on respondent rather than operant conditioning (Jacobson & Holburn, 2004) and were intended to both teach new behaviors and reduce challenging behaviors (Wilkins & Matson, 2009), often through the use of punishment-based strategies.

The fundamentals of ABA have their origin in the seminal work of Ayllon and Michael in 1959. They employed techniques derived from behavioral principles to modify the environment to improve behavior in psychiatric patients, noting that attention from nursing staff was inadvertently reinforcing the challenging behaviors.

Thus, demonstrating that the behaviors served to gain the patients' attention in an overcrowded environment where attention typically was given for challenging behavior rather than for appropriate behavior. Ayllon and Michael observed that modification of the environment and the reinforcement pattern could result in changes in behavior.

Over time, the principles identified by Ayllon and Michael (1959) were applied to a variety of challenging behaviors presented by persons with intellectual disabilities (Jacobson & Holburn, 2004). ABA was described by Baer, Wolf, and Risley (1968) as a discipline that:

> *...will make obvious the importance of the behavior changed, the experimental manipulations which analyze with clarity what was responsible for the change, the technologically exact description of all procedures contributing to that change, the effectiveness of those procedures in making sufficient change for value, and the generality of that change (Baer et al., 1968, p. 97).*

In their influential article, Baer and colleagues identified seven basic dimensions that conceptualized the field of ABA. They suggested ABA must be applied, behavioral, analytic, technological, conceptually systematic, effective, and generalizable (Baer et al., 1968).

At the core of ABA is an adherence to systematic individualized analysis that would lead to a program to alter environmental factors to observe the effects the changes would have on behavior (Jacobson & Holborn, 2004). One of the first researchers to introduce a systematic method of individualized analysis was Edward Carr (1977). His work identified the specific functions that behavior served (positive reinforcement, negative reinforcement, and automatic reinforcement) from which individualized intervention plans were derived and based on the functional determination. Carr's work has been reported to be an important step in the evolution of functional analysis which is today the cornerstone of ABA (Sturmey & Bernstein, 2004). Functional behavioral assessment as an experimental analog assessment was originally described by Iwata, Dorsey Slifer, Bauman, & Richman (1982) but was later adapted for descriptive methods of analysis (Durand & Crimmins 1988; O'Neill et al., 1997).

Prior to the emergence of functional assessment, treatment for highly challenging behaviors had focused primarily on the use of aversive approaches, including faradic (electrical) stimulation. A huge debate began in the field throughout the next decade as illustrated in the classic text edited by Repp and Singh (1990), in which various perspectives on the use of nonaversive and aversive interventions for persons with developmental disabilities were expounded by leading experts in the field. Topics including the role of the environment, the role of skill building, least restrictive use of reductive procedures, treatment acceptability, and quality of life were explored. As a result, the field of ABA experienced a divergence within the discipline (Jacobson & Holburn, 2004) in which Positive Behavior Support (PBS) emerged.

Carr and Sidner (2002) suggested that the defining features of PBS are person-centred planning, functional assessment, positive strategies, multicomponent intervention, environmental focus, meaningful outcomes, ecological validity, and systems level analysis. PBS provided a link between empirical approaches to behavior such as functional assessment, and application to achieve socially valid changes in behavior

(Sugai et al., 2000). "Of significance is the adoption of system-wide models of behavior support, which are geared toward 'real world' settings, and implemented by relevant stakeholders" (Luiselli, 2004, p. 48).

Although based on behavioral principles, PBS integrated the philosophy of normalization and the process of person-centered planning (Wacker & Berg, 2002). Person-centred planning approaches were introduced as a way of reconceptualizing service systems to meet individual needs. Although variations have been called by various names (e.g., essential plans, lifestyle plans, personal futures plans) they share some core principles. Holburn, Jacobson, Vietze, Swartz and Sersen, (2000) suggested that the person-centred planning involves the person, those closest to the person, and natural community supports. It is a process that is collaborative and involves long-term commitment. Plans are based on personal preferences, involving real choice and decisions, and focused on incorporating natural community supports and creative opportunities to provide a life that is satisfying to the person. The marriage of person-centred planning with a positive behavioral approach results in what Risley (1996) has described as "getting a life."

The development of PBS from the foundation of ABA has been discussed extensively (i.e., Carr, 1997) and has not been without its detractors (Johnston, Foxx, Jacobson, Green, & Mulick, 2006). Whether PBS represents a different form of ABA or whether it just encompasses ABA has been debated in the field (Carr & Sidener, 2002). Nonetheless, this debate has been an important influence on how persons with intellectual disabilities who present with challenging behavior are provided with support and treatment.

Since the 1980s, the field also began to recognize the role that biological factors could play in the presentation of challenging behavior. Behavioral medicine began (e.g., Luiselli, 1989) and a recognition of the role that mental health (e.g., Reiss, 1994) and genetics could play in the presentation of challenging behavior (e.g., Griffiths, Condillac & Legree, 2014), as well as the role of a biopsychosocial approach (Gardner, Graeber & Cole, 1996).

The shift in behavioral application to persons with intellectual disabilities was, perhaps, best summarized in a quote from Scotti, Ujcich, Weigle, Holland, and Kirk (1996) who note that:

> *The time is well past for the behavioral intervention literature to merely focus on demonstrating the effects on circumscribed target behaviors of certain procedures implemented in carefully controlled (and often segregated) settings. Broader effects must not only be assessed but actively sought. These include not only assessing the effects of intervention on collateral behaviors but determining changes in lifestyle and quality of life that occur as a result of intervention (e.g., level of independence, choice making, living in typical homes in the community, meaningful employment and social roles, friendships and social networks). Furthermore, enhancing lifestyle and quality of life should be a crucial intervention component rather than simply an outcome of target behavior reduction (p. 133).*

IMPLICATIONS OF THE SHIFTING PARADIGMS IN BOTH SEXUAL OFFENDING TREATMENT AND ABA AS APPLIED TO THE TREATMENT OF PERSONS WITH INTELLECTUAL DISABILITIES WHO HAVE SEXUALLY OFFENDED

Prior to the 1970s, sexualized behavior of any type, expressed by persons with intellectual disabilities, was often met with sanctions that could include institutionalization and even sterilization (Scheerenburger, 1983). In the 1970s, both institutionalization and nontherapeutic sterilization fell out of favour. Normalization became the movement that swept through North America when Wolf Wolfensburger penned his epic work that was based on approaches that had begun in Scandinavia by Nirje (see Scheerenburger, 1983). In line with the changes occurring in the field of intellectual disabilities, in the 1970s institutions for persons with intellectual disabilities throughout North America began to systematically downsize, and community-based residential, vocation, and support services began to emerge. As the offenders were transferred to the community, there was a recognition that if deinstitutionalization were to be successful a range of therapeutic supports, that had been provided in the institutions, would need to be provided in the community.

One of the agencies that opened in the late 1970s was York Behavior Management Services (YBMS) in Ontario, Canada. The service provided a range of behavioral options to families, schools, and agencies in the community who supported persons with intellectual disabilities. In 1979, YBMS received a referral for a 16-year-old man in the community who had sexually molested a child in his neighborhood. YBMS was developed to provide behavioral treatment for persons with intellectual disabilities who were experiencing problems that interfered with their lives in the community. However, sexualized behavior was not a typical referral at that time. In fact, at that time, the prevailing response to such sexualized behaviors, particularly sexually offensive behavior, was to institutionalize the person with a disability. The behavior therapists from YBMS explored treatment options for this young man and found that none existed, either in their community or in the institution to which he would likely be sent. It was decided that a program of treatment for this young man would be developed in the community. With the aid of world-renowned experts such as Gene Abel and Vernon Quinsey, the first community-based program was established in Canada for the treatment of persons with intellectual disabilities who sexually offended.

Gene Abel had developed a community-based program for sex offenders in Atlanta. In consulting with YBMS, he suggested that many of the elements necessary for an effective treatment program were already being used by typical behavioral services, such as social skills training and anger management. With the introduction of sex education and relationship training, and adding the expertise of a psychologist skilled in approaches to reduce deviant arousal, he suggested that treatment for this young man could be conducted within a typical community setting. One of Canada's leading experts in sexual offending behavior, Vernon Quinsey, joined the team to provide much-needed expertise regarding the use of covert sensitization and was the supervising psychologist for this case. From that first case emerged a treatment approach that was published in 1985 by Griffiths, Hingsburger, and Christian then later elaborated in 1989 by Griffiths, Quinsey, and Hingsburger.

It is important to recognize that at that time, even though the normalization movement had called for services and approaches to be community-based and to provide persons with intellectual disabilities the most normalized of life experiences, the one area that even Wolfensberger (1972) hesitated to normalize was sexuality. He reported that his Scandinavian counterparts encouraged persons with intellectual disabilities to engage in socio-sexual relationships similar to those of the neurotypical population, including dating, marriage, and access to erotica. However, he proposed that there were too many challenges associated with sexuality, including sociopolitical realities of the North American culture of the time. He wrote, "Maybe tomorrow, I can write of not only another but even a different sexual frontier for the impaired, but today I can see it no more than I could see the present one some years back" (Wolfensberger, 1972, p. 174).

Murphy, Coleman, and Abel (1983), in their paper *Human Sexuality in the Mentally Retarded,* called for an end to the longstanding denial of the existence of sexuality in persons with intellectual disabilities. They noted that, "one sees a progression from a tentative limited approach seemingly designed to benefit the institution, rather than giving the individual [with an intellectual disability]a more global and liberal approach to deal with emotional and physical needs" (p. 596). Exceptions to this began to emerge with comprehensive socio-sexual training packages such as that published by Kempton, Hanson, and Adams (1978), and its later version Kempton (1988).

In 1983, Murphy, Coleman, and Haynes produced the classic article on the assessment and treatment of persons with intellectual disabilities who sexually offend; this paper merged the two fields of sexual offending and intellectual disability. They noted that, "many of the problems outlined for the offender [with an intellectual disability] are very similar to those for the [non-disabled] offender" (p. 40). Borrowing from the integrated model of behavioral assessment and treatment of sex offenders developed by Abel, Blanchard, and Becker (1978), Murphy and colleagues identified four key areas for assessment: sexual arousal that is either excessive to deviant stimuli or deficient in arousal to non-deviant stimuli; social skills; sexual knowledge and function; and cognitive factors including perceptions, attitudes, and discrimination. They suggested that from clinical experience, sex offending behavior committed by persons who have mild or borderline levels of intellectual disability would be able to benefit from techniques such as covert sensitization and satiation, social skills training, and sex education. In a further chapter, Murphy Coleman, and Abel (1983) suggested that where covert sensitization and possibly satiation may exceed the cognitive abilities of persons with intellectual disabilities, odor aversion or exposure may be more appropriate.

The first review of behavioral treatments for sexually deviant behavior related to persons with intellectual disabilities was published shortly thereafter by Foxx, Bittle, Bechtel, and Livesay (1986). In their extensive review of the literature, they noted 13 articles stemming back to Fookes' (1960) paper on the treatment of exhibitionism, homosexuality, and fetishism-transvestism using contingent Faradic stimulation (shock). The range of behaviors described in the articles included exhibitionism, fetishism, pedophilia, public masturbation, sexual aggression, and promiscuity. The contingencies described in the Foxx et al. review were primarily aversive and included Faradic stimulation, aversive imagery, contingent confinement, contingent lemon juice, and facial screening. Teaching appropriate and prosocial sexual skills was notably absent, resulting in their call for an increase in socio-sexual training for both the prevention of inappropriate sexual behavior and as part of treatment. They noted that "the gap in literature may indicate our failure to acknowledge the maladaptive sexual behavior of [intellectually disabled] persons rather than the absence of such behavior" (Foxx et al., 1986, p 315). They hoped that by identifying the gap in the research that more behaviorally-based research would develop.

By the late 1980s, 40 treatment programs had been identified in the literature (Knopp & Lackey, 1987). In 1990, Haaven, Little, and Petre-Miller described their institutionally-based treatment program for offenders with developmental disabilities. However, treatment founded within the field of ABA did not emerge as Foxx and colleagues (1986) had encouraged.

Although there has been significant interest and research focused on forensic issues related to persons with intellectual disabilities in the last 20 years, the field has relied on adaptation of advances in work with nondisabled sex offenders. Assessment approaches that were being employed with the nondisabled sexual offending population were explored for relevance with offenders with intellectual disabilities:

- Kolton, Boer, and Boer (2001) revised the *Abel and Becker Cognition Scale* for offenders with intellectual disabilities.
- Keeling and Rose (2005) explored whether the pathways to offense as elaborated by Ward and Hudson (2000) could be applied to persons with intellectual disabilities. They concluded that a sexual offender with an intellectual disability may be more likely to offend using an approach-automatic pathway or an avoidant-passive pathway. However, their work was based on a literature review and requires empirical exploration as to its application to treatment.
- Lindsay, Steptoe, and Beech (2008) further explored the application of the offense pathways model of Ward and Hudson to offenders with intellectual disabilities. In their research, they found that allocation to specific pathways was highly reliable and suggested that the use of the pathways model might enhance treatment to reduce recidivism.
- Harris and Tough (2004) explored and concurred that it was appropriate to use risk assessment tools such as the RRASOR and STABLE-2000 with people with intellectual disabilities, as mentioned earlier.
- Camilleri and Quinsey (2011) re-evaluated their data on the modified VRAG with persons with low verbal-IQ skills and determined that the VRAG had sufficient predictive accuracy to enable it to be employed until specialized risk assessments for this population have been validated.

Models of treatment also began to be applied to offenders with intellectual disabilities:

- Keeling, Rose and Beech (2009) explored the application of the three classifications theory of Ward and Hudson (1998) to offenders with an intellectual disability. They suggested that this model appears to have relevance to offenders generally but argued for a more complete exploration of the theory for the intellectually disabled population.
- Griffiths (2002) expanded upon the biopsychosocial model, widely used with persons with mental health needs and with persons with dual diagnosis (persons with an intellectual disability and a mental health/behavioral challenge) and stated it

could be applied to the sexual offending behavior of persons with an intellectual disability.

Unfortunately, research and intervention using ABA principles has been sparse over the years, albeit with some notable exceptions. Assessment approaches used as standard practice in ABA to assess challenging behavior of persons with intellectual disabilities began to be applied to persons with intellectual disabilities who sexually offended. In line with the shift in behavioral treatment for persons with intellectual disabilities and the emphasis on functional assessment, Fredericks and Nishioka-Evans (1999) proposed functional assessment for the treatment of adolescents with intellectual disabilities who sexually offended. They identified methods to assess the conditions under which a person was more likely to sexually offend and to determine behavioral variables that can play a role in sexual offending behavior. Fyffe, Kahng, Fittro, and Russell (2004) used functional communication training and extinction to significantly reduce inappropriate sexual behavior that was maintained by social positive reinforcement. Similarly, a response interruption/time out (RI/TO) procedure was used to successfully eliminate public masturbation displayed by a male with intellectual disability (Dozier, Iwata, & Worsdell, 2011).

Vollmer, Reyes, and Walker (2012) discussed behavioral approaches to the assessment and treatment of persons with intellectual disabilities who had sexually offended. Their chapter provided an important comprehensive discussion on various assessment and treatment approaches for offenders with intellectual disabilities where there has been such limited research in this area. One tenet of ABA is that treatments identified in one context should be generalized to a target environment. Thus, a goal of sex offender treatment is to test and ensure efficacy in settings other than the clinical laboratory. A notable area lacking in sex offender treatment work is generalization of treatment skills over time. Vollmer and associates acknowledged that generalization and maintenance is a main tenet of ABA – one that can be confidently applied to enhance treatment skills in persons with intellectual disabilities who have sexually offended. Generalization will be discussed more fully in Chapter 11.

Some more recent literature has suggested a multi-component ABA approach to the treatment of persons with intellectual disabilities who had sexually offended. Pritchard and colleagues (2011) did a functional behavior assessment (FBA) with a 16-year-old male with mild intellectual disability who displayed aggression, property damage, and sexually offensive behavior. Their assessment determined that the sexually offensive behaviors were socially and automatically reinforced through attention received from peers and stimulation from sexual arousal. The authors used an intervention that consisted of differential reinforcement of other behavior (DRO) through restricting community visits, cognitive behavior therapy (CBT), a reinforcement token economy system, social stories, and staff training. Through a period of 80 weeks, they found that his challenging behaviors decreased in frequency and intensity, and his sexually offensive behavior occurred zero to one time per week, suggesting the utility of long-term, multi-component treatment plans for sexually offensive behavior (Pritchard et al., 2011). One notable criticism of this study however, is the apparent lack of a functional replacement for the automatic reinforcing properties of the sexually offensive behavior. Without this, the long-term maintenance of these results is questionable.

Pritchard and colleagues (2016) utilized another multi-component behavioral intervention to treat a 17-year-old youth on the autism spectrum who displayed physical aggression, property damage, self-harm, eloping, and various forms of sexually offensive behavior. Prior to starting the intervention, the adolescent had a conviction of sexual assault and was living in a residential school with restricted community access. Through the use of a reinforcement system, behavior contract, socio-sexual education, CBT, and staff training, the adolescent showed an absence of all problem behavior for the last 36 weeks of the intervention (Pritchard et al., 2016). It is not clear if an FBA was conducted on the sexual behavior. Based on this logical functional model the authors would recommend doing an assessment of the sexual behavior to determine if it was socially mediated or deviant in order to ensure functional replacements of behavior and precisely targeted treatment.

An obvious limitation of the previous two studies is sample size since they are both case studies, as often is the literature on sex offender treatment for people with intellectual disabilities. Another limitation is that neither study appears to incorporate a functional replacement for the sensory function of the sexual behavior. From the authors' clinical experience, this is often missed in ABA approaches to sexually offending behavior in persons with intellectual disabilities and therefore will be addressed frequently throughout this book.

Lastly, in a review of effective intervention techniques for inappropriate masturbation (i.e., in public, interfering with aspects of daily life) by people with intellectual disability, every intervention utilized components of contingency management (notably differential reinforcement) and were able to demonstrate either a decrease or elimination of the behavior (Tarnai, 2006). Such information can be obtained via three features of a behavioral assessment, including indirect methods (e.g., interviews and record reviews to identify the age, gender, and characteristics of victims as well as the stimulus context of the offense), preference assessments, including phallometric testing, and direct measures of sexual interest (e.g., visual reaction time).

Current practice in working with persons with intellectual disabilities who have mental health challenges, including those with sexual offending behavior (SOB), takes a holistic, strength-based, and multi-component approach. To date, there remains a lack of consensus in the field about which tools are most effective in determining the appropriate intervention path for a particular person, although we are certainly getting closer to agreement. For a thorough review of the literature and best practice on persons with intellectual disabilities who have sexually offended, see the informational packet developed by Blasingame, Boer, Guidry, Haaven and Wilson (2014).

SUMMARY

This chapter reviewed emerging and changing approaches to the behavioral treatment of sex offenders, the shifts in services and treatment of persons with intellectual disabilities over the last fifty years, and the integration of those changes as they pertain to the behavioral treatment of persons with intellectual disabilities who have sexually offended. In the chapter that follows, the authors will present another foundational chapter on the sexually offensive behavior of persons with intellectual disabilities, which sets the stage for the emergent logical functional model that will be introduced in Chapter 3.

REFERENCES

Abel, G. G., Becker, J. V., & Cunningham-Rathner, J. (1984). Complications, consent, and cognitions in sex between children and adults. *International Journal of Law and Psychiatry, 7,* 89-103.

Abel, G.G., & Blanchard, E.B. (1974). The role of fantasy in treatment of sexual deviation. *Archives of General Psychiatry, 30,* 467-475.

Abel, G.G., Blanchard, E.B., Barlow, D.H., & Flanagan, B. (1975, December). *A controlled behavioral treatment of a sadistic rapist.* Paper presented at a meeting of the Association for the Advancement of Behavior Therapy, San Francisco.

Abel, G.G., Blanchard, E.B., & Becker, J.V. (1978). An integrated program for rapists. In R.R. Rada (Ed.), *Clinical aspects of the rapist.* New York: Greene & Stratton.

Abel, G. G., Gore, D. K., Holland, C. L., & Camp, N. (1989). The measurement of the cognitive distortions in child molesters. *Annals of Sex Research, 2,* 135-153.

Andrews, D. A. & Bonta, J. (2010). *The psychology of criminal conduct* (5th ed.). Cincinnati, OH: Anderson.

Ayllon, T., & Michael, J. (1959). The psychiatric nurse as a behavioral engineer. *Journal of the Experimental Analysis of Behavior, 2,* 323–334.

Baer, D. M., Wolf, M. M., & Risley, T. R. (1968). Some still-current dimensions of applied behavior analysis. *Journal of Applied Behavior Analysis, 1,* 91–97.

Blasingame, G.D., Boer, D.P., Guidry, L., Haaven, J., & Wilson, R.J. (2014). *Assessment, treatment, and supervision of individuals with intellectual disabilities and problematic sexual behaviors: Informational packet.* [Education & Training Committee Report] Beaverton, OR: Association for the Treatment of Sexual Abusers.

Boer, D. P., Haaven, J., Lambrick, F., Lindsay, W. R., McVilly, K. R., Sakdalan, J. A., & Frize, M. (2013). *ARMIDILO-S* [Psychology Test website]. www.armidilo.net: Boer, Haaven, Lambrick, Lindsay, McVilly, Sakdalan & Frize. Retrieved September, 6, 2018 from http://www.armidilo.net/

Bond, I. K., & Hutchinson, H. C. (1960). Application of reciprocal inhibition therapy to exhibitionism. *Canadian Medical Association Journal, 83,* 23-25.

Camilleri, J. A., & Quinsey, V. L. (2011) Appraising the risk of sexual and violent recidivism among intellectually disabled offenders. *Psychology, Crime & Law, 17*(1), 59-74.

Carr, E. G. (1977). The motivation of self-injurious behavior: A review of some hypotheses. *Psychological Bulletin, 84,* 800–816.

Carr, E. G. (1997). The evolution of applied behavior analysis into positive behavior support. *Journal of the Association for Persons with Severe Handicaps, 22,* 208-209.

Carr J. E, & Sidener T.M. (2002). On the relation between applied behavior analysis and positive behavioral support. *The Behavior Analyst, 25,* 245–253.

Cautela, J. R. (1967). Covert sensitization. *Psychological Reports, 20,* 459-468.

Cautela, J. R., (1970). Covert reinforcement. *Behavior Therapy, 1,* 33-50.

Cautela, J. R. (1971). Covert extinction. *Behavior Therapy, 2,* 192-200.

Dozier, C. L., Iwata, B. A., & Worsdell, A.S. (2011). Assessment and treatment of foot-shoe fetish displayed by a man with autism. *Journal of Applied Behavior Analysis, 44,* 133-137.

Durand, V. M., & Crimmins, D.B. (1988). Identifying the variables maintaining self-injurious behavior. *Journal of Autism and Developmental Disorders, 18,* 99-117.

Fookes, B. H. (1960). Some experiences in the use of aversion therapy in male homosexuality, exhibitionism, and fetishism-transvestism. *British Journal of Psychiatry, 115*, 339-341.

Foxx, R. M., Bittle, D. R., Bechtel, D. R. & Livesay, J. R. (1986). Behavioral treatment of the sexually deviant behavior of mentally retarded individuals. *International Review of Research in Mental Retardation, 14*, 291-317.

Fredericks, B. & Nishioka-Evans, V. (1999). Functional assessment for a sex offender population. In A.C. Repp & R.H. Horner (Eds.), *Functional analysis of problem behavior: From effective assessment to effective support* (pp. 279-303). Belmont CA: Wadsworth Publishing.

Freund, K. (1965). Diagnosing heterosexual pedophilia by means of a test for sexual interest. *Behavior Research and Therapy, 3*, 229-234.

Fuller, P.R. (1949). Operant conditioning of a vegetative human organism. *American Journal of Psychology, 62*, 587-590.

Fyffe, C. E., Kahng, S., Fittro, E., & Russell, D. (2004). Functional analysis and treatment of inappropriate sexual behavior. *Journal of Applied Behavior Analysis, 37*, 401-404.

Gardner, W. I., Graeber, J. L. & Cole, C. L. (1996). Behavior therapies: A multimodal diagnostic intervention model. In J. Jacobson & J. Mulick (Eds,), *Manual of diagnosis and professional practice in mental retardation* (pp. 355-369). Washington DC: American Psychiatric Press.

Griffiths, D. (2002). Sexual aggression. In Wm. I. Gardner (Ed.), *Aggression and other disruptive behavioral challenges: Biomedical and psychosocial assessment and treatment* (pp.325-398). New York: National Association for Dual Diagnosis.

Griffiths, D. M., Condillac, R., & Legree, M. (2014). *Genetic Syndromes and Applied Behavior Analysis*. UK: Jessica Kingsley Publishing.

Griffiths, D., Hingsburger, D., & Christian, R. (1985, December). Treating developmentally handicapped sexual offenders. *Psychiatric Aspects of Mental Retardation Review, 4*, 49-52.

Griffiths, D. M., Quinsey, V. L., & Hingsburger, D. (1989). *Changing inappropriate sexual behavior: A community-based approach for persons with developmental disabilities*. Baltimore, MD: Paul H. Brookes Publishing.

Guthrie, E. R. (1935). *The psychology of learning*. New York: Harper.

Haaven, J., Little, R., & Petre-Miller, D. (1990). *Treating intellectually disabled sex offenders: A model residential program*. Orwell, VT: Safer Society Press.

Hanson, R. K., Harris, A. J. R., Scott, T. L., & Helmus, L. (2007). *Assessing the risk of sex offenders on community supervision: The Dynamic Supervision Project* (User Report 2007-05). Ottawa, ON: Public Safety Canada.

Hanson, R. K., Sheahan, C. L., & VanZuylen, H. (2013). STATIC-99 and RRASOR predict recidivism among developmentally delayed sexual offenders: A cumulative meta-analysis. *Sexual Offender Treatment, 8*(1).

Hanson, R. K., & Thornton, D. (2000). Improving risk assessments for sex offenders: A comparison of three actuarial scales. *Law and Human Behavior, 24*, 119-136.

Harris, A. J. R. & Tough, S. (2004). Should actuarial risk assessments be used for sex offenders who are intellectually disabled. *Journal of Applied Research in Intellectual Disabilities, 17*, 235-41.

Harris, G. T., Rice, M.E, Quinsey, V. L., & Cormier, C.A. (2015). *Violent offenders: appraising and managing risk* (3rd ed.). Washington, DC: American Psychological Association.

Holburn, S., Jacobson, J. W., Vietze, P.M., Schwarz, A.A. & Sersen, E., (2000). Quantifying the process and outcomes of person-centred planning. *American Journal of Mental Retardation, 105,* 402-416.

Hudson, S.M., Ward, T., & McCormick, J.C. (1999). Offence pathways in sexual offenders. *Journal of Interpersonal Violence, 14,* 779-798.

Iwata, B. A., Dorsey, M. F., Slifer, K. J., Bauman, K. E., & Richman, G. S. (1982). Toward a functional analysis of self-injury. *Analysis and Intervention in Developmental Disabilities, 2,* 3–20.

Jacobson, J. W., & Holburn, S. (2004). History and current status of applied behavior analysis in developmental disabilities. In J. L. Matson, R. B. Laud, & M. L. Matson (Eds.), *Behavior modification for persons with developmental disabilities: Treatments and supports* (Vol. 1, pp. 1–32). Kingston, NY: NADD Press.

Johnston, J. M., Foxx, R.M., Jacobson, J. W., Green, G., & Mulick, J. A. (2006). Positive behavior support and applied behavior analysis. *Behavior Analysis, 29,* 51-74.

Keeling, J. A., & Rose, J. L. (2005). Relapse prevention with intellectually disabled sexual offenders. *Sexual Abuse, 17,* 407-23.

Keeling, J. A., Rose, J. L., & Beech, A.R. (2009). Sexual offending theories and offenders with intellectual disabilities. *Journal of Applied Research in Intellectual Disabilities, 22,* 468-476.

Kelly, R. J. (1982). Behavioral re-orientation of pedophiliacs: Can it be done? *Clinical Psychology Review, 2,* 387-408.

Kempton, W. (1988). *Life horizons.* Santa Monica, CA: Stanfield Film Associates.

Kempton, W., Hanson, G., & Adams, B. (1978). *Sexuality and the mentally handicapped.* Santa Monica CA: Stanfield Film Associates

Kinsey, A. C., Pomeroy, W. B., & Martin, C. E. (1948). *Sexual behavior in the human male.* Philadelphia: Saunders.

Klee, R. (1997). *Introduction to the philosophy of science: Cutting nature at its seams.* New York: Oxford University Press.

Knopp, F. H., & Lackey, L. B. (1987). *Sexual offenders identified as intellectually disabled: A summary of data from forty treatment providers.* Orwell, VT: Safer Society Press.

Kolton, D.J.C., Boer, A., & Boer, D.P. (2001). A revision of the Abel and Becker Cognition Scale for intellectually disabled sex offenders. *Sexual Abuse, 13,* 217-223.

Laws, D. R. (1995). Verbal satiation: Notes on procedure, with speculations on its mechanism of effect. *Sexual Abuse, 7,* 155-166.

Laws, D. R., & Marshall, W. L. (2003). A brief history of behavioral and cognitive behavioral approaches to sexual offenders: Part I. Early developments. *Sexual Abuse,* 15, 75-92.

Lindsay, W. R. (2009). *The treatment of sex offenders with developmental disabilities: A practice workbook.* Chichester, UK: Wiley-Blackwell.

Lindsay, W. R., Steptoe, L., & Beech, A.T. (2008). Ward and Hudson Pathways Model of the sexual offense process applied to offenders with intellectual disability. *Sex Abuse, 20,* 40, 379-392.

Luiselli, J.K. (1989). Behavioral treatment of pediatric feeding disorders in developmental disabilities. In M. Hersen, R. Eisler, & P.M. Miller (Eds.), *Progress in behavior modification* (pp.91-131). Newbury Park, CA: Sage.

Luiselli, J.K. (2004). Behavior support and intervention: current issues and practices in developmental disabilities. In J. L. Matson, R. B. Laud, & M. L. Matson (Eds.), *Behavior modification for persons with developmental disabilities: Treatments and supports* (Vol. 1, pp. 33-53). Kingston, NY: NADD Press.

Mann, R. E., Hanson, R. K., & Thornton, D. (2010). Assessing risk for sexual recidivism: Some proposals on the nature of psychologically meaningful risk factors. *Sexual Abuse, 22,* 191–217.

Marks, I. M., & Gelder, M. G. (1967). Transvestism and fetishism: Clinical and psychological changes during faradic aversion. *British Journal of Psychiatry, 113,* 711-730.

Marks, I. M., Gelder, M. G., & Bancroft, J. H. J. (1970). Sexual deviants two years after electric aversion therapy. *British Journal of Psychiatry, 117,* 173-185.

Marks, I. M., Rachman, S., & Gelder, M. G. (1965). Methods for assessment of aversion treatment in fetishism with masochism. *Behaviour Research and Therapy, 3,* 253-258.

Marquis, J. N. (1970). Orgasmic reconditioning: Changing sexual object choice through controlling masturbation fantasies. *Journal of Behavior Therapy and Experimental Psychiatry, 1,* 263-271.

Marshall, W. L. (1971). A combined treatment method for certain sexual deviations. *Behavior Research and Therapy, 9,* 292-294.

Marshall, W. L. (1979). Satiation therapy: A procedure for reducing deviant sexual arousal. *Journal of Applied Behavior Analysis, 12,* 10-22

Marshall, W.L. (1989). Intimacy, loneliness, and sex offenders. *Behavior Research and Therapy, 27,* 491–504.

Marshall, W. L., & Barbaree, H. E. (1990). An integrated theory of the etiology of sexual offending. In W. L. Marshall, D. R. Laws, & H. E. Barbaree (Eds.), *Handbook of sexual assault: Issues, theories, and treatment of the offender* (pp. 257 – 275). New York: Plenum.

Marshall, W. L., & Williams, S. (1975). A behavioral approach to the modification of rape. *Quarterly Bulletin of the British Association for Behavioral Psychotherapy, 4,* 78.

McGuire, R. J., Carlisle, J. M., & Young, B. G. (1965). Sexual deviations as conditioned behavior: A hypothesis. *Behavior Research and Therapy, 3,* 185-190.

McGrath, R. J., Livingston, J. A., Falk, G., & Erickson Warfield, M. (2007). Community management of sex offenders with intellectual disabilities: Characteristics, services, and outcome of a state-wide program. *Intellectual and Developmental Disabilities, 45,* 391-398.

Meichenbaum, D. (1974). *Cognitive Behavior Modification.* General Learning Press.

Murphy, W. D., Abel, G. G., & Becker, J. V. (1980). Future research issues. In D.J. Cox & R.J. Daitzman (Eds.), *Exhibitionism: Description, assessment, and treatment* (pp. 339-392). New York: Garland.

Murphy, W.D., Coleman, E.M., & Abel, G.G. (1983). Human sexuality in the mentally retarded. In J.L. Matson & F. Andrasnik (Eds.), *Treatment issues and innovations in mental retardation.* New York: Plenum.

Murphy, W.D., Coleman, E.M. & Haynes, M.R. (1983). Treatment and evaluation issues with the mentally retarded sex offender. In J. G. Greer & I. R. Stuart (Eds.), *The sexual aggressor: Current perspectives on treatment* (pp. 22-41). New York: Van Nostrand Reinhold.

O'Neill, R.E., Horner, R.H., Albin, R.W., Sprague, J.R., Storey, K., & Newton, J. S. (1997). *Functional assessment and program development for problem behavior: A practical handbook.* Pacific Grove, CA: Brookes/Cole.

Pithers, W.D., Kashima, K.M., Cummings, G.F., Beal, L.D., & Buell, M. (1988). Relapse prevention of sexual aggression. *Annals of New York Academy of Sciences, Human Sexual Aggression: Current Perspectives, 528*(1), 244-260.

Pritchard, D., Graham, N., Ikin, A., Penney, H., Kovacs, L., Mercer, D., Edwards, R., Jones, D. (2011). Managing sexually harmful behavior in a residential special school. *British Journal of Learning Disabilities, 40,* 302-309.

Pritchard, D., Graham, N., Penney, H., Owen, G., Peters, S., & Mace, C.F. (2016). Multi-component behavioral intervention reduces harmful sexual behavior in a 17-year-old male with autism spectrum disorder: a case study. *Journal of Sexual Aggression, 22*(3), 368-378.

Quinsey, V. L., Chaplin, T. C., & Carrigan, W. F. (1980). Biofeedback and signaled punishment in the modification of inappropriate sexual age preferences. *Behavior therapy, 11,* 567-576.

Quinsey, V. L., & Earls, C. M. (1990). The modification of sexual preferences. In W. L. Marshall, D. R. Laws, & H. E. Barbaree (Eds.), *Handbook of sexual assault: Issues, theories, and treatment of the offender* (pp. 279-295). New York: Plenum.

Quinsey, V.L., Harris, G.T., Rice, M E., & Cormier, C.A. (1995). *Sexual Offender Risk Appraisal Guide*-SORAG. Washington, DC: American Psychological Association.

Quinsey, V. L., & Marshall, W. L. (1983). Procedures for reducing inappropriate sexual arousal: An evaluation review. In J. G. Greer & I. R. Stuart (Eds.), *The sexual aggressor: Current perspectives on treatment* (pp. 267-289). New York: Van Nostrand Reinhold.

Reiss, S. (1994). *Handbook of challenging behavior: Mental health aspects of mental retardation.* Worthington, OH: IDS Publication.

Repp, A. C., & Singh, N. N. (1990). *Perspectives on the use of nonaversive and aversive intervention for persons with developmental disabilities.* Sycamore: IL: Sycamore Publishing.

Risley. T. (1996). Get a life! Positive behavioral intervention for challenging behavior through life arrangement and life coaching. In L. K. Koegel, R. L. Koegel, & G. Dunlap (Eds.), *Community, school, family and social inclusion through positive behavioral support* (pp. 425-437). Baltimore, MD: Brookes.

Scheerenberger, R. C. (1983). *A history of mental retardation.* Baltimore: Paul. H. Brookes.

Scotti, J. R., Ujcich, K. J., Weigle, K. L., Holand, C. M., & Kirk, K. S. (1996). Interventions with challenging behavior of persons with developmental disabilities: a review of current research practices. *Journal of the Association for Persons with Severe Handicaps, 21,* 123-134.

Skinner, B. F. (1938). *The behavior of organisms: An experimental analysis.* Acton: Copley, MA.

Steptoe, L., Lindsay, W. R., Murphy, L., & Young, S. J. (2008). Construct validity, reliability and predictive validity of the dynamic risk assessment and management system (DRAMS) in offenders with intellectual disability. *Legal and Criminological Psychology, 13,* 309-321.

Stevenson, I., & Wolpe, J. (1960). Recovery from sexual deviations through overcoming nonsexual neurotic responses. *American Journal of Psychiatry, 116,* 737-742.

Sturmey, P., & Bernstein, H. (2004). Functional analysis of maladaptive behaviors: Current status and future directions. In J. L. Matson, R. B. Laud, & M. L. Matson (Eds.), ***Behavior modification for persons with developmental disabilities: Treatments and supports*** (Vol. 1, pp. 1–32). Kingston, NY: NADD Press.

Sugai, G., Horner, R. H., Dunlap, G., Hieneman, M., Lewis, T.J., Nelson,... Reuf, R. (2000). Applying positive behavior support and functional assessment in schools. *Journal of Positive Behavior Interventions, 2,* 131-143.

Tarnai, B. (2006). Review of effective interventions for socially inappropriate masturbation in persons with cognitive disabilities. *Sex Disability, 24,* 151-168.

Thornton, D., Mann, R., Webster, S., Blud, L., Travers, R., Friendship, C., & Erikson, M. (2003). Distinguishing and combining risks for sexual and violent recidivism. *Annals of New York Academy of Science, 989,* 225-35,

Tough, S. E. (2001, November). *Validation of two standard risk assessments (Rapid Risk Assessment for Sex Offense Recidivism, 1997; Static–99, 1999) on a sample of adult males* ***who are developmentally disabled with significant cognitive deficits.*** Paper presented at the Association for the Treatment of Sexual Abusers 20th Annual Research and Treatment Conference, San Antonio.

Vollmer, T. R., Reyes, J. R., & Walker, S. F. (2012). Behavioral assessment and intervention for sex offenders with intellectual and developmental disabilities. In. J.K. Luiselli (Ed.), *A handbook of high-risk challenging behaviors in people with intellectual and developmental disabilities (pp. 121-144).* Baltimore, MD: Paul H. Brookes.

Wacker, D. P., & Berg, W. K. (2002). PBS as a service delivery system. *Journal of Positive Behavior Interventions, 4,* 25-28.

Ward, T. & Beech, A. (2006). An integrated theory of sexual offending. *Aggression and Violent Behavior, 11,* 44–63.

Ward, T. & Gannon, T. A. (2006). Rehabilitation, etiology, and self-regulation: The comprehensive good lives model of treatment for sexual offenders. *Aggression and Violent Behavior, 11,* 77–94.

Ward, T., & Hudson, S. M. (1996). Relapse prevention: A critical analysis. *Sexual Abuse, 8,* 177-200.

Ward, T., & Hudson, S. M. (1998). A model of the relapse process in sexual offenders. *Journal of Interpersonal Violence, 13,* 700-725.

Ward, T., & Hudson, S. M. (2000). A self-regulation model of relapse prevention. In D. R. Laws, S. M. Hudson, & T. Ward (Eds.), *Remaking relapse prevention with sex offenders: A sourcebook* (pp. 79–101). Thousand Oaks, CA: Sage.

Ward, T., Hudson, S. M., & Siegert, R.J. (1995). A critical comment on Pithers' relapse prevention model. *Sexual Abuse, 7,* 167-175.

Ward, T., Melser, J., & Yates, P. M. (2007). Reconstructing the Risk Need Responsivity Model: A theoretical elaboration and evaluation. *Aggression and Violent Behavior, 12,* 208–228

Wilkins, J. & Matson J. L. (2009). A comparison of social skills profiles in intellectually disabled adults with and without ASD. ***Behavior Modification, 33,*** 143–155.

Willis, G.M., & Grace. R.C. (2008). The quality of community reintegration planning for child molesters: effects on sexual recidivism. *Sex Abuse,* 20(2),218-40.

Willis, G. M., & Grace, R. C. (2009). Assessment of community reintegration planning for sex offenders: Poor planning predicts recidivism. *Criminal Justice and Behavior, 36*(5), 494-512.

Wilson, R. J., Prescott, D. S., & Burns, M. (2014). People with special needs and sexual behavior problems: Balancing community and client interests while ensuring effective risk management. In K. McCartan & H. Kemshall (Eds., Special Issue), Sex offender (re)integration into the community: Realities and challenges, *Journal of Sexual Aggression, 21,* 86-99.

Wilson, R. J. & Yates, P. M. (2009). Effective interventions and the Good Lives Model: Maximizing treatment gains for sexual offenders. *Aggression and Violent Behavior, 14,* 157–161.

Wolfensberger, W. (1972). *Normalization.* Toronto, ON: National Institute on Mental Retardation.

Wolpe, J. (1958). *Psychotherapy by reciprocal inhibition.* Stanford, CA: Stanford University Press.

Chapter Two

Sex Offending Behavior and Persons with an Intellectual Disability

A century ago, persons with intellectual disabilities were considered sexually dangerous to society (Simmons, 1982). This attitude, best exemplified in the Eugenics Movement, led to mass institutionalization and sterilization of persons with intellectual disabilities. The belief that persons with an intellectual disability were dangerous and promiscuous has been, at times, countered by the belief that persons with intellectual disabilities were child-like innocents who should be protected from all things sexual (Griffiths & Fedoroff, 2008). Although apparently opposing perspectives, both beliefs achieved the same outcome, which was to stereotype the sexuality of persons with intellectual disabilities as atypical and out of the range of normal. These beliefs allowed the sexual expression of persons with intellectual disabilities to be censured and controlled either through the lens of protecting society or the person with a disability.

PREVALENCE OF ABUSE IN OFFENDERS AND EXPERIENCES WITH THE LEGAL SYSTEM

A review of the literature related to persons with intellectual disabilities and sexual offending behavior indicated that persons with intellectual disabilities may be overrepresented among those committing crimes, including those of a sexual nature (Langevin, 1992; Shapiro, 1986; Steiner, 1984) and may be more prevalent than previously recognized (Timms & Gorecczny, 2002). However, Lindsay, Hastings, Griffiths, and Hayes (2007) have suggested that studies have been conducted in different settings and, as a result, have illuminated different prevalence rates of offenders and the types of offenses. These data, however, require further investigation to determine if or why these findings are occurring. The following section will explore this phenomenon and the factors that may affect it.

Early research suggested that the incidence of sexual offenses committed by persons with intellectual disabilities ranged from 3-4% to 43-51% (Mohr, Turner & Jerry, 1964; Selling, 1959). Later research narrowed the range from 15 to 33%, when based on data from sex offenders with intellectual disabilities who had been charged with an offense (Shapiro, 1986; Steiner, 1984). Empirically controlled research such as that conducted by McEachron (1979) reported offense rates of only .6 -2.3%, which resembled that of the general population. Hayes (1991) also found that based on rates of conviction, the rate was only 3.7%.

The apparent overrepresentation of persons with intellectual disabilities in the criminal justice system for sexual offenses may relate in part to increased vulnerabilities associated with the intellectual disability, such as impaired judgment, lack of adaptive abilities, or the risk factors potentially associated with the lifestyle of a person with an intellectual disability including poverty, clustered living, lack of education, and abusive experiences (Griffiths, 2002). It has been reported that persons with intellectual disabilities are twice as likely to experience sexual abuse as the non-disabled population (Sobsey, 1994). McCarthy and Thompson (1997) reported that the prevalence rate of abuse among persons with intellectual disabilities differed by gender: women (61%) and men (25%). Although the statistics vary, the field presents a uniform message that sexual abuse is overrepresented in the population of persons with intellectual disabilities (see McCarthy & Thompson, 1997).

The high rates of sexual abuse experienced by persons with intellectual disabilities have been hypothesized to play a role in the later commission of a sexual offense (Firth et al., 2001). Lindsay, Law, Quinn, Smart, and Smith (2001) conducted a comparison of the sexual abuse histories of sexual and non-sex offenders with intellectual disabilities and found that 38% of the sex offenders had been abused while only 12.7% of the non-sex offenders had been abused. Their study added weight to the concept that some offenders may be re-enacting their own sexual abuse (traumagenic re-enactment). Caution should be taken, however, to not interpret this to mean that if a person has been abused that they will necessarily go on to abuse others (Briggs & Hawkins, 1996). For the definitive article on this topic see Jespersen, Lalumière, and Seto (2009). In the absence of appropriate education or therapy however, an abused person may fail to learn that certain behaviors are inappropriate, a violation of the rights of others, and illegal. If persons with intellectual disabilities have not been afforded appropriate socio-sexual education and are more likely to experience sexual abuse and/or have their sexuality abused (Griffiths, Quinsey & Hingsburger, 1989), then the person may be living in a moral vacuum without understanding that what was done to them was wrong and is, therefore, something that they should not do to others.

Alternatively, other researchers have suggested that the data may underestimate the actual incidence of offending, noting that many persons with an intellectual disability who commit sexual offenses have been diverted from the criminal justice system into institutions for persons with intellectual or psychiatric disabilities (Day, 1994). Therefore, persons with intellectual disabilities may not be charged for a sexual offense because of their disability or, if charged, may be diverted from the justice system because of their disability. Additionally, McBrien and Murphy (2006) have suggested that there is often an assumption that persons with intellectual disabilities are already being cared for within the social service systems, that they need to be provided with understanding more than punitive approaches, and, as such, should not be charged or prosecuted. They further noted that agencies supporting persons with intellectual disabilities often do not report an incident for fear of being criticized or because a lack of direction in protocol and policy. This has led to difficulties in establishing consequential learning for many persons with intellectual disabilities who sexually offend.

At this point, perhaps the clearest message on the comparative incidence of sexual offending among persons with intellectual disabilities was stated by Lindsay in 2002. In a thoughtful review of the research and literature on persons with intellectual disabilities who had sexually offended, he concluded there was no clear evidence that there is either an over- or under-representation of people with intellectual disabilities. Lindsay (2002) suggested that a valid prevalence rate of sexual offense amongst persons with intellectual disabilities is difficult to ascertain because study samples are based on people who have been incarcerated or hospitalized, in addition to being based on varying methods of diagnosing intellectual disability (Lindsay, 2002; Lindsay et al., 2007). Griffiths, Watson, Lewis, and Stoner (2004) cautioned that because research is often based on prison data or arrest/conviction rates, the data may be less indicative of an over representation of higher rates of sexual offenses among this population, but rather a higher rate of arrest, confession, and conviction (see also Murphy, Coleman & Haynes, 1983; Santamour & West, 1978). People with intellectual disabilities present with an increased risk of apprehension, incrimination, suggestibility, confession, pleading guilty (whether guilty or not), and waiving of legal rights because of a lack of understanding of the process and potential outcomes and are less likely be represented by counsel or have options presented for plea bargain or appeal judgment (Abel & Rouleau, 1990; Brown & Courtless, 1971; McGee & Menolascino, 1992; Moschella, 1982; Murphy et al., 1983; Santamour & West, 1978). Moreover, persons with intellectual disabilities also represent a segment of population that is often financially unable to obtain and afford appropriate legal assistance in their interactions with the criminal-justice system (Abel & Rouleau, 1990).

There is a wealth of research demonstrating that the typical path for an accused person with an intellectual disability who engages with the legal system is fraught with challenges. Griffiths, Taillon-Wasmund, and Smith (2002) noted that from arrest to trial, offenders who have intellectual disabilities are more likely to be disadvantaged in police interrogations because of their impaired understanding of their legal rights to legal counsel upon detention. Persons with intellectual disabilities are often victims of acquiescence bias; they are also more likely to confess (even if innocent), concede to pressure to seek approval from authority figures, and incriminate themselves. Studies conducted in the US reported that accused persons with intellectual disabilities were also more likely to be detained pre-trial because they failed to meet bail or personal recognizance requirements and when held in custody prior to trial their likelihood of conviction increases (Toberg, 1992). Additionally, they often do not have power or means to effectively interact in the courts or to be represented by counsel other than that provided by the courts. Moreover, persons with intellectual disabilities often enter the judicial system without evaluation or consideration as to how the nature of their disabling condition may have affected the commission of the crime, their understanding of rights, pre-trial testimony, understanding of possible outcomes, or their ability to provide consistent and accurate testimony (Marinos, Griffiths, Fergus, Stromski, & Rondeau, 2014).

Persons with intellectual disabilities are also more likely to be declared unfit to stand trial, which may result in long term commitment to a psychiatric facility with the assumption that fitness will be achieved; however, since many of the criminal codes were designed for mental health issues, they do not apply equally to persons with intellectual disabilities whose fitness is not related to mental incompetency due to a temporary condition, but is pervasive and lifelong. Research has further shown that if convicted they often receive longer sentences than similar offenders without disabilities (Laski, 1992). In the United States, 22 states and the federal government have established sexually violent predator/person (SVP) laws to allow for the post-sentence, involuntary, and indeterminate placement of designated SVPs in sex offender civil commitment centers (SOCC – see Brandt, Wilson, & Prescott, 2015). These centers are essentially secure treatment facilities that outwardly resemble high security prisons but appear more like a hospital inside the secured perimeter, with a higher ratio of clinical staff than typically found in penitentiary settings. Statutory criteria for sex offender civil commitment typically includes a history of sexual offending, a "mental abnormality or personality disorder" (as diagnosed by psychologists or psychiatrists hired by the state), and a lack of volitional control to inhibit future sexually violent offenses. SOCC placement requires a court procedure not entirely dissimilar to prosecution for sexual offenses in the first place – in that the person's personal and offense histories are examined prior to judgment. It is reasonable to conclude that whatever difficulties persons with intellectual disabilities might face in criminal court, these difficulties are likely to apply in civil proceedings.

Clinical observation by Robin Wilson, one of the authors, has been that between 10% and 15% of persons in such civil commitment centers would meet a working definition of intellectual disability (or other brain-based cognitive limitation). Although some SOCC facilities provide treatment and case management services specifically tailored to persons with intellectual disabilities, this is certainly not the standard, and several state SVP programs have been subject to class action lawsuits (Canupp et al. v. Liberty Behavioral, et al., 2009; Karsiens v. Piper, 2017) due to their failure to address client needs according to the responsivity principle (see Andrews & Bonta, 2010). However, even in those jurisdictions where responsive treatment options are available, SVPs with intellectual disabilities face additional challenges in demonstrating to the court that, following completion of treatment, they are ready for release.

In Canada, there was a famous case of Simon Marshall, dubbed the "Ste.-Foy rapist." Mr. Marshall was a 23-year-old man with an intellectual disability and behavioral challenges. When arrested he plead guilty, was convicted, and was imprisoned for a series of sexual assaults in Quebec. While in prison from 1997 to 2003, he was brutalized by other inmates. Upon his release, he again confessed to sexual assaults that were publicized in the news; however, this time DNA evidence confirmed he was not guilty of the crimes to which he was confessing. A later reconstruction of the original cases to which he had confessed revealed he had not committed the original offenses either (CBC News, 2005). The DNA evidence from the first offenses had never been tested, leading the Quebec Court of Appeal to rule that Mr. Marshall had been a victim of police misconduct. Accordingly, the verdict was overturned by the Quebec Court of Appeal, his record was expunged, and he was awarded $2.3 million for the wrongful conviction (CBC News, 2009).

Thus, in some cases the natural legal consequences that persons with intellectual disabilities may receive if accused or convicted of a sexual offense may be skewed because of an unequal opportunity for justice. Conversely, persons with intellectual disabilities have often been diverted from prisons to be placed in other long-term settings, such as an institution for persons with intellectual disability or even a psychiatric facility (Day, 1997), although there is a shift emerging where prisons are becoming the new hospitals (See Torrey, Kennard, Eslinger, Lamb & Payle, 2010). Some case law principles leading to this type of decision are based on the premise that the accused person with an intellectual disability may cope poorly in prison or is viewed as less reprehensible and, as such, the principles of general or specific deterrence are not relevant. Unlike jail sentences, these placements in alternative settings, like hospitals or institutions, can often result in longer incarcerations than persons would have received if they had been found guilty and sent to jail. Moreover, the diversion is often based on the mistaken belief that the person will receive appropriate support and treatment in a non-judicial facility or will at least be out of the community thereby ensuring public safety. However, being placed in a facility for persons with intellectual disabilities or a psychiatric facility does not always equate to effective offender treatment. In fact, opportunities for effective treatment are often unavailable.

In addition to possible legal sanctions, the additional naturally occurring aversive consequences that occur following the commission of a sexual offense often include losses regarding access to family, friends, and the greater community, activities the person enjoyed, and opportunities for employment and leisure. As a result, the commission of sexually inappropriate or offending behavior often results in the person with disability being denied experiences that might provide an enriched life; these are elements that are described in a therapeutic approach known as the Good Lives Model that has emerged as a foundation for proactive and preventative approaches to reducing recidivism by ensuring that human needs, as well as criminogenic needs, are met in therapy (See Ward and Stewart, 2003). This will be elaborated in later chapters.

COMMON THEORIES OF THE SEXUAL OFFENDING BEHAVIORS IN PERSONS WITH INTELLECTUAL DISABILITY

PARAPHILIA

Paraphilia is a derived from the Greek word implying "love of the unusual." It was popularized by John Money (1999) to be a non-pejorative label for sexual behaviors that were not the ideal or norm. However, the term has come to denote and categorize various forms of sexual deviance as described in the *Diagnostic and Statistical Manual of Mental Disorders* (DSM) since the 1980s. Soon, paraphilia came to be commonly described as "intense sexually arousing fantasies, sexual urges, or behaviors generally involving non-human objects, suffering or humiliation of oneself or others, children or other nonconsenting persons" (American Psychiatric Association, 1987).

In the most recent version, DSM-5 (American Psychiatric Association, 2013), paraphilias were defined as "any intense and persistent sexual interest other than sexual interest in genital stimulation or preparatory fondling with phenotypically normal, physically mature, consenting human partners." As such, the only sexual interests considered non-paraphilic are genital stimulation or fondling with a partner who is consenting and age appropriate (Griffiths, Fedoroff, Richards, & Lindsay, 2016).

The DSM-5 is the first edition to precisely distinguish between *paraphilias* and *paraphilic disorders,* noting that presence of a paraphilia does not require or justify psychiatric treatment unless it causes distress (harm or risk of harm) to the person or another, thereby making it a disorder. Paraphilic disorders cause harm directly or indirectly to the afflicted person or a direct or indirect victim. A paraphilia, denoting an unconventional interest or preference, is not sufficient to be a paraphilic disorder and as such may not require clinical intervention. It is only when it becomes a disorder that it is now considered a psychiatric disorder. For example, a person who experiences strong or preferential sexual interest in prepubescent children but is able to inhibit acting on those interests to the extent that he/she can live a relatively normal life without being unduly troubled by those interests would be diagnosed as having pedophilia. However, as long as the person in question continues to inhibit urges to act on those interests and the mere possession of the interests does not cause undue hardship to the person or others, he/she would not be suffering from pedophilic disorder.

The DSM-5 lists eight paraphilic disorders that were deemed as the most common and forensically important, namely voyeuristic disorder, exhibitionistic disorder, frotteuristic disorder, sexual masochism disorder, sexual sadism disorder, pedophilic disorder, fetishistic disorder, and transvestic disorder. Other paraphilias that cause distress can be diagnosed as disorders but under the categories of other specified paraphilic disorder or unspecified paraphilic disorder. These two diagnostic options replaced the earlier formulation Paraphilia Not Otherwise Specified (or Paraphilia NOS)

According to the DSM-5, paraphilias represent either *anomalous activity preferences* (e.g., courtship disorders and algolagnic disorders) *or anomalous target preferences.* These are described in Table 2.1: Paraphilic Disorders below.

Table 2.1: ***Paraphilic Disorders***

<table>
<tr><td colspan="3">Anomalous Activity Preferences</td></tr>
<tr><td rowspan="3">Courtship Disorders</td><td>Frotteuristic Disorder</td><td>Rubbing up or touching a nonconsenting person</td></tr>
<tr><td>Exhibitionist Disorder</td><td>Exposing genitals</td></tr>
<tr><td>Voyeuristic Disorder</td><td>Spying on others engaged in private activities</td></tr>
<tr><td rowspan="2">Algolagnic Disorders</td><td>Sexual Masochism Disorder</td><td>Undergoing humiliation, bondage, or suffering</td></tr>
<tr><td>Sexual Sadism Disorder</td><td>Inflicting humiliation, bondage, or suffering</td></tr>
<tr><td colspan="3">Anomalous Target Preferences</td></tr>
<tr><td rowspan="3"></td><td>Pedophilic disorder</td><td>Sexual interest in pre-pubescent children</td></tr>
<tr><td>Fetishistic disorders</td><td>Inanimate objects (e.g., leather, lingerie, shoes) or non-genital body parts (e.g., feet, hands, ears – sometimes referred to as partialism)</td></tr>
<tr><td>Transvestic Disorders</td><td>Sexually arousing cross-dressing</td></tr>
</table>

The DSM-V notes that:

> *Some paraphilias primarily concern the individual's erotic activities, and others primarily concern the individual's erotic targets. Examples of the former would include intense and persistent interests in spanking, whipping, cutting, binding, or strangulating another person, or an interest in these activities that equals or exceeds the individual's interest in copulation or equivalent interaction with another person. Examples of the latter would include intense or preferential sexual interest in children, corpses, or amputees (as a class), as well as intense or preferential interest in nonhuman animals, such as horses or dogs, or in inanimate objects, such as shoes or articles made of rubber* (American Psychiatric Association, 2013, p. 685).

Although paraphilic sexual disorders can be present in a subset of persons with intellectual disability, just as they exist in a subset of the general population, Day (1994) opined that actual paraphilia may be rare among persons with intellectual disability. However, this assertion has not been empirically tested, and it would stand to reason that there is little cause to believe that paraphilias should have a distinctly different prevalence in persons with intellectual disabilities. It may be, however, that diagnostics with persons with intellectual disabilities are complicated by the nature and consequences of the disability. Differential rates of sex offending between persons with and without intellectual disabilities might imply a higher prevalence of paraphilia in one group or the other, but it would be important to take into account other factors that may relate to the experiences of persons with intellectual disabilities. These different experiences may contribute to the commission of offenses that may not be related to the *actual* presence of paraphilia, such as a lack of opportunity to learn or engage in appropriate socio-sexual experiences or punitive practices related to the expression of their sexuality. For example, a person who exposes their genitals in public may appear to have exhibitionist disorder, but upon further examination, the behavior may be a result of other underlying, non-paraphilic factors (i.e., a person with severe cognitive limitations who needs to go to the bathroom).

Deviance and Counterfeit Deviance

In *Changing Sexually Inappropriate Behavior*, Griffiths, Quinsey, & Hingsburger (1989) described a community-based model at York Behavior Management Services (now Centre for Behavior Health Sciences) for treatment and risk management of persons with intellectual disabilities who had sexually offended. They highlighted the importance of evaluating the person's history and environment, as well as the circumstances of the offense. They further suggested that assessment should include determining the person's socio-sexual knowledge; social skills; coping skills; relationships; knowledge of responsibility; and assessment of sexual interests, preferences, and arousal. After evaluation, an individualized program was designed that focused both on teaching appropriate and alternative skills and providing coping strategies for deviant arousal or problematic behavior patterns. They noted that some of the persons presented with behaviors that were consistent with the DSM criteria involving arousal to unusual or intrusive sexualized images and fantasies; however, some people did not, suggesting that individualized treatment and supports needed to match the needs of the person, rather than apply a single protocol (one size fits all approach to treatment) for all offenders.

In a later paper, these same authors (Hingsburger, Griffiths & Quinsey, 1991) made a further distinction between persons with intellectual disabilities who sexually offended that presented with paraphilic tendencies, from other individuals with intellectual disabilities who had also committed a sexual offense, but who presented without the interests or urges related to a paraphilia. They coined the term 'counterfeit deviance' to describe clinical cases that appeared topographically paraphilic (which at the time implied deviance), but on closer examination proved to not fit the prevailing definition of paraphilia and, as such, required a different course of treatment (Hingsburger et al., 1991). Based on 10 years of clinical data (including cases involving exposure, assault, and child molestation), they identified that while some of the persons in their treatment program evidenced paraphilia as an underlying factor in commission of their offense(s), for other persons the presenting sexually offensive behaviors were the product of different diagnostically significant factors (e.g., a lack of sexual problem-solving, poor interpersonal boundaries, difficulty in age discrimination, problems with impulse control, and disinhibition). Accordingly, these different factors demanded differential treatment approaches.

There has been a degree of controversy in the clinical literature as to the veracity of the counterfeit deviance theory (see Lunsky, Frijters, Watson, Willison, & Griffiths, 2007; Michie, Lindsay, Martin, & Grieve, 2006; Talbot & Langdon, 2006). Notwithstanding these observations, it is important to recognize that this theory never denied the presence of paraphilia in some offenders with intellectual disabilities. Just as in the typically developing population, some persons with intellectual disabilities develop sexualized interests that meet the diagnostic criteria of paraphilia. However, Hingburger and associates (1991) have cautioned against making assumptions of paraphilia based solely upon behavior and identified the need for enhanced assessment to ensure that deviance (deviant fantasies or urges) was a factor in commission of the sexual offense rather than just assumed.

The underlying caution proposed in the theory of 'counterfeit deviance' was later echoed in the DSM-IV-TR (American Psychiatric Association, 2000), noting that persons with intellectual disabilities might have a "decrease in judgment, social skills, or impulse control that, in rare instances, leads to unusual sexual behavior" that is distinguishable from paraphilia (p. 568).

Hingsburger and colleagues (1991) posed eleven hypotheses as possible explanations for inappropriate sexual behavior observed among their clinical population that were deemed as not sexually deviant as noted in Table 2.2: Counterfeit Deviant Hypotheses.

Table 2.2: *Counterfeit Deviant Hypotheses*

Hypothesis	Explanation
Structural	Contextual factors including attitudes, practices, and protocols that render some environments highly restrictive of appropriate sexuality. Any sexual behavior in these settings may be deemed inappropriate and even punished. If appropriate sexuality was forbidden, persons might seek inappropriate sexual outlets such as engaging in sexual behavior in a public place but away from care providers.
Modelling	Some inappropriate expressions were modelled after care-provider behavior. In environments that did not model appropriate privacy when providing personal care, a person may have replicated touching without respect for boundaries.
Behavioral	Inappropriate sexual behavior is highly functional in either garnering attention or allowing the person to escape or delay an undesired situation. If the person cannot get a desired function in alternative means, acting in a sexually inappropriate manner is likely to receive attention or escape.
Partner selection	Living in a socio-sexual 'peer-void' because of a lack of opportunity or social skills to develop relationships can create a relationship vacuum. A person may attempt to fill the void with inappropriate partners such as care-providers, children, or others.
Inappropriate courtship	Lack of opportunities and education may lead to a lack of courtship skills. A person may be overly direct, blunt, or aggressive in attempts at courtship.
Sexual knowledge	A lack of appropriate and comprehensive sexual knowledge, either formally or informally, may sometimes cause a person to seek sexual interaction inappropriately.
Perpetual arousal	A chronic state of sexual arousal and engaging in repeated masturbation due to inability to masturbate to completion. A person may be unable to masturbate to completion and thus remain in a constant state of arousal, possibly due to prescription of certain medications, being afforded no privacy or time to complete the act, or because of a specific physical disability or a history of punishment when engaging in masturbation.
Learning history	A non-normative learning history that may include sexual abuse or having one's sexuality abused through harsh negative sexual messages (e.g., a case of coprophilia described by Hingsburger (1989) in which feces was used as a lubricant to expedite sexual release and avoid punishment).
Moral vacuum	In congregate settings, *private* activities such as dressing and even masturbation were often conducted in *public* given the constant presence of staff and co-residents, regardless of gender. Considering the sexual life experiences of many persons with intellectual disabilities regarding societal values around sexuality and disability, some people with disabilities may not have developed standards by which to judge their own behavior or that of others.
Medical	A person may exhibit sexually offensive behavior when experiencing a medical or mental health challenge (i.e., mania).
Medication side-effect	Sexually inappropriate behavior prompted by frustration, in an attempt to gain sexual satisfaction when a medication has been added that altered their sexual functioning.

Although specific research into the hypotheses that fall within 'counterfeit deviance' has been rare, Griffiths, Hingsburger, Hoath, and Ioannou (2013) explored the basis for counterfeit deviance within the existing literature. They illustrated how some or part of the sexually offending behavior exhibited by persons with intellectual disabilities can be mitigated by non-deviant factors and serve alternate functions (and, hence, demonstrating a need for ABA). They highlighted that persons with intellectual disabilities often live in multi-bed environments that provide non-normative learning opportunities regarding sexuality and that are often typified by sexual segregation, a lack of privacy, a lack of appropriate partners, restrictiveness, and even punishment for any sexual behavior.

Lindsay (2009) suggested that there should be an additional counterfeit deviant hypothesis to explain why a person with an intellectual disability might sexually offend, other than for paraphilic reasons. He called for assessment of the offender's understanding of laws and society rules, suggesting that some people with intellectual disabilities may not have learned self-control with regard to their sexual behavior nor social mores regarding appropriate relationships. He cautioned that while not being "completely naïve about the fact that their behavior is inappropriate, they have not internalized the extent to which it is against the conventions of society" (p. 98). Craig and Lindsay (2010) further suggested "although they may also understand something of the illegality or inappropriate sexual behavior, they may not have a full comprehension of the extent of which such practices are condemned by society. This relative lack of understanding may interact with a wish or need for sexual contact or indeed deviant sexual interest resulting in episodes of inappropriate sexual behavior." (p.16)

A further need for contextual assessment was highlighted by Day's observation that often the sexual offenses of persons with intellectual disabilities involved more "minor or nuisance offenses" (p. 279) which might represent an inappropriate expression of sexual feelings rather than sexual deviance, *per se* (Day, 1994). This implies some people with intellectual disabilities may lack the opportunity and skills to develop normative relationships.

A lack of socio-sexual knowledge has been identified as pervasive among people with intellectual disabilities (McCabe, 1999). However, research has shown that sex offenders in treatment programs were not lacking in sexual knowledge (Michie, et al., 2006). This apparent discrepancy was clarified by Lunsky et al. (2007) who found that Type 1 offenders with intellectual disability (pedophiles, rapists, or those exhibiting repeated or forced sexual assaults) indeed had greater sexual knowledge then the general group of nonoffenders with intellectual disabilities. They also identified a second group of people with intellectual disabilities who sexually offended, who they called Type 2 offenders (people who engaged only in inappropriate touching, public exhibitionism or public masturbation). The Type 2 group showed no significant differences in their knowledge compared to a non-offender group. Hence, building on McCabe's work, the Type 2 group had significantly lower levels of sexual knowledge than the Type 1 group. These findings support the work of Day (1994), who suggested that there are two types of persons with intellectual disabilities who offend sexually. The naïve or Type 2 offender may, but not necessarily, have committed an offense because of a lack of sexual knowledge. Thus, a lack of sexual knowledge may play a role in a sexual offense for Type 2 offenders (those not motivated by deviant imagery) and, therefore, should be assessed as a possible contributing factor. Craig and Lindsay (2010) further asserted that "although sexual offenders with ID may have a higher level of sexual knowledge and more liberal sexual attitudes than non-offenders, their sexual knowledge remains at a stage where it is considerably poorer than that required by non-handicapped men" (p.16).

To explicitly clarify this point, which has often been misunderstood in the literature, the theory of counterfeit deviance *does not suggest* that all persons with intellectual disabilities who have offended sexually have poor sexual knowledge. In fact, the research, as noted above, reported that those with pervasive sexual offending tendencies often have greater knowledge than their peers with intellectual disabilities (Lunsky et al., 2007). This increased knowledge may be a consequence of previous exposure to either sexualized behavior or previous education provided as part of treatment for some sexual incident. As a result, it is indeed possible that a person with an intellectual disability may have good sexual knowledge and deviant arousal; although they too may have gaps or misunderstandings because of the nature of training (or lack thereof) that is often provided. Day (1994) similarly does not deny the existence of paraphilia within the population of intellectual disabilities; rather, he recommends caution in differentiation.

Further, the theory of counterfeit deviance does not imply that someone with an intellectual disability and poor sexual knowledge *will* sexually offend; a lack of sexual knowledge does not *ipso facto* imply that a person will act in a way contrary to social mores. What the theory does suggest, however, is that a person with an intellectual disability *could possibly* sexually offend because of poor sexual knowledge and that if an inappropriate sexual behavior has occurred, an assessment should be conducted to determine if the lack of sexual knowledge played a part in the commission of an offense by the person. Thus, as part of a comprehensive clinical investigation, the person's sexual knowledge should be examined, and only then can it be determined if a lack of knowledge potentially played a role in the offense role and as such for this person there is a benefit to providing sexual education as an element of treatment. As Griffiths et al. (2013) noted, "The wrong question is often asked in research and practice. The question is not 'Do persons with intellectual disabilities offend sexually because of a lack of sexual knowledge?' but 'Has ***this*** particular individual acted in a sexually inappropriate way because of poor knowledge?'" (p. 476).

Since the original theory of counterfeit deviance, additional counterfeit deviance theories have been added in the literature. Hingsburger, Dalla Nora and Tough (2011) observed that a person may be re-enacting a previous abuse situation and suggested that it was a means of communication (i.e., behavioral reporting of abuse). They further observed that some persons with disabilities may engage in sexual behavior to please or access social attention (i.e., Malicious Peer Pressure theory, Hingsburger et al., 2011). Wulfert, Greenway, and Dougher (1996) noted that some persons may engage in "pedophilic" behaviors not because of a sexual attraction to children, but because of a lack of access to age appropriate sexual expression or, possibly, as a means of reducing sexual stress. And, as stated above, Lindsay (2009) has suggested that ignorance of the laws and social mores of society may also play a role in the offenses of some people. Other theorists have suggested that some sexually inappropriate behaviors could be related to behavioral phenotypes or psychiatric challenges, such as touching of genitals as a tic disorder (Griffiths et al., 2007). As Griffiths et al. (2007) noted, the idea of counterfeit deviance does not represent a static list, but one that emerges as time goes on. The hypotheses do not represent a standard diagnostic tool; rather, they represent potential areas of consideration in a holistic assessment based upon examination of the experiences of those with intellectual disabilities and to look beyond topography.

GOING BEYOND TOPOGRAPHY FOR ABA ASSESSMENT

In the 1980s, there was an "if/then" approach to treatment that was pervasive among many behavior therapists in the field. Prior to development of standardized functional assessments, behavior therapists would often rely on the latest research to guide them in effective practice. If a person with intellectual disability was engaging in a challenging behavior, the therapist would search through the *Journal of Applied Behavior Analysis*, the ultimate journal for ABA, to see what the experts reported as most effective strategies. It led to a very simplistic, if/then consequence-based approach: if self-injury then...; if aggression then...; if toileting accidents then.... Although the field has moved a long way from the simplistic if/then consequence driven approach of the 1980s to today's reliance on functional behavior assessment as a means of determining context and function, there is often a devolution to earlier strategies when the challenging behavior is sexual, and in particular a sexual offense. However, just as we have learned that effective treatment follows comprehensive assessment with behaviors such as self-injury and aggression, so too must it apply to sexualized behavior.

Let us take a simple example of someone who has been accused of masturbating in public. Based solely on the topography of the behavior, one might assume it is sexually driven. However, there is a host of hypotheses that could be generated for the same behavior, some biomedical, some social, and others psychological. Here are only a few of many actual examples from the casefiles of our authors.

BIOMEDICAL HYPOTHESES

Case I: Peter was a young man who began to act-out sexually by touching himself and others. The behavior was described as "coming out of the blue" along with other behaviors such as not sleeping, pacing, pressured speech, and increased distractibility. An assessment showed that he was experiencing a ***manic episode*** that was treated with medication, and the sexual indiscretions went away. The behavior was the result of an episodic psychiatric condition.

Case II: Alice was on a bus and began to grab at her genital area. The bus driver called the police, and she was arrested when the bus stopped. The police asked her what she was doing on the bus. Alice said, "I didn't do anything wrong, I just had a bad itch." Alice's group home supervisor was called, and when she arrived and spoke to Alice she found out that Alice had developed a rash and that she was merely trying to ease the discomfort. Cases of vaginitis, a sexually transmitted disease, an allergy to fabrics or soaps, or similar causes could cause extreme ***medical discomfort*** that if handled indiscriminately by the person might be misunderstood as sexual. Alice's situation was treated by both attention to her medical need and education to ensure she understood that she needed to: (a) inform staff if she had a medical issue that needed attention; and b) discriminate private and public places in which it would be appropriate to relieve her itch.

Case III: Paul displayed a range of inappropriate behaviors, such as throwing and breaking glass, spitting, hitting at things, and touching others in the groin area. Although all the behaviors were problematic, staff members were most concerned about the sexual behaviors and had referred him to a behavior therapist claiming he was sexually assaulting others. The therapist observed him over several occasions, documenting all of his behaviors and suggested that he be assessed for a ***tic disorder***. The assessment came back to indicate that he had Tourette's syndrome and that all of his behaviors including the sexualized one was related to this syndrome.

Psychological Hypotheses

Case IV: Ernie was a young man with moderate to severe intellectual disability. He was at the mall with a new staff member when he began to flail his hands in front of her face. She redirected him to keep his hands down several times. Then he began to grab at his genital area. The staff member immediately removed him from the mall and returned him home. Once there she wrote in the communication book that he had masturbated in the mall and that she felt he should not be allowed to engage in this type of social activity because of his inappropriate behavior. The supervisor was surprised because Ernie had never engaged in this type of behavior in public previously. The behavior therapist assigned to the home was asked to consult. In the discussion, the therapist explored the nature of the precursor behaviors (i.e., flailing hands). The new staff member imitated the hand motions as best as she could remember, but they were sufficient for both the therapist and the supervisor to understand that Ernie had been using sign language to ask for a bathroom. The new staff did not understand sign language. Ernie was desperate for a bathroom and was trying to ***communicate*** this to his new staff. In desperation, he tried to stop himself from voiding in public in a manner that appeared as public masturbation.

Case V: Robert was accused of sexual exhibitionism in front of a young boy when found masturbating in the bathroom of the local Walmart. Upon investigation, the therapist conducted a socio-sexual knowledge and attitude assessment with Robert and discovered that he had learned that it was acceptable to masturbate in his bedroom or a bathroom. His previous educational experience had failed to inform him that it was illegal to engage in sexual behavior in a public bathroom.

Social Hypotheses

Case VI: Enzo began to masturbate in the common areas of the group home when one of the staff members was on shift. There appeared to be nothing inappropriate in the manner in which the staff member interacted with him, but her presence appeared to stimulate him sexually. The staff decided that when he started to masturbate they would send him to his room, to engage in the self-stimulatory behavior in private. They were cautious to let him know that the behavior was fine, but it had to be done in his bedroom. However, two minutes after going into his room he would re-emerge and would soon resume his masturbation. The therapist surmised that the issue was related to the presence of the stimulus (staff member) in the common area and a lack of sexual stimulus in the bedroom. Aware of the concern to deal with the situation in the most ethically appropriate way, the staff were instructed to purchase a non-pornographic poster of a woman (such as posed in a bathing suit) that could be posted on the back of his door. When he was sent to his room, the door would be shut, and he would then have an alternative stimulus to assist him to remain in his room and satisfy himself. The hypothesis here was that he was unable to sustain the stimulus arousal in memory when he returned to his room and required a stimulus to be present in his room. After repeated trials and consistent instruction that the behavior was not appropriate in the common area, the masturbation in public discontinued. His behavior was inappropriate because he was engaging in the behavior in a public place, motivated by the ***presence of a stimuli.*** When given an alternative, appropriate sexual stimuli, in an appropriate private location, his behavior changed.

Case VII: Mark was a student in a segregated school for students with intellectual disabilities. A behavior therapist was called in because Mark was engaging in masturbation in public. The therapist had never been to the school before and asked directions to the home room. Walking down the hall, looking side to side for the classroom, the therapist was surprised to see a door open and a young man sitting on a toilet exposed for all to see. Arriving at the home room, the therapist felt compelled to say something. "I just came in and there was a young man on the toilet and the door had been held ajar with a brick to keep it open..." Without allowing the therapist to finish, the teacher said, "Yes, we have to do that because he flushes toilet paper down the toilet if we don't leave it open and then the plumber has to come." Aware of the behavior therapist's status as a guest and a first-time visitor to the school, discretion seemed in order, so the topic was changed. "I am here to visit Mark, I am the behavior therapist, and I understand he has a problem understanding the difference between public and private." The teacher nodded. "Yes, that was Mark you saw." "Ahh," the therapist thought, "the person who cannot discriminate public and private is the same person everyone who has walked down the hall has seen partially naked." How could Mark learn private and public, when the setting made no distinction with regards to privacy? Mark's behavior was a product of a lack of education regarding issues of private/public and sexual behavior and ***an environment that provided inconsistent messages*** regarding that issue.

Case VIII: Staff members at a group home were concerned because Reggie was engaging in masturbation in public areas. The behavior therapist was called in to consult. One of the first questions the therapist asked was, "What do you do when he masturbates?" The staff indicated that they redirect him but added further that this was not working and that the behavior appeared to be occurring more frequently. The therapist set appointments to visit the home to observe the context of the behavior and how staff managed the situation. Surprisingly, when the behavior occurred the therapist noted that the staff did redirect him, but not to his bedroom or a private place where he could engage in this behavior but to an activity of macramé. The therapist asked why they chose to redirect to this activity rather than his room. The staff member proudly said that she had attended a course that said that if someone is doing something inappropriate with their hands, that you should redirect them to an activity that is incompatible and, "You cannot masturbate and do macramé at the same time," she declared. The therapist praised the staff for having attended so well to what the instructor had told them about introducing incompatible behaviors but asked if the instructor had also talked about functionality. The staff member said, "I think they did that, but I had to leave early." This represents an example of a good staff member with only limited knowledge who was trying to redirect the behavior without understanding that ***macramé and masturbation do not share the same function!***

Case IX: Brian was placed in a nursing home when he came down with an illness that was presumed to require long term nursing care. He quickly recovered, but unfortunately his space in his group home had been given to someone else. There was nowhere for him to go in the near future. The nursing home environment was designed to care for people with extreme medical needs, not for active persons with intellectual disabilities who were more likely to seek engaging activities and social interaction. Brian started engaging in attention seeking behaviors according to the nurses' reports. They complained they had no time to be with him to do the things he might like to do. One day he was found masturbating outside the administrator's office. Quickly, the nursing staff found things for him to do and people to engage with him. Masturbation served as an excellent way to gain the ***desired attention*** in an environment that was bereft of interaction appropriate to his needs.

Case X: The staff members in a group home were concerned about Ralph's incessant masturbation in public. They said he was constantly masturbating in the common areas of the house. The therapist visited the home and observed the following: After dinner, a staff member instructed Ralph to clear the table and fill the dishwasher. Ralph began to masturbate and was sent to his room. The staff then did the dishes. Later that evening the staff member asked Ralph to do his laundry; Ralph began to masturbate and was sent to his room again. The staff member finished his laundry. The therapist asked the staff to do some data collection in terms of what came before (antecedents), the behavior, and what came after (consequences) for three days, just to ensure the observations were consistent over time. The chart revealed a consistent pattern: Staff request Ralph to do something undesirable, Ralph masturbated. Once Ralph was sent to his room, the staff member completed the chore. Ralph had found an ***effective strategy to escape undesired activities.***

Throughout the examples provided above, examples of counterfeit deviance have been illustrated. However, it is important to recognize that the concept of counterfeit deviance was not designed to explain all incidents of sexual misconduct or offenses by people with intellectual disabilities. The theory only poses areas of investigation to rule out the possibility that someone may be misdiagnosed with a paraphilia when none exists. For example, Frank masturbated in public because he liked the reaction that he received from others. He liked the shock factor and gained sexual satisfaction from engaging in public exposure. His arousal was linked to his exhibitionism. You don't know what you are dealing with until you investigate; you cannot treat until you know what you should be treating. Determination of paraphilia or counterfeit deviance can only be accomplished by a comprehensive evaluation of the person in relation to the behavior in question.

SUMMARY

The main messages from this chapter are twofold: First, a sexual offense committed by a person with intellectual disability may occur for many reasons. Some may be motivated by a deviant interest and some for other reasons. Second, assessment and treatment for sexual offense behaviors must follow a comprehensive examination of the context of the behavior relating to that person. Just as in the assessment and treatment of any other behavior, the antecedents, consequences, motivating operations, and, ultimately, function(s) of the behavior must be explored if treatment is to match the needs of the person and produce efficacious outcomes. There are, however, some differences in the assessment and treatment of sex offenders that require variations on a typical behavioral analytic approach to behavior. The pivotal one of course is that, above all, prevention of a future offense must be paramount. Additionally, the assessment and treatment approach may require the behavior analyst to use a wider lens that examines all possible biopsychosocial influences in order to ensure that a holistic approach is taken. In the chapter that follows, the logical functional model for assessing persons with intellectual disabilities who sexually offend will be presented.

REFERENCES

Abel, G. G. & Rouleau, J. (1990). The nature and extent of sexual assault. In W.L. Marshall, D.R. Laws, & H.E. Barbaree (Eds.), *Handbook of sexual assault* (pp. 9-21). New York: Plenum Press.

Andrews, D.A. & Bonta, J. (2010). *The psychology of criminal conduct* (5th Edition). New York, NY: Elsevier.

American Psychiatric Association (2013). *Diagnostic and statistical manual of mental disorders* (5th ed.). Washington, DC: Author.

American Psychiatric Association (1987). *Diagnostic and statistical manual of mental disorders* (3rd ed., text revision). Washington, DC: Author.

American Psychiatric Association (2000). *Diagnostic and statistical manual of mental disorders* (4th ed., text revision). Washington, DC: Author.

Brandt, J., Wilson, R. J., & Prescott, D. S. (2015). Doubts about SVP programs: A critical review of sexual offender civil commitment in the US. In B. Schwartz (Ed.), *The sex offender*, Vol. 8. Kingston, NJ: Civic Research Institute.

Briggs, F. & Hawkins, R. M. F. (1996). A comparison of the childhood experiences of convicted male child molesters and men who were sexually abused in childhood and claimed to be non-offenders. *Child Abuse and Neglect, 20*, 221-233.

Brown, B. S., & Courtless, R. F. (1971). *Mentally retarded offender.* Washington, D.C.: National Institute of Mental Health, Center for Studies of Crime and Delinquency.

Canupp, et al. v. Liberty Behavioral, et al. (2009) No. 2:2004cv00260 - Document 318 (M.D. Fla. 2009). Retrieved 04/09/2018 from https://law.justia.com/cases/federal/district-courts/florida/flmdce/2:2004cv00260/4847/318/.

CBC News Posted: Aug 10, 2005 Man confessed to sex crimes he didn't commit http://www.cbc.ca/news/canada/man-confessed-to-sex-crimes-he-didn-t-commit-1.536266

CBC News (Aug 06, 2009) *Canada's wrongful convictions: Cases where the courts got it wrong.* Retrieved from http://www.cbc.ca/news/canada/canada-s-wrongful-convictions-1.783998#marshall

Craig, L. & Lindsay, W. R. (2010). Sexual offenders with intellectual disabilities: Characteristics and prevalence. In L. Craig, W.R. Lindsay, W.R., & K.D. Browne (Eds.),

Assessment and treatment of sexual offenders with intellectual disabilities (13-36). Chichester, UK: Wiley-Blackwell.

Day, K. (1994). Male mentally handicapped sex offenders. *British Journal of Psychiatry, 165*, 630-639.

Day, K. (1997). Clinical features and offense behavior of mentally retarded sex offenders: A review of research. In R.J. Fletcher & D. Griffiths (Eds.), *Congres Proceedings: International Congress II on the Dually Diagnosed* (pp. 95-99). Kingston, NY: NADD.

Firth, H., Balogh, R., Berney, T., Bretherton, K., Graham, S., & Whibley, S. (2001). Psychopathology of Sexual Abuse in Young People with Intellectual Disability. *Journal of Intellectual Disability Research 45*, 244-252.

Griffiths, D. (2002). Sexual aggression. In W. I. Gardner (Ed.), *Aggression and other disruptive behavioral challenges: Biomedical and psychosocial assessment and treatment* (pp.525-398). New York: National Association for Dual Diagnosis.

Griffiths, D., & Fedoroff, P. (2008) Persons with intellectual disabilities who sexually offend. In F.M. Saleh, A.J. Grudzinskas, J.M., Bradford, & D.J. Brodsky (Eds.), *Sex offenders: Identification, risk, assessment, treatment, and legal issues* (pp. 352-374). New York: Oxford University Press.

Griffiths, D., Fedoroff, P., Richards, D., Cox-Lindenbaum, D., Langevin, R., Linsday, W. D., ... Goldman, M. (2007). Sexual and Gender Identity Disorders. In R. Fletcher, E. Loschen, S. Stavrakaki, & M. First (Eds.). *Diagnostic manual - intellectual disability (DM-ID): A textbook of diagnosis of mental disorders in persons with intellectual disability* (pp. 411-457). Kingston, NY: NADD Press.

Griffiths, D., Fedoroff, P., Richards, D. & Lindsay, W. (2016). Paraphilia. In R. Fletcher, J. Barnhill, & S.A. Cooper (Eds.), *Diagnostic manual- Intellectual disabilities: A textbook of diagnosis of mental disorders in persons with intellectual disability* (2nd ed.; pp.637-666). Kingston, NY: NADD.

Griffiths, D., Hingsburger, D., Hoath, J., & Ioannou, S. (2013). 'Counterfeit deviance' revisited. *Journal of Applied Research in Intellectual Disabilities, 26*, 471-480.

Griffiths, D.M., Quinsey, V. L., & Hingsburger, D. (1989). *Changing inappropriate sexual behavior: A Community based approach for persons with intellectual disabilities.* Baltimore, MD: Paul H. Brookes Publishing.

Griffiths, D., Taillon-Wasmund, P. & Smith, D. (2002). Offenders who have a developmental disability. In D.M. Griffiths, C. Stavrakaki, & J. Summers, *Dual diagnosis: An introduction to the mental health needs of persons with developmental disabilities* (pp. 387-418). Sudbury, ON: Habilitative Mental Health Resource Network.

Griffiths, D., Watson, S., Lewis, R., & Stoner, K. (2004). Research in sexuality and intellectual disability. In E. Emerson, C. Hatton, T. Parmenter, & T. Thompson (Eds.), *Handbook of methods of research and evaluation in intellectual disabilities (pp. 311-334).* London, UK: Wiley.

Hayes, S. (1991). Sex offenders. *Australian and New Zealand Journal of Developmental Disabilities, 17*, 221-7.

Hingsburger, D. (1989). Motives for coprophilia: working with individuals who have been institutionalized with developmental handicaps. *Journal of Sex Research, 26*,139-140.

Hingsburger, D., Dalla Nora, M., & Tough, S. (2011). *The key: assessment and treatment of sex offenders with intellectual disabilities who live in community settings.* Barrie, ON: Diverse City Press.

Hingsburger, D., Griffiths, D., & Quinsey, V. (1991). Detecting counterfeit deviance: differentiating sexual deviance from sexual inappropriateness. *The Habilitative Mental Healthcare Newsletter, 10,* 51-54.

Jespersen, A. F., Lalumière, M. L., & Seto, M. C. (2009). Sexual abuse history among adult sex offenders and non-offenders: A meta analysis. *Child Abuse and Neglect, 33*(3), 179-192.

Karsjens v. Piper, (2017) US District Court for Minnesota, Civil No. 11-3659 (DWF/JJK). Retrieved 04/09/2018 from https://mitchellhamline.edu/sex-offense-litigation-policy/2017/07/20/karsjens-v-piper/.

Langevin, R. (1992). A comparison of neuroendocrine abnormalities and genetic factors in homosexuality and in pedophilia. *Annals of Sex Research, 6,* 67-76.

Laski, F. J. (1992). Sentencing the offender with mental retardation: Honoring the imperative for immediate punishments and probation. In R. W. Conley, R. Luckasson, & G. N. Bouthilet (Eds.), *The criminal justice system and mental retardation* (pp.137-152). Baltimore: Brookes.

Lindsay, W. R. (2002). Research and literature on sex offenders with intellectual and developmental disabilities. *Journal of Intellectual Disabilities Research, 46 (Suppl. 1),* 74-85.

Lindsay, W. R. (2009). *The treatment of sex offenders with developmental disabilities: A practice workbook.* West Sussex, UK: Wiley Blackwell.

Lindsay, W. R., Hastings, R. P., Griffiths, D. M., & Hayes, S. C. (2007). Trends and challenges in forensic research on offenders with intellectual disability. *Journal of Intellectual & Developmental Disability, 32,* 55–6.

Lindsay, W. R., Law, J., Quinn, K., Smart, N., & Smith, A. H. (2001). A comparison of physical and sexual abuse: histories of sexual and non-sexual offenders with intellectual disability. *Child Abuse & Neglect, 25,* 989-995.

Lunsky, Y., Frijters, J., Watson, S., Willison, S., & Griffiths, D. (June 2007). Sexual knowledge and attitudes of men with intellectual disabilities who sexually offend. Special issue on offenders with ID/DD. *Journal of Intellectual and Developmental Disabilities, 32,* 74-81.

Marinos V. Griffiths, D., Fergus, C., Stromski, S., & Rondeau, K. (2014). Victims and witnesses with intellectual disability in the criminal justice system. *Criminal Justice Quarterly, 61,* 517-530.

McBrien, J. A., Murphy, G. (2006) Police and carers' views on reporting alleged offenses by people with intellectual disabilities. *Psychology, Crime and Law 12,* 127-144

McCabe, M. (1999). Sexual knowledge, experience and feelings among people with disabilities. *Sexuality and Disability, 17,* 157-170.

McCarthy, M. & Thompson, D. (1997). A prevalence study of sexual abuse of adults with intellectual disabilities referred for sex education. *Journal of Applied Research in Intellectual Disabilities, 10,* 105-124.

McEachron, A. E. (1979). Mentally retarded offenders: Prevalence and characteristics. *American Journal of Mental Deficiency, 84,* 165-176.

McGee, J., & Menolasino, F. J. (1992). The evaluation of defendants with mental retardation in the criminal justice system. In R. W. Conley, R. Luckasson, & G. N. Bouthilet (Eds.) *The criminal justice system and mental retardation: Defendants and victims* (pp. 55-78). Baltimore, MD: Paul. H. Brookes.

Michie, A. M., Lindsay W. R., Martin, V., & Grieve, A. (2006). A test of counterfeit deviance: a comparison of sexual knowledge in groups of sex offenders with intellectual disabilities and controls, *Sex Abuse, 18,* 271-8.

Mohr, J., Turner, R. E., & Jerry, M. (1964). *Pedophilia and exhibitionism.* Toronto, ON: University of Toronto Press.

Money, J. (1999). *Principles of developmental sexology continuum.* New York; Continuum.

Moschella, S. (1982). The mentally retarded offender: Law enforcement and court proceedings. In M. B. Santamour & P. S. Watson (Eds.), *The retarded offender* (pp. 195-204). New York: Praeger.

Murphy, W. D., Coleman, E. M., & Haynes, M. (1983) Treatment and evaluation issues with the mentally retarded sex offender. In J. Greer & I. Stuart (Eds.), *The sexual aggressor: Current perspectives on treatment* (pp. 22-41). New York: Van Nostrand Reinhold.

Santamour, W., & West, B. (1978). *The mentally retarded offender and corrections.* Washington, DC: U.S. Department of Justice.

Selling, L. S. (1959). Types of behavior manifested by feeble-minded sex offenders. *Proceedings from the American Association of Mental Deficiency, 44,* 178-186.

Shapiro, S. (1986). Delinquent and disturbed behavior within the field of mental deficiency. In A. V. S. deReuck & R. Porter (Eds.), *The mentally abnormal offender.* New York: Grune & Stratton.

Simmons, H. (1982). *From asylum to welfare.* Toronto, ON: National Institute of Mental Retardation.

Sobsey, D. (1994). Sexual abuse of individuals with intellectual disabilities. In A. Craft (Ed.), *Practice issues in sexuality and intellectual disability* (pp. 91-112). London, UK: Routledge.

Steiner, J. (1984) Group counselling with retarded offenders. *Social Work, 29,* 181-182.

Talbot, T. J., & Langdon, P. E. (2006). A revised sexual knowledge assessment tool for people with intellectual disabilities. *Journal of Intellectual Disability Research, 50,* 523–531.

Timms, S. & Goreczny, A. J. (2002). Adolescent sex offenders with mental retardation: Literature review and assessment considerations. *Aggression and Violent Behavior, 7,*1-19.

Toberg, M. A. (1992). *Pretrial release: A national evaluation of practice and outcomes,* McLean, Va. Lazar Institute.

Torrey, E. F., Kennard, A. D., Eslinger, D., Lamb, R., & Pavle, J. (2010). *More mentally ill persons are in jail and prisons than hospitals: A Survey of the states.* National Sheriffs Association and Treatment Advocacy Center. Retrieved October 25, 2013 from http://www.sheriffs.org/userfiles/file/FinalJailsvHospitalsStudy.pdf.

Ward, T., & Stewart, C. (2003). Criminogenic needs and human needs: A theoretical *model. Psychology, Crime & Law,* 9, 125-143.

Wulfert, E., Greenway, D. E., & Dougher, M. J. (1996). A logical functional analysis of reinforcement-based disorders: alcoholism and pedophilia. *Journal of Consulting and Clinical Psychology, 64,* 1140-1151.

Chapter Three

Towards a Multi-Component Decision Model for Assessment and Treatment of Sexual Offending Behavior of Persons with an Intellectual Disability

In this book, the authors propose a multi-component decision model based on Wulfert, Greenway and Dougher (1996) and many years of well-established behavioral assessment and treatment methodologies. Hence, the proposed model is not new; it is a refinement and application of current models that are used with the neurotypically developing population. Although this book attempts to describe the nuances involved in applying the proposed model to people with intellectual disabilities and sexual offending behavior, it is important for readers to keep in mind the following two points that were noted in the previous chapter:

1) *With whom the model should be applied.* The proposed model is discussed in relation to persons with intellectual disabilities who have sexually offended versus violent offenders in the typically developing population. This distinction is important, as there are very important differences in both the person and environmental variables such as culture, history, etc. that may contribute to differences in assessment methods and treatment outcomes for these two populations. This model is described in relation to the population of people with intellectual disabilities whose offenses may (but not always) be less a sexual offense and more an inappropriate expression of sexual behaviors. This is an important distinction considering the drastically different life experiences, cultural mores, learning styles, and personal histories experienced by people with intellectual disabilities. These factors may have a major impact on how clinicians approach and respond to sexually offensive behavior.
2) *Applying the model will take time and resources.* The resources and time necessary to apply the model may vary according to the person or group applying the model, as well as the person to whom the model is being applied. Although this book attempts to describe the model in as straightforward a manner as possible, given the complex nature of the population and the behavior, the process will take careful consideration and resources in terms of training and expertise. Background in behavior analytic principles should be considered necessary.

Current practice recommends a holistic, multi-factorial, and strength-based approach in working with persons with intellectual disabilities and concurrent mental health challenges, including those with sexual offending behaviors. However, there is no real consensus in the field as to which methods are most effective for determining the appropriate intervention path for a particular person with sex offending behavior. As such, the value of comprehensive behavioral assessment in that process cannot be underestimated. A comprehensive behavioral assessment is vital in understanding the conditions under which the behaviors are more or less likely to occur (i.e., the antecedent events that may occasion the behavior) and the function that the behaviors serve for the person (i.e., the consequences that maintain the behavior).

To aid in identifying and intervening to address the full range of potential causal factors, Wulfert and colleagues (1996) suggested that if functional clusters of behavior could be identified for sexually offensive behavior (specifically, pedophilia), then a stronger link could be formed between assessment and treatment. Wulfert and colleagues (1996) suggested that the logical functional analysis, based on Hayes and Follette (1992), which lays out a decision model to organize the assessment and subsequent targeted treatment, might potentially provide the basis for developing treatment guidelines founded on understanding the function of the sexual offending behavior. This approach has been accomplished with other challenging behaviors such as aggression and self-injury when displayed by persons with an intellectual disability (e.g., Gardner, Cole, Davidson, & Karan, 1986). We agree with Wulfert et al. and argue that a comprehensive and functional behavioral assessment is vital for understanding the conditions under which sex offending behaviors are, more or less, likely to occur and which factors in the environment precipitate and maintain behavior. This information is necessary for guiding effective intervention.

The authors propose a six-component decision model (see Figure 3.1), based on Wulfert and colleague's model (1996), to serve as a basis for behavior analysts to assess and intervene for persons with intellectual disabilities with sexual offending behavior or alleged problem sexual behaviors. The six components fall into three areas: 1. *Assessment,* which includes determining the antecedents and consequences (Chapter 4), motivating operations (Chapter 5), and function (Chapter 6), which then serves as a foundation for a decision about a path for 2. *Treatment,* which includes teaching alternative or coping skills (Chapter 9), and providing remedial consequences (Chapter 10), and finally 3. *Generalization and Maintenance* (Chapter 11), which aims to ensure that any favorable behavioral outcomes maintain over time and occur across various conditions, people, settings, etc. Each of the six components will be summarized in this chapter and addressed in more detail throughout the remaining chapters in the book.

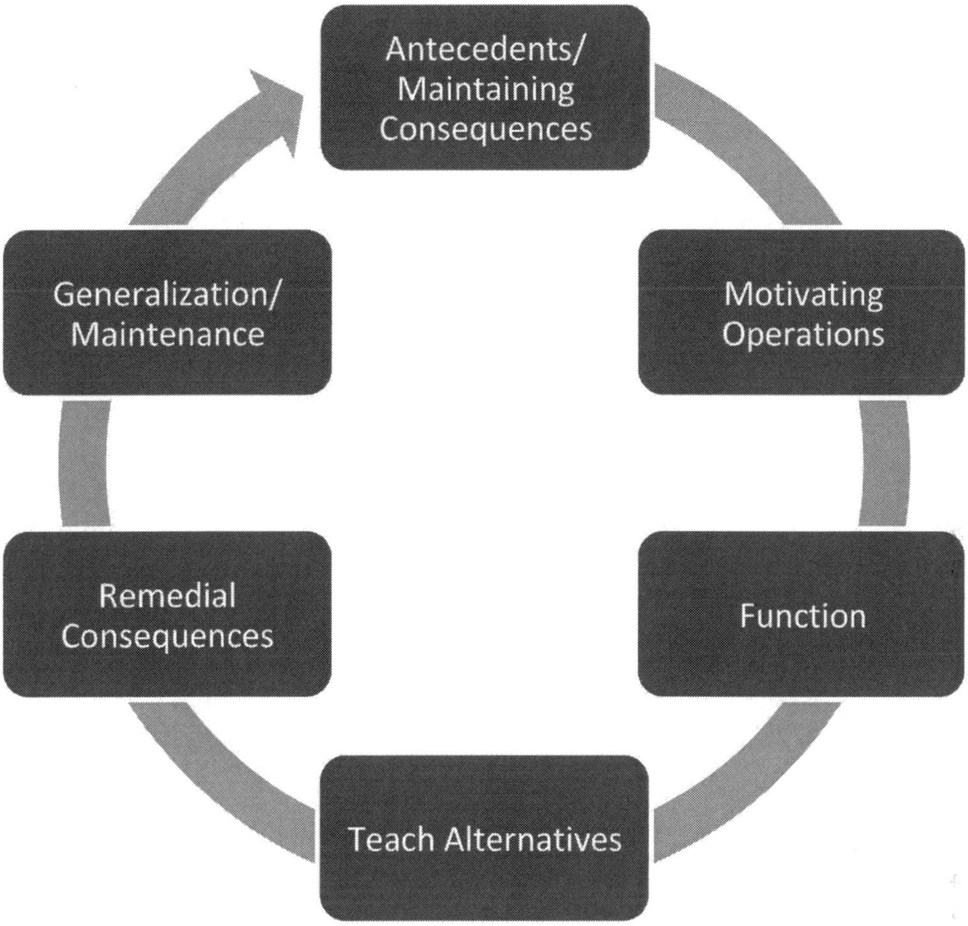

Figure 3.1. **Components of the decision model for assessment and intervention for sexualized offending behavior.**

ASSESSMENT (Model Components 1-3)

The first three components of the proposed model pertain to assessment. A comprehensive functional behavior assessment takes into consideration the antecedent events or motivational states that may occasion the behavior as well as the consequent events that may maintain the behavior (i.e., the function that the behavior serves for the person). This approach does not attempt to intervene based on the topography of behavior (i.e., what a behavior looks like) or a specific behavior disorder or syndrome, but rather addresses the underlying causes of behavior or what is maintaining it. To do this, one must consider the environment, as well as the person and all of the variables that are continuously interacting between the two. Just because one variable (e.g., early sexual abuse) may be shown to be a predictive or correlative factor with later sexual offending behavior at a population level for the majority of persons with intellectual disability who sexually offend, it may not be the case for every person. A person's constant state of interaction with the environment may cause slight or large deviations from the population mean, which has important implications for treatment. If intervention is based on the population average, then important individual variables may not be considered. As such, a variable orientation (e.g., relying on statistical averages to make predictions, guide treatment, etc.) definitely serves a valuable purpose but is strengthened by an individual approach that attempts to directly determine function of behavior for the individual (Magnusson & Bergman, 1988). The proposed functional model also takes this perspective – an individualistic, yet comprehensive, function-based, and person-centred approach. Chapter 4 discusses how to assess antecedents and maintaining consequences, Chapter 5, summarizes the importance of motivating operations in the assessment of sexual offending behavior, and Chapter 6 discusses functions of sexual offending behavior.

An important distinction in the terminology involved in a comprehensive functional behavioral assessment is between *assessment* and *analysis*. Functional *assessment* is a process of gathering information to form hypotheses about what variables are potentially maintaining a behavior, whereas functional *analysis* is experimentally testing those hypotheses in a systematic way by manipulating variables in the environment. Attempts to determine *why* behavior occurs goes back to the early days of behavior analysis with the works of Skinner, Lovaas, Carr, Bijou, and others. Originally, the term functional analysis referred to attempts to demonstrate a cause-effect relationship (Baer, Wolf, & Risley, 1968) or potential ways in which the environment-controlled behavior (Skinner, 1953). Skinner preferred experimental analyses over descriptive assessment, and, currently, functional analysis has come to imply an experimental manipulation of variables to test hypotheses about causal factors (Dixon Vogel, & Tarbox, 2012). Given the present-day use of functional analysis, technically any assessment activities that do not include the systematic manipulation of variables should be referred to most accurately as functional *assessment* (Cone, 1997). Wulfert and colleagues (1996) use the term functional analysis in the more traditional sense: attempting to determine cause and effect of behavior not necessarily with experimental manipulations of variables.

Carr was among one of the first to promote forming hypotheses about the function of behavior and then matching interventions to the function. Carr and colleagues (1976) specified three questions that could be raised to identify the conditions associated with problem behavior of children. That is, to determine whether the behavior increases under any of the following circumstances: (1) when it is attended to, (2) when the client no longer receives reinforcement for other behaviors, and (3) when the child is in the company of adults. His important work demonstrating functional relationships between environmental variables and the occurrence of self-injurious behavior contributed greatly to the development of functional analysis methods (Carr, Newsom, & Binkoff, 1980)

Mace (1994) argued that the introduction of the experimental functional analysis of behavior is what prompted the transition from "behavior modification" to "applied behavior analysis" in the 1960s. Before clinicians attempted to experimentally confirm the history of reinforcement, or what was maintaining a challenging behavior, reinforcement and punishment contingencies were superimposed in attempts to alter the behavior. The logic was that if more potent contingencies were applied, they would "override" the existing contingencies of reinforcement that were responsible for maintaining the challenging behavior, the functions of which were often unknown. This approach sometimes led to an over-reliance on default (punishment) technologies (Mace, 1994). Further, interventions were often matched to disorders or syndromes or specific maladaptive behaviors as opposed to matching interventions to the operant function of the behavior, which varied among persons with the same behavioral disorder or maladaptive behavior and could also change over time. In 1989, the National Institutes of Health (NIH) Consensus Conference on the treatment of destructive behaviors associated with developmental disabilities recommended that treatment of severe behavior disorders be based on the results of a pre-treatment functional analysis (National Institutes of Health, 1989). Since then, experimental functional analysis methodology has been well established in the literature (e.g., Iwata, Dorsey, Slifer, Bauman, & Richman, 1982/1994) for determining the function of various challenging behaviors. Determining the cause or function of behavior before applying treatment is now considered best practice (Dixon et al., 2012). Ultimately, the results garnered from the functional behavior assessment process (including experimental functional analyses) are meant to guide effective treatment.

Experimental Analysis of Function of Sexual Offending Behavior

The traditional functions of behavior evaluated in experimental functional analyses that have been empirically supported in the literature include: (1) socially mediated positive reinforcement (e.g., maintained by access to desired stimuli such as attention – see Carr, 1977); (2) negative reinforcement (e.g., maintained by escape or avoidance of aversive stimuli/situations – see Carr et al., 1980); and (3) automatic reinforcement (e.g., behavior is maintained by the reinforcement that is produced automatically when the behavior occurs – see Skinner, 1953). There are other potential functions including tangible (e.g., maintained by preferred item or activity), and controlling the environment (e.g., maintained by the opportunity to control a situation). It is also possible and quite common for behavior to be maintained by a combination of functions or, in other words, to be multiply controlled. Behavior can also be under the control of idiosyncratic variables such as the presence of certain stimuli in the environment (e.g., attention from a specific individual vs. attention from any individual).

When it comes to sexual offending behavior, functional categories are complex, and although there are some theoretical explanations for sexual offending behavior they often do not take into consideration contextual variables and, therefore, do not directly determine function. For example, it has been argued that persons with autism spectrum disorder may engage in sexual offending behavior due to misunderstanding social cues, lacking empathy and understanding of societal norms, having poor impulse control, and being vulnerable to manipulation into criminal acts by others (Allen et al., 2008). Basic operant assessment of sexual arousal behavior in general, and sexual offending behavior specifically, is sparse in the behavior analytic literature with the exception of a handful of studies that have focused on reverting unwanted sexual arousal through ethically questionable methods (Roche & Barnes, 1998). For example, some of the early studies evaluated methods such as aversion and desensitization for treating homosexuality (e.g., Bancroft, 1970). Further research is needed in novel application of experimental functional analyses including sexual offending behavior.

Experimental functional analyses are most often conducted in research settings versus clinical settings. For just one exception see Feldman, Condillac, Tough, Hunt, and Griffiths (2002). The experimental functional analysis methodology may need to be adjusted based on the environment. Recent methodological advancements such as brief, trial-based, single-function, latency, and precursor functional analyses make the process more doable with limited time and resources and more amenable to conducting in complex clinical environments (Iwata & Dozier, 2008). The aim of a functional analysis is to determine the cause of behavior, so the process involves manipulating antecedent/motivating operations and subsequent events/stimuli to actually evoke the target behavior to determine which variables are maintaining the behavior. The seminal article by Iwata and colleagues (originally 1982, republished in 1994) demonstrated the powerful experimental functional analysis methodology in the following conditions: (1) a play (control) condition, in which no demands were placed on the person, preferred items were available, brief attention was provided, and no consequences were provided to the person contingent on the target behavior; (2) an academic (demand/escape) condition in which demands were placed on the person and then removed contingent on the occurrence of the target behavior; (3) a social disapproval (attention) condition, in which social attention was withheld and delivered contingent on the person engaging in the target behavior in the form of disapproving statements contingent on the behavior such as "Don't do that" in combination with physical attention such as a pat on the shoulder; and (4) an alone (automatic reinforcement) condition in which the person was alone without toys or social attention and no consequences were provided contingent on the target behavior (Iwata et al., 1982/1994).

Despite the empirical support for the reliability of outcomes of experimental functional analyses, it is important to note that not *all* causal variables can be systematically manipulated, and at times functional analyses may not be ethical or appropriate since they involve evoking the challenging behavior to determine what is maintaining it. Although it is best practice to determine function of behavior before applying an intervention, sexual offending behavior is not always amenable to experimental functional analysis for obvious ethical considerations that are involved with evoking the behavior. In cases like these, the methodology may need to be adapted to an experimental analysis of precursor behaviors or other assessment methods may need to be applied.

Other Components of the Functional Behavior Assessment Process

Cone (1997) outlined three stages of functional behavior assessment: descriptive, interpretation, and verification. Iwata, Vollmer, and Zarcone (1990) classified similar stages: informant (indirect) assessment, observation (direct), and functional or experimental analysis. In general, the functional behavior assessment process can reveal important information about what may be maintaining behavior, which can be accomplished through various means such as:

- Explore and rule out biomedical influences (pain, discomfort, psychiatric conditions, medication side effects). A physical examination by a qualified medical

professional should precede behavioral interventions in some cases.
- Review historical files and previous reports to assess for any patterns in behavior occurring before or after the target behavior.
- Conduct interviews with people from the person's past who were involved when sexually offending behavior occurred and individuals who are currently familiar with the person (e.g., staff, therapists, family, others).
- Utilize self-reports to determine what the person was thinking, feeling, doing, who was present, and what the setting was, prior to the target behavior.
- Utilize scatterplot and/or descriptive assessment data to determine what antecedent and consequent variables are occurring and look for patterns to hypothesize what is contributing to/maintaining the behavior.
- Systematically manipulate controlling variables identified in the descriptive assessment in an experimental functional analysis to verify the hypothesized function(s) if appropriate and feasible.

Biomedical

Axelrod (1987) argued that behavioral intervention should not be completed before a physical exam is conducted to rule out any underlying medical causes for the behavior. In line with a comprehensive functional behavior assessment and the biopsychosocial model of assessment, biomedical influences contributing to the problematic behavior must be thoroughly examined and ruled out first. Baker, Blumberg and Freeman (2002) suggested that current behavioral assessments should be adapted to also evaluate the role that biomedical issues may play in presenting a behavioral symptom. They suggested, for example, that physiological arousal might be seen as an antecedent event for many problem behaviors. Gardner (2002) cautioned, however, that physical, psychiatric, or physiological challenges do not trigger the occurrence of a challenging behavior; rather, they represent a vulnerability that may contribute to the behavior in the presence of other environmental stimuli (such as specific social triggers). However, as Baker and colleagues (2002) suggested, adaptations to the traditional behavioral assessment could be made to expand the observations to include these factors.

Direct and Indirect Assessment

A clinician can assess the antecedents (including motivating operations) and consequences using direct and indirect measurement strategies. Direct measurement can include descriptive assessment such as antecedent-behavior-consequence (ABC) data collection, which attempts to reveal events or environmental variables that are correlated with a behavior. Antecedent-behavior-consequence data provides details of a person's behavior in the natural context and summarizes the antecedents and consequences for each instance of a target behavior in temporal sequence. Therefore, it is useful for giving a structural description of *what* behaviors are occurring but not useful for determining a functional reason for *why* the behaviors are occurring. Thompson and Iwata (2007) suggested that caution should be used when interpreting the results of descriptive assessment alone due to poor correspondence of the results with experimental functional analyses (Hall, 2005; Lerman & Iwata, 1993).

Scatterplots can be useful for determining during which time periods or with whom the target behavior is occurring. The scatterplot can be used to estimate the rate of behavior at different times in a day. It can be determined when the rate is at highest levels and then more systematic assessment procedures can take place during those times (Touchette, MacDonald, & Langer, 1985). Although the above process outlines a means of gathering information about when the target behavior is present, it is equally valuable to use the same process to examine under which settings, conditions, and with whom the target behavior is *not* present. This provides a useful comparative analysis that can sometimes lead to replicating variables that are present when the target behavior does not occur in an intervention. It is important to note that this information helps to form hypotheses about why the behaviors are occurring but does not confirm function of the behavior.

Indirect measurement is different from direct measurement in that it is accomplished through reviewing anecdotal documents, interviewing people who know the person best, and interviewing the person to give a self-report of the problematic behavior. Interviews can be open-ended or structured and are relatively easy to administer, time effective, and do not require as many resources as direct observation. Indirect and direct assessment procedures are described in more detail in Chapter 6.

The assessment components, as they are used to assess sexually offending behavior in persons with intellectual disabilities, are elaborated in the following Chapters: Chapter 4, The Antecedents and Consequences related to Behavior (ABCs), Chapter 5, Motivating Operations, and Chapter 6, Function.

TREATMENT (Model Components 4-5)

The fourth and fifth components of the model pertain to treatment. Once the function of behavior has been determined, intervention strategies must be implemented to address whatever is maintaining the problem behavior. In the case of sexually offending behavior it may include getting a sexual need met in a non-offending way (McGuire, 2001). Consequences for behavior can be reinforcement or punishment based, natural or contrived. Treatment should consider all environmental variables to which the individual is exposed. When attempting to decrease any challenging behavior, it is most desirable and ethical to first attempt the least intrusive and/or reinforcement-based intervention strategies. However, it is important to note that for very severe problem behavior, a punishment-based procedure such as response cost (e.g., loss of privileges) can be the most ethically justified treatment option since punishment strategies (which do not necessarily mean aversive) lead to more immediate decreases in behavior. Punishment procedures have been and continue to be misapplied by many professionals in attempts to reduce challenging behaviors (Evans & Meyer, 1985). The reality is no different for sexual offending behaviors, which raises important ethical considerations such as the use of psychotropic intervention, isolation, etc. (Ioannou, 2013). Chapter 10 discusses the ethical considerations of consequence-based treatment for sexual offending behavior in more detail.

An important consideration when designing intervention programs for sexual offending behavior is that since the behavior is sexual in nature it may involve a complex interaction of respondent and operant conditioning. Therefore, an intervention must assess and address each form of conditioning accordingly. It is also most effective to teach alternative functional replacement behavior in any behavior reduction program

(Evans & Meyer, 1985). That is, simply reducing the problem behavior is not sufficient and will likely not maintain or generalize. Therefore, clinicians need to ensure that any punishment procedures are supplemented with other reinforcement-based strategies as non-contingent reinforcement, differential reinforcement, and extinction in addition to teaching alternative, more appropriate functionally equivalent behavior. Chapter 9 reviews teaching alternative behavior in further detail.

The chapters that apply to treatment of offenders who have an intellectual disability are: Chapter 9: Teach Alternatives and Chapter 10: Corrective and Remedial Consequences.

GENERALIZATION AND MAINTENANCE (MODEL COMPONENT 6)

The final component of the model pertains to generalization and maintenance of behavior change (i.e., reduction of challenging behavior and maintenance of alternative, more appropriate behaviors). Behavior change is considered generalized if it occurs at other times and other places than the intervention setting, without being retrained, or if a behavior that is functionally equivalent to the target behavior emerges untrained (Cooper, Heron, & Heward, 2007). A challenging goal of any behavioral treatment program is to produce desirable outcomes that generalize across people, environments, and behaviors (Stokes & Baer, 1977). This is a particularly difficult outcome to achieve in persons with intellectual disabilities and sexually offending behavior since the risks for recidivism must be minimized while the treatment gains are maximized. Although it is important for any generalized behavior change to maintain after an intervention is terminated or faded out, it is especially important for any reduction/elimination of sexual offending behavior as it is vital to the person's future and the safety of others.

General strategies to promote generalization and maintenance of treatment gains in any behavior reduction program include selecting target behaviors that will meet naturally occurring contingencies of reinforcement, specifying all desired variations of the behavior and the settings and situations where it should and should not occur, teaching the full range of relevant stimulus conditions and response requirements, making the instructional setting similar to the generalization setting, and maximizing the person's contact with reinforcement in the generalization setting, among others (see Cooper, Heron, & Heward, 2007, Ch. 28).

Application of strategies for generalization and maintenance in the community following treatment will be elaborated in Chapter 11. In that chapter, some of the strategies to promote generalization and maintenance of treatment gains for persons who sexually offend specifically include: transitional planning, capitalizing on the abative and evocative effects of motivating operations, creating a life worth living (Good Lives Model; Ward & Stewart, 2003; Yates, Prescott, & Ward, 2010), supporting contingencies in the natural environment, and moving toward community access.

SUMMARY

In summary, a logical functional model built on solid behavioral principles suggests a process that answers the following questions for each person: What are the antecedents and consequences surrounding the sexual offending behavior that serves to inform the maintaining contingencies? What are the motivating operations that make the sexual offending behavior more or less likely to occur? What function(s) does the behavior serve, in addition to sexual gratification, or automatic reinforcement? How do these assessment variables integrate to inform a treatment plan? What environmental changes can be made to set the stage for success to prevent relapse or to promote positive behavioral change? What skills and behaviors can be taught that can serve as replacement or alternative behaviors to the sexual offenses or that can promote coping, self-regulation, or reinforcement-enhancement? What consequences, either corrective or remedial, need to be put in place? What maintenance and generalization strategies are essential in ensuring that there is transfer of skills within a culture or that ensures the safety and protection of all? In the chapters that follow, assessment, treatment, and generalization/maintenance strategies will be explored in relation to persons with intellectual disabilities who have sexually offended.

REFERENCES

Allen, D., Evans, C., Hider, A., Hawkins, S., Peckett, H., & Morgan, H. (2008). Offending behavior in adults with Asperger syndrome. *Journal of Autism and Developmental Disorders, 38,* 748-758.

Axelrod, S. (1987). Functional and structural analyses of behavior: Approaches leading to reduced use of punishment procedures? *Research in Developmental Disabilities, 8,* 165-178.

Baer, D.M., Wolf, M.M., & Risley, T.R. (1968). Some current dimensions of applied behavior analysis. *Journal of Applied Behavior Analysis, 1,* 91-97.

Baker, D.J., Blumberg, R., & Freeman, R. (2002). Considerations for functional assessment of problem behavior among persons with developmental disabilities and mental illness. In J. Jacobson, S. Holburn, & J. Mulick, (Eds.), *Contemporary dual diagnosis: MH/MR – Service models Volume II: Partial and supportive services* (pp. 51-66). Kingston, NY: NADD Press.

Bancroft, J. (1970). A comparative study of aversion and desensitization in the treatment of homosexuality. In L. E. Burns & J. L. Worsley (Eds.), *Behavior therapy in the 1970s: A collection of original papers* (pp. 1-22). Bristol, England: John Wright and Sons.

Carr, E.G. (1977). The motivation of self-injurious behavior. A review of some hypotheses. *Psychological Bulletin, 84*(4), 800-816.

Carr, E.G., Newsom, C.D., & Binkoff, J.A. (1976). Stimulus control of self-destructive behavior in a psychotic child. *Journal of Abnormal Child Psychology, 4,* 139–153.

Carr, E.G., Newsom, C.D., & Binkoff, J.A. (1980). Escape as a factor in the aggressive behavior of two retarded children. *Journal of Applied Behavior Analysis, 13,* 101–117.

Cone, J.D. (1997). Issues in functional analysis in behavioral assessment. *Behavior Research and Therapy, 35,* 259-275.

Cooper, J.O., Heron, T.E., & Heward, W.L. (2007). *Applied behavior analysis.* Upper Saddle River, NJ: Pearson/Merrill-Prentice Hall.

Dixon, D.R., Vogel, T., & Tarbox, J. (2012). A brief history of functional analysis and applied behavior analysis. In J. L. Matson (Ed.), *Functional assessment for challenging behaviors* (pp. 3-24). New York: Springer Science and Business Media.

Evans, I.M., & Meyer, L.H. (1985). *An educative approach to behavior problems: A practical decision model for interventions with severely handicapped learners.* Baltimore, MD: Paul H. Brookes.

Feldman, M., Condillac, R.A., Tough, S., Hunt, S., & Griffiths, D. (2002). Effectiveness of community positive behavioral inervention for persons with developmental disabilities and severe behavior disorders. *Behavior Therapy, 33 (3),* 377-399.

Gardner W.I. (2002). *Aggression and other disruptive behavioral challenges: biomedical and psychosocial assessment and treatment* (pp. 325-398). Kingston, NY: NADD Press.

Gardner. W.I., Cole, C.L., Davidson, D.P., & Karan, O.C. (1986). Reducing aggression in individuals with developmental disabilities: An expanded stimulus control, assessment, and intervention model. *Education and Training of the Mentally Retarded, 21, 3-12.*

Hall, S.S. (2005). Comparing descriptive, experimental and informant-based assessments of problem behaviors. *Research in Developmental Disabilities, 26,* 514–526.

Hayes, S.C., & Follette, W.C. (1992). Can functional analysis provide a substitute for syndromal classification? *Behavioral Assessment, 14,* 345-365.

Ioannou, S. (2013). *Managing risk in a culture of rights: Providing support and treatment in community-based settings for persons with intellectual disabilities who sexually offend.* (Unpublished master's thesis.) Brock University, St. Catharines, Ontario, Canada.

Iwata, B.A., Dorsey, M.F., Slifer, K.J., Bauman, K.E., & Richman, G.S. (1982). Toward a functional analysis of self-injury. *Analysis and Intervention in Developmental Disabilities, 2,* 3-20.

Iwata, B.A., Dorsey, M.F., Slifer, K.J., Bauman, K.E., & Richman, G.S. (1994). Toward a functional analysis of self-injury. *Journal of Applied Behavior Analysis, 27,* 197-209.

Iwata, B.A., & Dozier, C.L. (2008). Clinical application of functional analysis methodology. *Behavior Analysis in Practice, 1,* 3-9.

Iwata, B.A., Vollmer, T.R., & Zarcone, J.R. (1990). The experimental (functional) analysis of behavior disorders: Methodology, applications, and limitations. In A. C. Repp & N. N. Singh (Eds.), *Perspectives on the use of nonaversive and aversive interventions for persons with developmental disabilities* (pp. 301-330). Sycamore, IL: Sycamore.

Lerman, D.C., & Iwata, B.A. (1993). Descriptive and experimental analyses of variables maintaining self-injurious behavior. *Journal of Applied Behavior Analysis, 26*(3), 293-319.

Mace, F.C. (1994). The significance and future of functional analysis methodologies. *Journal of Applied Behavior Analysis, 27,* 385-392.

Magnusson, D., & Bergman, L.R. (1988). Individual and variable-based approaches to longitudinal research on early risk factors. In M. Rutter (Ed.), *Studies of psychosocial risk: The power of longitudinal data* (pp. 45-61). New York, NY: Cambridge University Press.

McGuire, T. (2001). Sex offending: Behavioral analysis perspective. *Advances in Psychology Research, 6,* 129-155.

National Institutes of Health (1989). *NIH consensus development conference on the treatment of destructive behaviors in persons with developmental disabilities.* Bethesda, MD: Author.

Roche, B., & Barnes, D. (1998). The experimental analysis of human sexual arousal: Some recent developments. *The Behavior Analyst, 21,* 37-52.

Skinner, B.F. (1953). *Science and human behavior.* New York: The Macmillan Company.

Stokes, T.F., & Baer, D.M. (1977). An implicit technology of generalization. *Journal of Applied Behavior Analysis, 10,* 349-367.

Thompson, R.H., & Iwata, B.A. (2007). A comparison of outcomes from descriptive and functional analyses of problem behavior. *Journal of Applied Behavior Analysis, 40,* 333-338.

Touchette, P.E., MacDonald, R.F, & Langer, S.N. (1985). A scatterplot for identifying stimulus control of problem behavior. *Journal of Applied Behavior Analysis, 18*(4), 343-351.

Ward, T., & Stewart, C.A. (2003). The treatment of sex offenders: Risk management and good lives. *Professional Psychology: Research and Practice, 34,* 353-360

Wulfert, E., Greenway, D.E., & Dougher, M.J. (1996). A logical functional analysis of reinforcement-based disorders: alcoholism and pedophilia. *Journal of Consulting and Clinical Psychology, 64,* 1140-1151.

Yates, P. M., Prescott, D.S., & Ward, T. (2010). *Applying the good lives and self-regulation models to sex offender treatment: A practical guide for clinicians.* Brandon, VT: Safer Society Press.

PART II:

ASSESSMENT

Chapter Four

Exploring the Antecedents and Consequences Related to Sexual Offending Behavior of Persons with an Intellectual Disability

UNDERSTANDING BEHAVIORAL CONTINGENCIES

External contingencies are constantly operating and affecting our behavior, even without our awareness. Unlike other variables such as genetics, behavioral contingencies can be assessed and then modified. Skinner (1957) argued that, in order to assess contingencies that control behavior we need to analyze three components: the environmental events that precede behavior (antecedents), the behavior of interest, and environmental events that follow behavior (consequences). This three-term contingency, or the ABC analysis of behavior, is the basis for studying operant conditioning. A fourth term (motivating operations) must also be considered and is described in Chapter 5.

Skinner (1957)distinguished operant conditioning (behavior that is controlled by its consequences) from respondent (or Pavlovian) conditioning, which includes reflexes or automatic responses to previously neutral antecedent stimuli due to pairing. An example of operant conditioning may be a green light serving as a cue (discriminative stimulus) that driving through the light will lead to reinforcement (e.g., the first time you saw a green light and drove through it on your driver's exam, you were reinforced), and, therefore, you are more likely to drive through green lights in the future. Whereas, when you saw a red light during your driver's test and you drove through it, your behavior was likely punished. A red light became a cue that driving through the light would not pay off, and you are more likely to stop at a red light, be reinforced for doing so (or avoid being punished), and be more likely to do the same in the future. Respondent conditioning occurs when a neutral stimulus (e.g., tone) is paired with a potent unconditioned stimulus (e.g., food) which typically elicits an unconditioned (or unlearned) response such as salivation. After subsequent pairings, the neutral stimulus becomes a conditioned stimulus in that it comes to elicit the same response (salivation) in the absence of the potent stimulus.

Both operant and respondent conditioning can contribute to sexual behavior and the complex nature of sexual offending behavior. In this chapter we attempt to analyze sexually deviant behavior in terms of both operant and respondent conditioning. We also attempt to interpret a self-regulation model of offending from a behavioral perspective.

THE ROLE OF ANTECEDENTS IN SEXUALLY OFFENSIVE BEHAVIOR

As mentioned, an *antecedent* is anything in an individual's environment that precedes behavior. If the individual has the opportunity to offend, for example, through a lack of supervision or access to their target victim group, these are identifiable antecedents that can be modified in order to impact behavior. When an antecedent evokes behavior, it is said that the antecedent has acquired *stimulus control.* An antecedent has stimulus control when the behavior in the presence of a certain stimulus (known as a discriminative stimulus, or S^D) produces reinforcement more often than when the behavior occurs in the absence of that particular stimulus (Cooper, Heron, & Heward, 2007). In other words, an S^D is any antecedent stimuli that acts as a cue that a particular behavior will pay off (Martin & Pear, 2015). Behavior can change in rate, duration, intensity, or amplitude based on specific stimuli in the environment. For example, an adult male pulls his pants down exposing his genitals in front of his respite worker but never in front of his parents, siblings, or peers. Sometimes, when the topography of the behavior is described as "pulling down pants exposing genitals," it is common to assume that he is sexually deviant or exhibits this behavior for his own sexual arousal. Instead, the case may be that the individual is highly motivated by attention and receives the most attention from his respite worker when he pulls his pants down. For exhibitionists there is a further reinforcing component in terms of the reaction of the victim. The victim's reaction (startle, fear, etc.) is directly related to how reinforcing the behavior is and how large of an effect the sensory component will be. Sexual behaviors can in fact serve a behavioral purpose outside of the sensory (or automatic) sexual function, which supports the need for teaching functionally equivalent replacement behavior.

Some sexual behaviors deemed problematic are not necessarily behavior problems, but a result of engaging in the behavior in inappropriate places, at inappropriate times, or with inappropriate people. This demonstrates a problem with stimulus control, known as *faulty stimulus control.* A behavior that is appropriate in one setting may be inappropriate in another. For example, masturbating in the privacy of one's own bedroom is acceptable, whereas masturbating in the public area of the living room is not. Similarly, a behavior that is appropriate with one individual may not be appropriate with other individuals. It may be acceptable for an adult to kiss his/her mother on the cheek, but not his/her supporting staff members. These examples indicate problems with stimulus control and also point to the learning history and environments unique to individuals with intellectual disabilities, which are recognized in the theory of counterfeit deviance (Griffiths, Hingsburger, Hoath, & Ioannou, 2013). An individual may engage in sexually offensive behavior for reasons other than deviant arousal, and, therefore, the deviant behavior may be altered with antecedent manipulations. For example, an individual who is living in a restrictive environment that does not allow for privacy or opportunity for appropriate sexual expression, or who experiences provocation from a peer, may exhibit a behavior that is sexually offensive because of environmental conditions that challenge the appropriate behavior (Griffiths et al., 2013). Thus, some persons with intellectual disability may commit a sexualized crime that appears topographically rooted in sexual deviance/automatic reinforcement; however, they may commit the offense for other reasons. As noted in earlier chapters, "Counterfeit deviance" can be the product of experiential, environmental, or medical factors. Sexual offending behaviors such as these are the result of lack of privacy in the environment (structural), modeling by others, inappropriate partner selection or courtship, lack of sexual knowledge or moral training, a maladaptive learning history, medical disorders, or medication effects (Griffiths et al., 2013; Hingsburger, Griffiths, & Quinsey, 1991). Counterfeit deviance is important to understand as behaviors that are topographically similar to sexual offenses, but not motivated by deviant or sensory functions, may be due to various antecedent conditions or consequences. Although several studies have questioned the validity of the counterfeit deviance hypothesis (Lunsky, Frijters, Griffiths, Watson, & Williston, 2007; Michie, Lindsay, Martin, & Grieve, 2006; Talbot & Langdon, 2006), the concept highlights a couple of important considerations. First, individuals with intellectual disabilities often lack an awareness of the extent to which their acts are socially unacceptable (Lindsay, 2009), and, second, it is important to evaluate the influence environmental factors may have regarding the degree to which those factors increase risk for sexual offending.

As with any other problem behavior, such as hitting or property destruction, antecedent analysis can be used to assess inappropriate sexual behavior. It is also important to consider the impact of *setting events,* which "are antecedent events that are removed in time and place from the occurrence of behavior, but are functionally related to that behavior" (Gresham, Watson, & Skinner, 2001, p. 160). Setting events can vary in their temporal extent; they can be either *distal* or *proximal* events that are functionally related to behavior. Proximal events may be at play immediately before or at the same time as problem behavior and can include lack of sleep, a headache, or a change in routine. Distal setting events encompass broader and more complex antecedent factors and can include the behavior of others as well as learning history. Setting events are relevant to sexual offending behavior, and are described in the sexual offending literature as risk factors (to be discussed in this chapter). For example, if staff members are distracted by something that takes their attention away from a client in a group home who is at high risk of offending behavior, and the individual is deprived of reinforcement, this may serve as a setting event for the individual to engage in inappropriate sexual behavior in the presence of certain antecedent events (e.g., the presence of a female in the home may be an S^D for engaging in inappropriate sexual behavior).

From the authors' clinical experiences, common setting events and/or antecedents to inappropriate sexual behavior can include emotional states (e.g., feeling angry, depressed), knowledge and attitudes, physiological states (e.g., sexual arousal), and changes in routine that lead to an opportunity to engage in the behavior such as a lack of supervision and close proximity to their target group (including living with people against whom they are likely to offend). Various environmental conditions and restrictions can also precede inappropriate sexual behavior. If an individual is restricted from expressing sexual behavior in acceptable ways, through anti-sex or anti-masturbation policies and beliefs in their environment, or a lack of opportunities to develop relationships, the individual may resort to engaging in inappropriate sexual behavior.

The role of emotional state has been described as a setting event to sexually offending behavior in a self-regulation model (Yates, Prescott, & Ward, 2010). As mentioned, a setting event increases the likelihood that an antecedent will trigger behavior and may vary across individuals. In other words, if each time an individual sexually offended they were angry immediately before the offense, this suggests that anger may be one setting event to sexual offending and that the individual may have difficulty with emotional regulation.

Emotional regulation has long been cited in the literature as implicated in problematic behavior, and can be defined as, "the extrinsic and intrinsic processes responsible for monitoring, evaluating, and modifying emotional reactions, especially their intensive and temporal features, to accomplish one's goals" (Thompson, 1994, pp. 27-28). The same can be said about other emotional or physiological states such as depression or arousal. If an individual commonly exhibits depression or arousal prior to an offense, it can be hypothesized that these are antecedents that contribute to the offending behavior and, therefore, could be considered as important factors in an intervention. If the offending behavior leads to a decrease in the anxiety (consequence), then the behavior may be strengthened through negative reinforcement.

We have established that a number of different variables may contribute to offending behavior. These variables may be unobservable (e.g., private events such as deviant interests) or observable (e.g., access to potential victims) and provide us with information about what may increase the likelihood that an offense may occur. Essentially, what are the conditions that lead to reoffending? Although the research is relatively young, there has been work done to determine what conditions are relevant specifically for individuals with intellectual disabilities who sexually offend.

The Dynamic Supervision Project (Hanson, Harris, Scott, & Helmus, 2007) yielded information on the factors most related to general sexual offender recidivism; these factors were generally divided into one of two categories: static and dynamic. Tools associated with this project are the popular Static-99R and the Stable-2007 and Acute-2007 – the latter two of which address dynamic risk factors or criminogenic needs. Static factors are those that do not change (such as age of first offense) or only go in one direction (number of charges). They essentially answer the question, "What has the individual done in the past?" Dynamic factors are those that are changeable and fluid; these factors reflect a shorter term and malleable form of risk. They essentially answer the question, "Who is the individual today?" or, from a behavioral lens, "what may impact the individual today." The dynamic factors are those events or situations that occur within a short time of the offense; essentially, they are the setting events that increase the likelihood that an offense will occur.

Many of these factors were adapted for the ARMIDILO-S (Boer et al., 2013), a risk assessment designed for individuals with an intellectual disability who have sexually offended. The ARMIDILO-S is, in many ways, an analogue to the Stable-2007 and Acute-2007 in that it looks at stable and acute dynamic traits. An interesting extension of this framework found in the ARMIDILO-S is the inclusion of factors related to the individual's environment, over and above factors specific to the individual. This is important given that many persons with intellectual disabilities have lived or are living in care facilities (e.g., multi bed settings which could include institutions or group homes). Factors include attitudes towards supervision and treatment, knowledge of cognitive distortions, socio-sexual knowledge, self-management and coping strategies, control of mental health issues, and common acute changes in social support, relationships, routines, emotional state, access to victims or increased rumination regarding deviant interests. Unlike the actuarial assessments, this clinical tool known as the ARMIDILO-S, guides the clinician to make observations and to determine on a case-by-case basis what factors could influence the probability of a re-offense for that person (e.g., if the person is approaching a particularly vulnerable time of year, shifts in mood or aggressiveness, or there is a change in the application of treatment integrity such as a change in staff or program protocols).

Additionally, the factors of the ARMIDILO-S can be rated as being either risk-enhancing or protective. Collectively, these variables assist evaluators in measuring how difficulties in these domains contribute to, or potentially prevent, future offending behavior. In being specific to persons with an intellectual disability, the ARMIDILO-S tries to capture the unique contributors to case management and treatment that traditional risk assessments might miss, including the role of supervision and front-line staff. Environmental supports and skills may be considered protective factors, which are strategies and features that mitigate risk. Importantly, unlike many other risk assessments, the presence of charges is not necessary to perform the assessment, only a history of sexually offending behavior.

Regardless of the assessment framework used, the relevance for clinicians is in determining what dynamic factors are currently contributing to risk, pointing to areas for possible intervention. Setting events occur before a behavior occurs and increase its likelihood; the goal should be isolating those events that are critical in increasing risk and mitigating them based on whether they are dynamic or static. Risk domains that are environmental (dynamic) including supervision and staff knowledge of the individual; a lack of supervision and understanding of the individual's unique features can contribute to offending. These factors can be moderated through training and environmental modifications. Static risk factors that are unique to the individual and cannot be changed, such as their past offenses or sexual deviance, can provide important historical information and assist in risk management. It is important to address both skill-based and environmental needs together in a comprehensive treatment package; providing someone with the skills to change behavior without ensuring an environment that allows and fosters that change ultimately sets the individual up for failure. Assessment of contributing variables and setting events is a critical step in determining both current risk and the means of reducing it through behavioral strategies such as skill teaching and environmental modifications.

Another factor that may be a setting event for sexual offending behavior is cognitive distortions, or the individual's attitudes that facilitate and support offending. Cognitive distortions have been conceptualized as self-statements that operate as rules that come to exert control over behavior (Plaud & Newberry, 1996). These self-statements could be both distal or proximal setting events that stem from an individual's learning history which may impact likelihood of offending. Cognitive distortions can be considered private events such as self-statements or faulty rule statements made by an offender that allow them to deny, minimize, rationalize, and justify their behavior (Maruna & Mann, 2006). Research has shown that cognitive distortions increase the risk of sexual offending (Lindsay, Whitefield, Carson, 2007), meaning they can be explored as being functionally related to offending behavior. For example, if an individual sees a potential victim and has self-statements that support offending (e.g., faulty rule statements) and then immediately follows through and is reinforced by the act, this can be seen as a reinforcement contingency that maintains not only the sexually offending behavior, but also the faulty rule. Specific rules may represent attitudes consistent with offending and increase the likelihood of behaviors associated with offending. Finkelhor (1984) has suggested that for sexual aggression to occur the offender must overcome the internal resistance that would normally inhibit sexual assault.

Cognitive distortions have also been described as a type of operant antecedent where the person is responding to their own verbal rationalization (Wulfert, Greenway, & Dougher, 1996). According to Skinner's analysis of verbal behavior, our own private verbal events can exert control over our behavior and are subject to the same operant contingencies as our overt behavior (Skinner, 1957). Although no solid operational definition exists, "cognitive distortions and attitudes which support sexual offending are considered fundamental to the processes in which individuals who offend deal with their internal inhibitions and establish a series of thoughts which might be considered permissive of or consistent with actions which result in sexual offending" (Lindsay, 2009, p. 179). As noted above, individuals who offend may be aware of the social taboos of the fantasies or behaviors that are resulting in pleasure. Their motivation to offend has been found to undermine their belief in these social taboos (Lindsay, 2009). If the individual experienced sexual abuse as a child, then their early understanding of these social taboos may have influenced the development of rules that do not coincide with social values. Since the rate of sexual abuse among persons with intellectual disabilities has been documented to be extremely high and since this abuse is often undetected, unreported, and untreated (Sobsey & Varnhagen, 1989), this may provide fertile ground for disinhibition regarding social mores. Disinhibition allows the individual to overcome personal inhibitions, which are most commonly cognitive distortions (see Ward, Hudson, Johnston, & Marshall, 1977). Cognitive distortions can reduce the dissonance associated with offending, thereby decreasing the internal factors that would otherwise cause discomfort.

Theory based on the work of Abel, Becker, and Cunningham-Rathner (1984) does not suggest that there is evidence to see cognitive distortions as precursors to the behavior. Indeed, current understandings of cognitive distortions are hampered by lack of an operational definition (Maruna & Mann, 2006) and research findings suggesting that denial and minimization (implicated in many cognitive distortions) may not be related to risk for reoffending (Hanson & Bussiere, 1998; Hanson & Morton-Bourgon, 2005). The term has been used to describe preoffense cognitions supporting engagement in sexually offensive conduct, as well as post-offense "excuse-making" (Friestad, 2012).

The *Abel and Becker Cognition Scale* (ABCS; Abel et al., 1984) was the first measure designed to measure cognitive distortions in the general population of persons convicted of sexual offenses. Later, Kolton, Boer, and Boer (2001) revised the measure for use with persons with intellectual disabilities, but it has yet to be assessed for validity. Until recently, no valid measure existed for use with individuals with an intellectual disability. However, Lindsay, Whitefield, and Carson (2007) developed the *Questionnaire on Attitudes Consistent with Sex Offending* (QACSO) to evaluate cognitions of persons with intellectual disabilities related to rape, voyeurism, exhibitionism, dating abuse, stalking, homosexual assault, and offenses against children. The Bumby RAPE and MOLEST Scales (Bumby, 1996) are measures of cognitive distortions that both relate to rape and child molestation that have been used clinically. The scales have demonstrated both test-retest reliability and internal consistency. The RAPE scale includes 38 items using a Likert scale to produce scores between 38 and 152. There are 36 items in the MOLEST scale, scored similarly and producing scores from 36-144. These questions may be modified as needed for the client's cognitive level, but the answers provide critical information into the motivation and attitudes behind the offending behavior. Even though the assessment may not be formally scored, given the lack of research for its use with persons with intellectual disabilities, the questions themselves yield valuable information and engage the client in a discussion of distortions that may be difficult to determine otherwise. The scales are not without limitations, however, such as susceptibility to social desirability (Arkowitz & Vess, 2003).

Additionally, Fredericks and Nishioka-Evans (1997) suggested that 'thinking errors' presented by the offender need to be identified, such as: (a) lying and making evasive or misleading statements; (b) blaming others for the offense, such as poor upbringing by parents or sexual abuse suffered as a child; (c) indicating that the victim wanted the sexual act to occur; (d) making excuses or justifying why the behavior occurred (indicating that he deserves to have sex and getting it is more important than anything else); and (f) minimizing the effects of the offense (p. 293).

The authors also note that,

> *Many offenders with disabilities are lacking in certain knowledge and skills, and because of this deficit, they have a tendency to not think clearly about their own sexuality and the sexuality of others. The functional deficits fall into two major categories: (a) a lack of sexual knowledge or experience, and (b) poor social skills (Fredericks & Nishioka-Evans, 1997, p. 291).*

In the *Diagnostic Manual – Intellectual Disability* (Fletcher, Loschen, Stavrakaki, & First, 2007), Griffiths (2007) suggested that, in addition to phallometric measures, there are four other areas of assessment regarding paraphilia in persons with intellectual disabilities: socio-sexual knowledge and attitudes (Griffiths & Lunsky, 2003), cognitions (Broxholme & Lindsay, 2003), viewing time measures (e.g., *Abel-Blasingame Assessment System for the Intellectually Disabled*: ABID – see Abel & Blasingame, 2005), and risk (Quinsey, Harris, Rice & Cormier, 2015).

As noted in Chapter 2, the role of sexual knowledge, or lack thereof, for persons with intellectual disabilities, as a factor in offending has been a source of debate in the field for the past decade. However, Lunsky and colleagues (2007) provided support to justify the need to assess sexual knowledge and attitudes and prior sexual education as part of the profile of potential factors that may be contributing to an offense to determine if it has relevance or not to the particular individual's offense pattern.

Although there are other notable socio-sexual assessments, such as the *Sexual Knowledge, Experience and Needs Scale for people with Intellectual Disability* (SexKen-ID;

McCabe, 1999), the authors of this manual employ the *Sociosexual Knowledge and Attitude Tool- Revised* (SSKAAT-R; Griffiths & Lunsky, 2003). The SSKAAT-R was developed to provide an assessment of a person's basic socio-sexual understanding and opinions regarding sexual issues. The tool assesses seven areas: anatomy, women's bodies and what women need to know about men's bodies, men's bodies and what men need to know about women's bodies, intimacy, pregnancy, childbirth and child rearing, birth control and STDs, and healthy socio-sexual boundaries. For each subscale, scores have been given in a Rasch-style scale and related to T-scores, allowing comparison of the test results to both scores between scales (something, that cannot be legitimately done using typical measures) and to a field-tested group of 276 persons with intellectual disabilities across North America. T-scores that exceed 60 are one standard deviation above the mean and scores of 70 are two standard deviations above the mean of 50. The latter score of 70 would indicate that the individual has significantly more knowledge than other individuals with the same functioning level, as evaluated as borderline, mild, moderate, or severe. These scores allow the administrator to evaluate how the individual compares to others who have similar cognitive abilities and to assess the relative weights of each of the subscales for strengths and challenges (see illustration of Graphic Profile of the Rasch Scale in Figure 4.1). In addition, although information regarding knowledge and attitudes in all areas can be informative, relative to offending behavior the attitudes questions provides targeted information to assist the assessor in examining issues related to cognitive distortions and misunderstandings.

Consent is often a difficult concept for individuals with intellectual disabilities because it is abstract. People wishing to engage in sexual activities must understand both the requirement to obtain consent from a potential partner and the need to provide consent in return. The SSKAAT-R (Griffiths & Lunsky, 2003) is often used to explore an individual's understanding of both consent and age appropriateness. The section on healthy boundaries was designed specifically to explore these concepts. This subtest contains 28 items and presents stimuli and questions related to appropriate activities to perform with children and with staff/caregivers, appropriate dating behavior, voyeurism, exhibitionism, rape, incest as well as sexual coercion by direct care staff, family, and other care providers. The materials require some verbal ability but mostly involve pointing to pictures or drawings and matching activities with settings. Problem solving scenarios are used to elicit answers that would highlight how a person might handle various situations. Gathering information on an individual's sexual knowledge is beneficial in identifying setting events, if lack of sexual knowledge and understanding of consent is hypothesized to be functionally related to the inappropriate sexual behavior.

Using the SSKAAT-R, it is possible to evaluate the relative understanding of these concepts in relation to others who have similar cognitive abilities to determine if their knowledge is above or below that of others who have similar cognitive functioning. This depiction is provided by plotting the individual's score and that of the average score of other individuals who have similar cognitive functioning on the assessment summary sheet as shown in Figure 4.1. However, in addition to assessing the individual's overall response on the assessment tool, it is often also valuable to explore the particular gaps in knowledge and also whether the individual is applying their knowledge in their day-to-day interactions. As such, interviews with family and support staff are often advised to complement the assessment.

Figure 4.1. **Socio-Sexual Knowledge and Attitude Test Revised Summary Sheet**

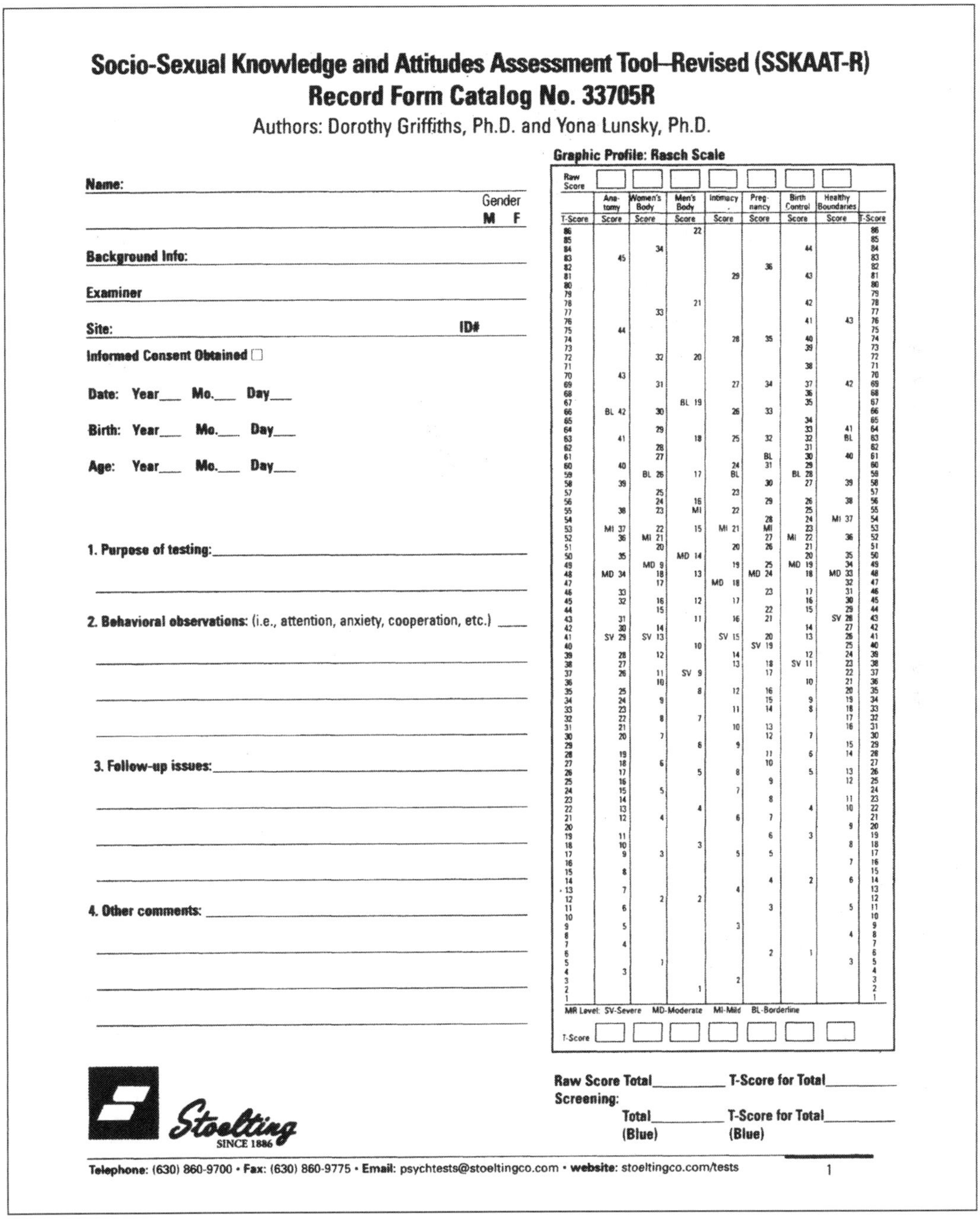
Socio-Sexual Knowledge and Attitudes Assessment Tool–Revised (SSKAAT-R)
Record Form Catalog No. 33705R
Authors: Dorothy Griffiths, Ph.D. and Yona Lunsky, Ph.D.

Name: ____________________
Gender **M F**

Background Info: ____________________

Examiner ____________________

Site: ____________________ **ID#** ________

Informed Consent Obtained ☐

Date: Year___ Mo.___ Day___

Birth: Year___ Mo.___ Day___

Age: Year___ Mo.___ Day___

1. Purpose of testing: ____________________

2. Behavioral observations: (i.e., attention, anxiety, cooperation, etc.) ____

3. Follow-up issues: ____________________

4. Other comments: ____________________

Graphic Profile: Rasch Scale

Raw Score

T-Score	Anatomy Score	Women's Body Score	Men's Body Score	Intimacy Score	Pregnancy Score	Birth Control Score	Healthy Boundaries Score	T-Score

MR Level: SV-Severe MD-Moderate MI-Mild BL-Borderline

T-Score

Raw Score Total________ **T-Score for Total**________
Screening:
Total________ **T-Score for Total**________
(Blue) **(Blue)**

Stoelting SINCE 1886

Telephone: (630) 860-9700 • **Fax:** (630) 860-9775 • **Email:** psychtests@stoeltingco.com • **website:** stoeltingco.com/tests

1

THE ROLE OF CONSEQUENCES IN SEXUAL OFFENDING BEHAVIOR

A *consequence* refers to what occurs directly after a behavior. Specifically, an environmental condition or stimulus change(s) that follows a behavior can have varying effects on the probability of the behavior occurring in the future, depending on the individual's current motivational state and the immediacy of the consequence (Cooper et al., 2007). In general, when a behavior continues to occur, it is helpful to think in terms of consequences and what is maintaining that behavior, either through adding or removing positive or aversive stimuli. In *positive reinforcement* a desirable consequence is added after the occurrence of behavior, whereas in *negative reinforcement* an aversive consequence is removed following behavior (e.g., termination of an aversive mood or feeling state, such as anger), and both lead to an increase in the likelihood that the behavior will occur in the future. *Positive punishment* adds an aversive stimulus following behavior, whereas *negative punishment* removes a desirable stimulus following behavior. Both positive punishment and negative punishment lead to a decrease in the probability of the behavior occurring in the future.

Consequences can be socially mediated or non-socially mediated. Other forms of consequences that can maintain sexual offending behavior may include automatic reinforcement (or "reinforcement that is not mediated by the deliberate action of another person"; Vaughan & Michael, 1982, p. 219). For example, an individual may experience pleasurable sensations when visualizing a violent sex act and, therefore, may be more likely to do so in the future. This is not controlled by consequences mediated by another person but by the sensory stimulation.

As discussed, from an operant perspective, an individual's offending behavior can be maintained by its consequences, such that engaging in behavior (e.g., approaching an attractive woman) that led to sexual reinforcement in the past is strengthened. The learning history of an individual can be explored through an operant lens, but it is important to state that there is no simple explanation of sexual offending behavior. Rather, there is an interconnected relationship between respondent and operant conditioning, such that "stimuli that have acquired arousing properties through classical conditioning can also have behavioral effects and contribute to the approach of those stimuli" (Hoffmann, Janssen, & Turner, 2004, p. 44). It is also important to consider that the contingencies maintaining these behaviors can be operating concurrently.

Like antecedents, monitoring consequences is also an important part of the assessment of sexual offending behavior to determine what variables may be maintaining the behavior (e.g., positive or negative reinforcement, positive or negative punishment, escape or avoidance). Assessing consequences provides valuable information about what may be maintaining the behavior (discussed further in Chapter 6: Function of Sexual Offending Behavior). Figure 4.2 provides a very simple example of a form to track antecedents and consequences to the sexual offending behavior. Both proximal and distal setting events have been included, factors that have been shown in the literature to be related to sexual offending in persons with intellectual disabilities. However, although not all of these factors may be relevant for the individual and their behavior, they should not be ignored or dismissed. Rather, the functional relevance of each setting event should be explored. Although this is a good place to start when forming hypotheses about what might be maintaining the behavior, function cannot be confirmed without more specific assessments such as an experimental functional analysis (described in Chapter 3). Once function is determined, various consequent strategies (such as reinforcing alternative functional behaviors, discussed further in Chapter 9) and consequences can be administered (discussed further in Chapter 10).

Figure 4.2. Sample Descriptive Assessment Data Collection Form

Data Sheet

Client: *JF* **Setting(s):** *Group Home* **Observer:** *KT*

Target Behavior: *Public masturbation*

Operational Definition: *Any time the client touches his genital area for more than 3 seconds in any location other than his bedroom or bathroom. Does not include itching.*

Date/Time									
Initials									
Setting Events (check all that apply)									
Distal (one check if applicable)									
Sexual deviance history									
Lack of sexual knowledge									
Sexual abuse history									
Cognitive distortions									
Other (specify):									
Proximal									
Medical (change in med, illness, etc.)									
Change/disruption in routine									
Lack of sleep									
Emotional states (angry, sad)									
Boredom/lack of activity									
Staff/caregiver complacency									
Low self-esteem									
Lack of assertiveness									
Other (specify):									
Antecedent(s)									
Demand placed									
Arousing stimuli present									
Target group present									
Free time/low demand activity									
Alone (i.e. lack of staff supervision)									
Other (specify):									
Consequence(s)									
Attempted to redirect to other activity									
Reminder of consequences									
Ignored the behavior									
Took individual to different location									
Other (specify):									

RESPONDENT CONDITIONING ALSO PLAYS A ROLE IN SEXUAL OFFENDING BEHAVIOR

In Chapter 2 we discussed sexual deviance, referred to as paraphilias in DSM-5 (American Psychiatric Association, 2013). Paraphilias are defined as "intense and persistent sexual interest other than sexual interest in genital stimulation or preparatory fondling with phenotypically normal, physically mature, consenting human partners" (p. 685). Sexual interest in paraphilias or paraphilic disorders is often expressed in urges and fantasies that involve a response to inappropriate stimuli, such as children or the use of aggression. For pedophilia, the stimulus that evokes sexual arousal is children; for sexual aggressors the stimuli involve violence and/or power and control. When it comes to sexual arousal and sexual offending behavior, it is difficult to separate the respective effects of operant (Skinnerian or instrumental) and respondent (classical or Pavlovian) conditioning. The role of respondent conditioning has been examined in the literature and evidence for this type of learning has been demonstrated in male sexual arousal in both humans and animals (Lalumiere & Quinsey, 1998; Plaud & Martini, 1999).

Respondent conditioning would suggest that offending behavior is elicited by antecedent events and is the result of stimulus-stimulus pairings. An example may be sexual arousal elicited by a male seeing someone he finds attractive, which might be paired with deviant sexual interests eventually leading to sexual offending behavior. These preferences, possibly formed in early childhood, gain strength through repeated pairings. McGuire, Carlisle and Young's conditioning theory (1965, p. 186) suggests that "any stimulus which regularly precedes ejaculation by the correct time interval should become more and more sexually exciting, and masturbation to a fantasy provides both the stimulus and the optimal setting for this conditioning to take place." The preferred stimulus can be very discrete involving specific ages, gender, and developmental characteristics (such as the budding sexuality of adolescents), all of which coalesce to form what Money (1986) called a 'love map.' The love map defines the specific characteristics of mate selection. This theory accounts for the ontogenic conditioning of specific deviant interests. These interests become part of the individual's fantasies and masturbatory repertoire, thereby forming a critical cognitive stimulus when external stimuli are not present. The love map and subsequent fantasies (inappropriate or not) may be a result of previous experience, which may include a history of abuse or lack of sexual education. Abel (1989) noted that the repeated use of these fantasies from an early age, combined with social mores that dictate that these fantasies are private, results in the strengthening and establishment of these fantasies to have strong erotic value as an antecedent for sexual pleasure by the time that the individual becomes aware that they are maladaptive. This awareness may come about as a result of further education or rules (e.g., children are not to be looked at in a sexual way) or may be the result of an experience in which the behavior was punished (e.g., the individual was charged for possession of child abuse images). This type of situation can lead to what cognitive psychologists refer to as "dissonance", in which the individual is engaging in behavior that is reinforcing (masturbating to child abuse images) which then becomes known to the individual as socially wrong and legally punishable.

From an operant conditioning perspective, the outcome in this situation may depend on the individual's history of reinforcement or punishment with rules (or the social and legal mores) compared to the conditioned sexual response. That is, if the sexual offending behavior resulted in a consequence that was aversive it may be successful in decreasing (i.e., punishing) future instances of the behavior. However, the matching law suggests that when there are two concurrent schedules of reinforcement, the rate of responding is typically proportional to the rate of reinforcement received from each choice alternative (Cooper et al., 2007). Therefore, if an individual has been receiving incentive for engaging in inappropriate sexual behavior, the payoff for engaging in alternative behavior must be of equal or greater value. If the aversive consequences do not outweigh the benefits, then the behavior will be more likely to continue. In the same sense, if the individual does not have positive replacement behaviors, or their positive behaviors do not work to get them what they want, then the offending behavior will continue. In Figure 4.3, a visual depiction of this has been shown through the Competing Behavior Model (O'Neill et al., 1997). It is important to remind readers that sexually offending behavior can occur in a variety of topographies for a variety of reasons; a simple example has been used in order to illustrate the concept. In the diagram, a clear contingency of the problem behavior is illustrated. By teaching the individual an appropriate functional replacement behavior, they can still get their desired outcome, but in non-offensive ways.

People with intellectual disabilities tend to live in a punitive and restrictive socio-sexual culture. Therefore, appropriate sexual behavior might be met with sanctions and, since it would not be covert, it would likely have a higher probability of being detected. Because the typical schedule of reinforcement for appropriate behavior would likely not be sufficiently frequent to match the reinforcement value acquired by engaging in the already established inappropriate fantasies and behaviors, then engaging in alternative behavior would result in a significant reinforcement trade-down. Later in this book, we will examine this principle of trade-down, illustrated by Hingsburger (1996), as it relates to consequences. For this chapter, we are examining it relative to the reinforcement value in establishing antecedents.

If the reinforcement values for engaging and not engaging in inappropriate sexual behavior match, or if the reinforcement value or frequency for nonoffending outweighs the value of offending, then the individual may not engage in the inappropriate behavior. If, however, the reinforcement value or frequency of reinforcement is greater for the inappropriate behavior, then the matching law would suggest that inappropriate sexual behavior would be more likely to occur. In that case, the condition is set wherein the inappropriate sexual behavior is likely to continue and to be strengthened over time by repeated reinforcement. This mismatching of the reinforcement value for offending and nonoffending also plays a major role in treatment and risk management, as will be discussed later in this book.

This further sets up the condition where in order to continue enjoying something that is considered socially wrong and punishable, the dissonance is resolved by establishing justifications for the behavior or private verbal behavior in the form of rules such as blaming the victim: "*I could see she wanted it (sex) because she came over and sat on my knee*" – a statement made in response to a 4-year-old who agreed to sit on the offender's knee when he offered her candy. These justifications form the rationale for the development of cognitive distortions (self-statements) as a way to reduce the dissonance connected with the behavior.

***Figure 4.3.* Competing Behavior Model for Sexually Offending Behavior**

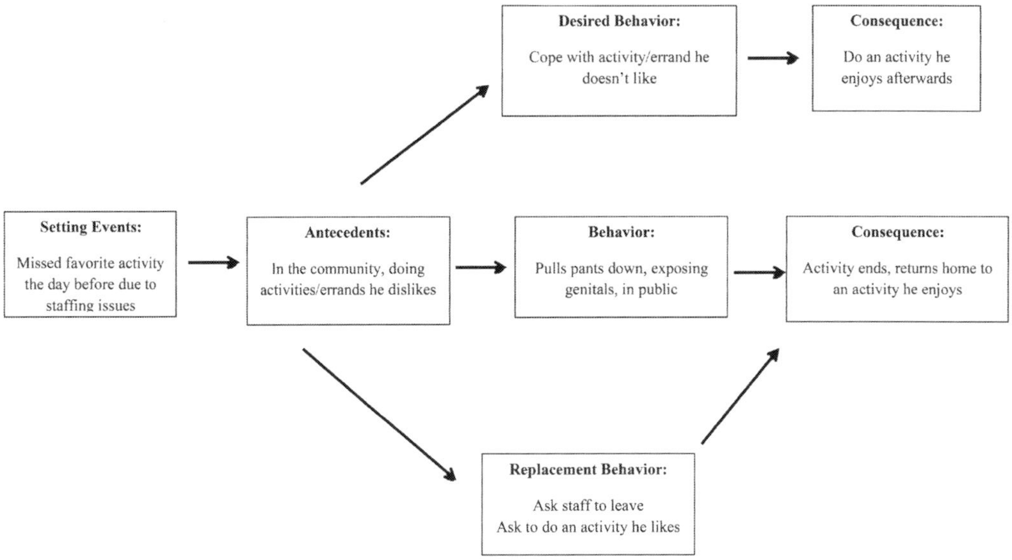

It would be ideal if an individual could effectively choose not to engage in the offending sexual response (whether realized or in fantasy). However, as demonstrated, we know that sexual offending behavior is impacted by a complex combination of operant and respondent conditioning processes. Therefore, it may be misleading to talk about an individual "choosing" to or "not choosing" to offend, especially for individuals with intellectual disabilities. Ward and Hudson (1998) suggested that there are four pathways to offending. For individual offenses that followed the *Avoidant Pathway* (passive or active), inhibiting desires to offend was attempted but there was a lack of effective coping skills or application of ineffective strategies. For offenses that followed the *Approach Pathway* (automatic or active), the individual did not try to inhibit their behavior and their offenses were often impulsive and situational or deliberate and strategic. The model proposes that the pathway to offending may differ based on the specific offense. The model also suggests that the consequences that maintain offending behaviors may differ across individuals. We will attempt to interpret this model from operant and respondent conditioning perspectives.

In looking at Table 4.1, start with the assumption that the function of the offending behavior is automatic (sensory) reinforcement. Men may be more biologically predisposed to increased sexual arousal to visual stimuli (Hamann, Herman, Nolan & Wallen, 2004; Rupp & Wallen, 2008; Stoleru, Fonteille, Cornelis, Joyal & Moulier, 2012), thereby increasing the likelihood that a stimulus will acquire sexual properties. For example, if a man encounters a child, a seemingly neutral stimulus, which is then paired with sexual arousal, the child may become a conditioned stimulus that elicits sexual arousal. From an operant conditioning perspective, if sexually offensive behavior has occurred with a child and was reinforced, the presence of children may become an S^D (i.e., a cue) that sexual offending behavior will pay off. Depending on which pathway an offense falls into, offending behavior can result from a dynamic relationship between antecedents (e.g., arousing stimuli), motivating operations (described in detail in Chapter 5), as well as consequences the individual has experienced in the past for sexual offending behavior. Presumably, approach-based individuals may experience sexual arousal and have experienced positive consequences for offending behavior in the past. Perhaps avoidant individuals have experienced punishment contingencies for offending, but those consequences were not strong enough to decrease the likelihood of the behavior. Contrary to their hypothesis, Lindsay, Steptoe, and Beech (2008) found that persons with intellectual disabilities who have sexually offended were more likely to be in the Approach Explicit category than the Avoidant Passive. Evaluating the sexual offending behavior from a behavioral perspective can help clinicians take into account the environmental factors that play a role and prevent faulty circular logic about cause of offending. For example, "Why did he offend? Because he was motivated to offend. How do you know he was motivated to? Because he offended."

Table 4.1: ***Self-Regulation Model – Pathways to Offending***

Pathway	Dynamics	Behavioral Explanation
Avoidant Passive	Persons whose offending behavior follows this pathway are motivated to refrain from offending, but do not actively attempt to do so, or simply attempt to deny urges or to distract themselves.	These individuals may engage in verbal behavior (in the form of rules) that may exert some stimulus control (e.g., presence of a stimulus leads to a response) over their behavior. However, the reinforcing consequences for the offending behavior may be more frequent and valuable than the consequences for not offending/alternative behavior. If the individual is also deprived of sexual stimulation this may serve as a motivating operation for engaging in sexual behavior of any kind.
Avoidant Active	Persons whose offenses follow this pathway have strategies and engage in behaviors other than offending and therefore avoid offending.	Engaging in non-offending prosocial behaviors may be maintained by negative reinforcement by way of escape (behavior leads to removal of) or avoidance (behavior prevents) aversive consequences such as extra security, punishment contingencies, etc.
Approach Automatic	Persons whose offenses follow this pathway engage in behavior that is ultimately related to offending, even if they do not actively seek to commit an offense. For example, an individual who is more likely to offend when he or she goes out drinking might decide to go out drinking late at night. This puts the individual at a greater risk of reoffending.	Respondent conditioning may play role when the individual has deviant sexual interests. Sexual arousal may have been previously paired with drinking and therefore drinking may elicit sexual arousal. The individual may also engage in the offending behavior because it has previously been reinforced; perhaps more frequently (or with more valuable reinforcement) than alternative behavior, and any aversive consequences that followed the offense may not have served as effective punisher.

Approach Explicit	By contrast, persons on the Approach Automatic Pathway, seek explicitly to commit a particular offense. The dynamics of offending within this pathway are associated with goals that explicitly support sexual offending, such as attitudes supporting sexual activity with children or hostile attitudes toward women.	The behavioral contingencies may be similar to an Approach Automatic offender in that sexual arousal has previously been paired with specific offending visualizations. Further reinforcement for offending may be more immediate and valuable than the consequences for an alternative, non-offending behavior. The individual may also have a long reinforcement history for engaging in sexual offending behavior.

(adapted from a reprint with permission from Wilson and Burns [2011])

ASSESSING AROUSAL TO DEVIANT STIMULI

To begin examining the antecedents and consequences for inappropriate sexual behavior, both indirect and direct data collection methods should be used. These are incorporated in a functional behavior assessment, which can include collecting descriptive assessment (antecedent, behavior, consequence) data, indirect assessment data (e.g., interviewing people in the individual's environment such as family and staff as well as reviewing medical records), and conducting an experimental analysis of the function of behavior (Iwata, Dorsey, Slifer, Bauman, & Richman, 1982/1994). Although function of behavior cannot be confirmed with certainty from descriptive or indirect assessments alone, an experimental functional analysis is not as amenable to sexual offending behavior as other challenging behaviors (Vollmer, Reyes, & Walker, 2012). Rather, experimental functional analysis can be conducted on the less risky precursor behaviors. This assessment process will be described further in Chapter 6.

Arousal to children encompasses deviant sexual interests that can be caused by a number of factors (Lindsay, 2009). Although a complicated relationship exists between developmental sexual abuse and later engagement in sexual offending, it appears that at least some groups of persons convicted of sexual offenses report a higher likelihood of having been sexually abused as children (Jespersen, Lalumière, & Seto, 2009). Individuals with intellectual disabilities are reported to experience a higher rate of sexual abuse than nondisabled persons (Sobsey, 1994). Lindsay (2009) has suggested that the early experiences of sexual abuse may serve to condition the individual to a basic arousal to children and also to disinhibit this interest. He further suggested that these early experiences might have involved pornography, which could further lead to the sexualization of children. Lindsay (2009) further suggested that people who have sexually offended may develop a "congruence with children" because of the power dynamic with children or because their own emotional development makes relationships with children more comfortable than with adults (p. 74). Individuals with offense histories also may experience a blockage in development of satisfying adult relationships, such as lack of social skills, intimacy or relationship problems, such that children become replacements.

When examining the respondent effects to various stimuli, it is important to determine through assessment what stimuli prompt arousal for the particular offender. Through a series of interviews, the interviewer wants to determine what type of sexual activities are preferred as well as the content of their fantasies. However, Griffiths, Quinsey, and Hingsburger (1989) caution that persons with intellectual disabilities may be less articulate in the description of their fantasies or preferred activities. This may be in part due to a history in which all sexual behavior has been punished or discouraged, or due to an attempt to give the response that is expected in order to please or appease the interviewer. This tendency, known as acquiescence bias, is often quite problematic in evaluating persons with intellectual disabilities, in that individuals may respond in the affirmative when they perceive that doing so might "please" the interviewer. Unfortunately, this bias is evident even when answering in the affirmative is not actually in the individual's best interests, such as during police interviews. There are many other clinical situations in which persons with disabilities are prejudiced by their tendency to "go with the flow" or fail to appropriately advocate on their own behalf, such as failing to request special programming consistent with their skills and responsivity concerns (Wilson & Burns, 2011). Several assessment methods have been developed to provide information in a nonverbal or minimally verbal and nonthreatening manner, such as the *Novaco Anger Scale* (Novaco & Taylor, 2004), and the *Card Sort* (Griffiths, Quinsey, & Hingsburger, 1989). However, it is up to clinical and supervisory professionals to ensure that they conduct interviews and other interactions with persons with intellectual disabilities in a fair and equitable manner.

Assessing the individual's arousal pattern is vital in determining key elements related to an individual's sexual offense, including the "age, gender and characteristics of the victim, as well as the stimulus context of the offense" (Vollmer et al., 2012, p. 129). The most common sexual preference assessments can be categorized into three methods: physiological, attentional (viewing time) assessments, and self-report techniques (Kalmus & Beech, 2005).

In recent years, there has been some discourse in the literature on measuring sexual arousal in persons who sexually offend. The research has been focused on the accuracy and utility of measuring sexual arousal directly using phallometric testing compared to the less intrusive sexual preference assessments. These various assessments will be discussed thoroughly, highlighting their utility and ethical considerations when assessing sexual deviance in persons who sexually offend.

I. Physiological

Phallometry is one of the most commonly used direct measurements for persons who have sexually offended (Freund, 1965). Phallometry is a reliable and valid means of measuring differential sexual arousal to a variety of stimulus categories (e.g., males vs. females, adults vs. children, or consenting vs. coercion) in examination of sexual preferences. The phallometric or penile plethysmograph (colloquially known as the PPG) assessment can provide a relatively clear indication of sexual preferences in individuals who do not try to interfere with the testing procedure (e.g., faking – see Wilson, 1998). PPG assessment involves measuring the individual's penile responses to slides or audiotaped descriptions of socially accepted sexual activities compared to responses to inappropriate or deviant sexual activities. The phallometric device measures physical changes in penile physiology (e.g., volume or circumference) as the individual is exposed to various sexually based stimuli. The stimuli vary depending on the test site and assessors; however, there are typically visual and auditory stimuli, involving prepubescent and pubescent children and adults. The stimuli might involve only pictures, only audio narration of a story, or both; the nature of the stories may be based on that individual's history. This measurement involves having the offender place a mercury-in-rubber strain gauge around the shaft of the penis, which is hooked up to a computer that determines the relative level of arousal to various stimuli. During this time an apparatus is fitted over the individual's penis that measures changes in volume or circumference based on what stimulus is present. The measure is either circumferential (girth) or volumetric (the overall volume of the penis) in nature. Baseline measures are taken and compared to size changes throughout the assessment; these changes are correlated with the stimuli on-screen at that time and provide an idea of putative sexual preference.

The use of phallometric measures has been highly researched in the typically developing population and requires specially trained technicians who know how to administer and interpret the measures in controlled laboratory conditions (Blanchard et al., 2012; Wilson & Miner, 2016). It also requires the development of appropriate stimuli sets (Laws & Osborn, 1983). However, despite its frequent use with this population, the PPG has yielded issues with reliability and validity in persons with intellectual disabilities (Wilson & Burns, 2011).

Fedoroff and Moran (1997) caution that phallometric testing does not provide a determination of guilt or innocence relative to a specific offense and must therefore not be assumed as predictive. A person who has deviant arousal may never act on that arousal; however, for people who have already acted on deviant arousal, research suggests that those individuals with deviant arousal patterns on phallometric testing are at increased risk to re-engage in similar behaviors (see Hanson & Bussière, 1998). Although a valuable measure, phallometry does not always account for the function served by the sexual offending behavior. For example, research has shown that persons with pedophilic arousal patterns may be motivated because of stronger arousal to children (preferential); however other individuals with child molestation histories (situational) demonstrate stronger arousal to adults but will engage in sexual interaction with children when specific conditions occur. Often this relates to proximal establishing operations (Wulfert et al., 1996). Proximal establishing operations have been described as factors that are physical (setting), social (who is present), and medical/biological (what happens in the body) (Southam-Gerow, 2013). For an offender who is attracted to children, although the most direct antecedent would be the presence of a child, other more proximal stimulus conditions can set the occasion for the trigger to be more or less likely to be acted on including: the physical setting (secluded vs. highly visible), the others in the environment (no other adult present that may serves as a discriminative stimuli for non-offense behaviors), and biological variables that can affect motivation to offend (presence or absence of sexual arousal). This creates a situation where a lack of external risk management and stimulus control, combined with an automatic sensory (arousal) function, make it more likely a behavior will occur, despite the potentially aversive social consequences.

Phallometric assessments are typically conducted under laboratory conditions; however, there have been recent advancements in development of procedures that may allow assessment of arousal in the natural environment using portable phallometric devices (Vollmer, 2014). Vollmer et al. (2012) suggest that "it is important to conduct arousal assessments under naturalistic conditions" (p. 130) given that this assessment procedure provides a more accurate assessment of an individual's deviant sexual interests *in situ*, while also ensuring the safety of the community via staff monitoring. Reyes, Vollmer, Whitehouse, and Jansen (2009) suggested that the arousal observed in a clinical setting with the standard penile plethysmograph is comparable to arousal seen in the community setting with the mobile plethysmograph. However, caution still needs to be used to ensure that all ethical steps have been examined and that the person evaluating the outcomes of the measure is appropriately qualified to administer and interpret the results.

Figures 4.4 and 4.5 below provide examples of phallometric profiles of a heterosexual male non-offender and an offender with pedophilic interests involving female prepubescent children. The charts show the average penile circumference magnitude, in standard of Z-score form on the vertical axes. The horizontal axes depict the categories of the slides presented: Neutral (Neu), which might be a picture of a tree, Adult Female (AF), Pubescent Female (PF), Child Female (CF), Adult Male (AM), Pubescent Male (PM), and Child Male (CM). The Neutral stimulus is presented to determine a baseline to ensure the person is either not responding to any stimuli or is responding to all stimuli.

Figure 4.4 depicts a person with high preference for age-appropriate sexual contact with adult females (AF), some response to pubescent females (FM), but no arousal to children or to males. The slight degree of attraction to pubescent females (PF) is commonly seen in most gynephilic men who have never engaged in sexual conduct with children (Blanchard et al, 2012). Notwithstanding this elevation, the response hierarchy clearly shows much higher arousal to female adults than to any other stimulus category.

***Figure 4.4.* Phallometric profile of a heterosexual male non-offender**

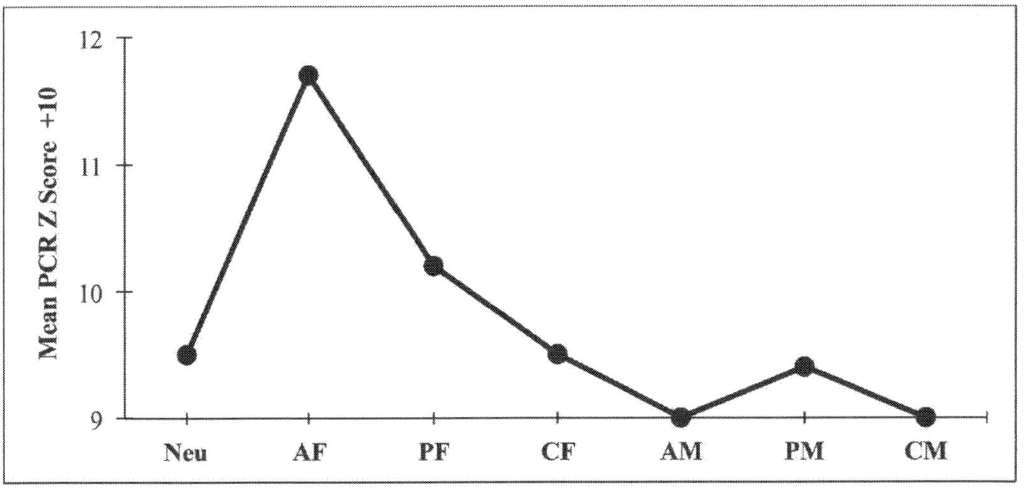

Let us contrast this with a phallometric data profile for an individual who has engaged in a serious sexual offense against a child (see Figure 4.5). In this chart it is clear that the person is showing more arousal to children and less to stimuli involving age-appropriate partners. The relative age of interest to children (i.e., children under 5, children 5-10, pubescent child) can be evaluated by differential presentation of stimuli of those potential target groups. As is also evident on the chart, the assessment can differentiate interest in hetero or homosexual sexual activity in addition to age preference.

***Figure 4.5.* Phallometric profile of an offender with pedophilic interests involving female prepubescent children**

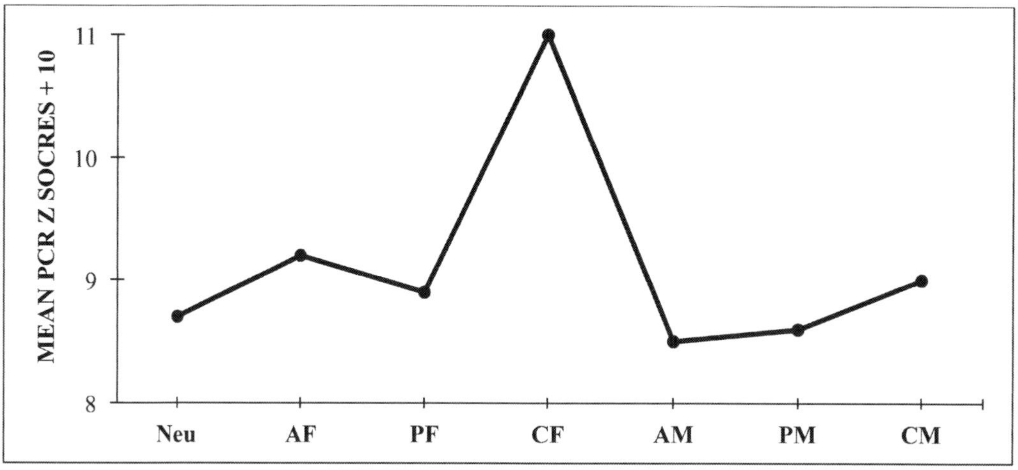

The use of the phallometric measurement with persons with intellectual disabilities has not been as widely researched; however, there are some recent emergent studies. The cautions that have been raised regarding the use of this type of measurement for persons with intellectual disabilities date back over two decades (Murphy, Coleman, & Haynes, 1983). Griffiths and Fedoroff (2009) suggested that although there is no contraindication to the use of phallometric measures with persons with intellectual disabilities, caution regarding interpretation is vital. There is a high risk that misinterpretation of results indicating inappropriate arousal might be used by agencies to deny services such as housing or day programming. As well, they suggest that a phallometric evaluation may be used to assess interest in children, but it will also reveal information about sexual orientation concerning adults, which has ethical implications in that the information could again be misused by supportive agencies. Furthermore, although the use of child stimuli has been shown to be one of the best predictors of re-offense (see Hanson & Morton-Bourgon, 2005), Marshall and Fernandez (2003) reported that some jurisdictions have laws that prohibit the use of sexually explicit materials, requiring adaptations using images of individuals in bathing suits, which may not produce as much arousal and increasing the likelihood of invalid results because of insufficient responding. Additionally, although the assessment is a measure of relative interest or arousal to either a particular age or gender, it does not mean the person will always act on that interest or arousal. This is where the power of self-regulation becomes evident or, from a behavioral lens, the reinforcing consequences for alternative behavior outweigh those for deviant behavior or the punishing consequences for deviant behavior outweigh the reinforcement. For example, at a time when homosexuality was frowned upon, both socially and legally, some homosexual individuals elected to live a life of heterosexuality or celibacy rather than violate the mores of society or incur the wrath of authorities. The reinforcing consequences for alternative behavior outweighed those for homosexuality behaviors.

Measuring arousal to determine deviant sexual interests is an important aspect of assessment as it can be an indicator of risk of reoffending, as well as a guide to individualized intervention. However, recent literature by Reyes, Vollmer, and Hall (2017) point out that assessing arousal alone does not include all variables involved; arousal encompasses the respondent aspects of sexual offending but in order to commit the offense, a variety of other behaviors must occur, ones that are operant in nature. For example, the person would need to choose a potential victim and then engage in behaviors that allow them to be alone with the victim. Assessing an individual's operant behavior may provide a more complete picture of sexual preference, rendering "operant-oriented" (p. 28) assessments more useful and less intrusive (Reyes et al., 2017).

In their study, Reyes, Vollmer, and Hall (2017) introduced a novel application of a behavior analytic assessment to measuring sexual preference in persons with intellectual disability and compared it to results of a phallometric arousal assessment. They adapted a paired stimulus preference assessment using still frame images taken from the phallometric assessment (which included images of males and females under and over 18). These images were presented in pairs on a computerized system with the individual selecting one image. Each image was presented with every other image, and the individual was asked to make a selection each time. Their results showed that the outcomes of the preference assessment corresponded with the phallometric assessment for 4 out of the 5 individuals. Although they acknowledge that preference assessments can be used for people with intellectual disabilities to determine age and gender preferences, the authors noted that it is too early to use preference assessments alone. Rather, preference assessments can add to the results of arousal assessments through information about operant behavior. For example, just because an individual showed arousal to an adult female does not mean he will not choose younger females if given the opportunity (Reyes et al., 2017).

Phallometry (Freund & Blanchard, 1989) is the most validated form of sexual arousal testing, but it possesses flaws, both ethical and clinical in nature. Although the phallometric shows high discriminatory power (Lalumiere & Quinsey, 1994), there remain issues regarding both utility and ethical implications. Some research has shown that the sexual arousal can temporarily be supressed or enhanced with basic instructions (Wilson, 1998), and other factors may play a role in the results, aside from arousal. As well, the intrusive nature of the assessment suggests that it should be used judiciously and, perhaps, only when all other measures of sexual preference or interest have been exhausted. As described earlier, operant behavior must also be measured, as arousal alone does not capture the complete picture of victim preference in sexual offending. Semi-structured interviews, such as the card sort, may be nearly as reliable and are far less intrusive to implement (Tough & Figliolia, 2007). Use of card sort methods may be particularly helpful in assessments of individuals in the ID population, who may be less able and likely to attempt deception during the assessment process.

II. Attentional (Viewing Time) Methods

Visual reaction time is one type of operant assessment used to measure sexual preference and it has received scientific support in the literature. In a study by Reyes (2009) an individual was presented with a choice between two pictures using stimuli standardized for phallometric assessments. Once the individual clicks on the selected picture, it enlarges and remains for five seconds then disappears. Following a period of blank screen, new pictures emerge for a cycle of 18 presentations per picture. Using this method Reyes (2009) found that there was a consistent pattern with preferred choice to the highest level of arousal by age category using a plethysmograph test.

The *Abel-Blasingame Assessment System for Individuals with Intellectual Disabilities* (ABID) is a viewing time tool used to assess sexual interest that collects information using three sources: a survey evaluating the individual's level of intellectual functioning, a self-report questionnaire, and visual reaction time (VRT; Blasingame, Abel, Jordan, & Wiegel, 2011). The ABID was validated on a large sample of persons with intellectual disability and sexual offense histories. It is an assessment tool that shows promise as it is the only one of its kind to examine sexual preference in persons with intellectual disabilities through VRT and self-report. It has, however, received criticism for relying too heavily on self-report disclosures (Reyes et al., 2017). The authors caution that more research is needed before it can be widely used (Blasingame et al., 2011).

Vollmer et al. (2012) noted that "[a]lthough indirect methods may have value under certain circumstances or when combined with other sources of information, it is not appropriate to rely on them solely" (p. 125). Miltenberger (2008) suggested that where possible direct assessment measures are preferable and have greater utility in ABA. However, as Vollmer and colleagues noted, direct observation of a sexual offense is very unlikely. Therefore, it is important to measure other responses to sexual offending but within conditions where potential for harm is minimized.

Viewing time measures (Harris, Rice, Quinsey, & Chaplin, 1996) are similar in many respects to the Card Sort assessment, which will be described more fully below. Individuals are shown different pictures of people that vary in a number of key aspects including: age, gender, race, and clothing. These pictures are shown on a computer and how long each picture remains on the screen is up to the individual. Unlike the card sort, only one picture is presented at a time and the individual does not need to comment on it. Instead, the program measures the amount of time spent looking at each picture before changing it, which theoretically correlates with level of attraction to the target. The longer you look at the picture, the more preferred the target or stimuli is. Viewing time measures are relatively easy to implement, and show strong convergent validity (Schmidt, Babchishin, & Lehmann, 2016), making them a practical clinical option. However, it is important to note that viewing time measures assess sexual interest and not sexual preference; although these two elements are correlated (Wilson & Miner, 2016).

III. Self-Report

There are numerous assessment methods for sexual preference that rely on the individual telling the assessor who they are sexually attracted to. This can be done through interviews, by simply asking the individual what their sexual preference is, or through developed assessment tools.

Preference assessments, such as the *Card Sort Test,* were introduced by Griffiths, Quinsey and, Hingsburger (1989) for use in combination with other measures to determine if the individual with an intellectual disability was able to discriminate age, sees himself as a person of that age, or to provide a nonthreatening way to address the individual's age preference for a sexualized partner. This Card Sort test assists the interviewer in gathering answers to three critical questions regarding age identification, self-identification, and sexual interest. This measure was developed in the earliest stages of work with persons with intellectual disabilities when no specific tools had been developed and as such was not standardized; however, it has been used extensively in the field. This measure was developed by taking pictures from magazines and catalogues of men, women, male and female adolescents, and male and female children. The pictures were each glued onto a card made of Bristol board. The pile of pictures is then presented to the examinee, who is asked to sort through the cards in response to different questions that aim to determine three critical areas of inquiry:

I. Can the individual categorize the photos by age? (Prompt: Put the cards into three piles – adult, teenager, child.)
II. Can the individual identify someone of their own age (peer)? (Prompt: Show me the cards that are most like you.)
III. What is their sexual preference? (Prompt: Show me the cards of people with whom you would like to have sex.)

These types of questions in the Card Sort however, are subject to acquiescence by the individual saying what the assessor wants to hear or what they know is the right answer.

The concepts of the Card Sort were later included in a standardized and widely field-tested assessments for socio-sexual knowledge and attitudes known as the SS-KAAT-R, developed by Griffiths and Lunksy (2003) and described earlier. The same areas of inquiry are addressed within the battery of questions used for general assessment of knowledge and attitudes but using standardized stimuli. It should, however, be noted that these nonverbal or minimally verbal assessments, although not conclusive, can be very helpful in building confirmatory information regarding the type of sexual stimuli the person finds arousing and are included within a comprehensive assessment profile. An unpublished review by Tough and Figliola (2007) showed that of those persons with an intellectual disability who were administered a Card Sort test and demonstrated sexual interest difficulties, 87% were later confirmed to have sexually deviant arousal using phallometry.

Worling (2006) developed a self-report sexual arousal graphing procedure that he uses in practice with typically developing adolescents who sexually offend. In a study comparing three sexual arousal approaches, he found that the self-report tools could distinguish adolescents who sexually assaulted children from adolescents who assaulted adults or peers. He found that the self-report measures, including the sexual arousal graphing procedure, could provide useful and accurate information on sexual interests in adolescents who sexually offend.

Arousal graphs (Worling, 2006) are a graphic and concrete means of illustrating abstract arousal patterns in a non-invasive way (See Figure 4.6). They are simple line graphs where the *x*-axis represents the variable or potential target in question and the *y*-axis represents level of arousal; the variable in question is typically age of preferred sexual partner. The clinician describes the age group being assessed (for instance: 1-5, 6-10, 11-15, 16-24, 25-35, 35-40, etc.) and the individual rates their preference on scale of 1-10 (1 being no sexual desire and 10 being extreme physical arousal). Additionally, other variables can be investigated simply by adjusting the *x*-axis; the gender of the target, use of force, and environment in which sexual activity takes place may be manipulated. There are some flaws with these graphs. By their nature, they are subjective and only provide information that the individual is aware of and willing to share. However, they do provide insight into the individual's awareness of their preferences and their willingness to discuss it in sessions.

Figure 4.6. **Example of Arousal Towards Females by Age (based on Worling, 2006)**

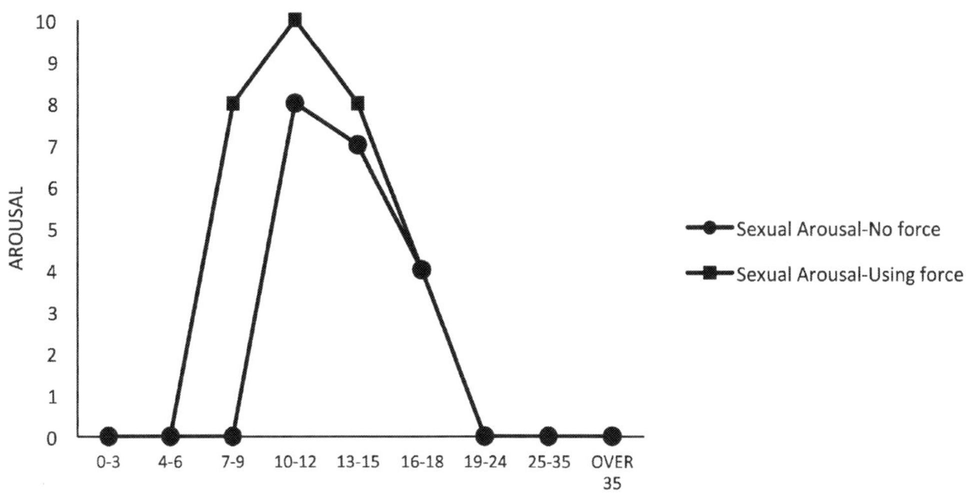

This particular arousal graph shows that the individual reports high arousal to females ages 7-15 using force. The individual reported some arousal to females aged 16-18 using force. They also reported high sexual arousal to females aged 10-15 without force.

It is noteworthy to mention that in typical practice, if an individual with an intellectual disability self-discloses sexual deviancy (e.g., arousal to children), then further testing would not necessarily be pursued. If an individual willingly admits to sexual deviancy, an extremely taboo disclosure, this is typically taken as truth, rendering more preference assessments unnecessary. However, as we noted earlier in this chapter, it is also important to be sure that the admission is being given freely, without inducement, as people with disabilities are commonly known to give affirmative answers when doing so is likely to incur favor from the assessor. Diagnostic profiles including such highly pejorative labels as "pedophilia" or "sexual deviance" can sometimes take on a life of their own.

Covert Observation

Due to the clandestine nature of most sexual offending behavior, researchers have suggested that evaluation of sexual preference can be done covertly through observing their behavior when they are unaware that observation is occurring. However, due to the dangerous nature of the behavior the therapist cannot ethically set the conditions to observe an offense. Vollmer and colleagues (2012) suggested that offense-related (i.e., approach) actions by persons with pedophilic interests may include watching children, approaching areas where children are present, and frequenting locations where children could be nearby. Although open to concern, an alternative method was suggested by Rea, DeBriere, Butler and Saunders (1998) whereby an individual at risk would be observed in a public place such as a shopping mall to witness the behavior in public. However, due to the potential risk and ethical concerns posed by placing individuals in the community, even if supervised and under surveillance, Vollmer and colleagues (2012) alternatively suggested that assessment could be conducted by creating baited situations in safe environments, such as having an audiotape of a child's voice playing to see if the person would enter the room, or leaving a group of magazines – some of which included images of children – to see if when people thought they were alone they would respond to these stimuli. The use of these procedures may result in effective ways of observing the individual engaging in behaviors that are associated with high-risk situations, without posing a risk of offense and in a seemingly unsupervised manner (Vollmer et al., 2012).

Utilizing Vollmer's ideas, more recent clinical practice has attempted to use experimental analysis procedures to simulate opportunity for offense while managing risk (Hoath, Lynn, & Miller, 2013). Situations are orchestrated to make it appear as though the offender has victim access by a variety of means, including manipulating the environment, bringing in perceptively new or untrained staff, or by making it appear as though a risky outing was possible. The individual's reactions and responses are assessed and gauged to determine motivation to succeed, use of skills and existence of pre-offending behaviors. Given these naturalistic settings, a much more accurate prediction and demonstration of risk is likely.

SUMMARY

Complex operant and respondent conditioning processes are involved in sexual behavior in general and especially in sexual offending behavior. Analyzing sexual offending behavior using Skinner's three-term contingency of behavior, as well as through a respondent lens of stimulus-stimulus pairings, is very important in helping clinicians to understand the environmental factors that impact cause of sexual offending behavior and help avoid circular logic or summary labels of causal factors such as "intention" to offend. Along with examining the antecedents and consequences to inappropriate sexual behavior, there must be equal consideration given to motivating operations, such as what the individual wants at that given time and automatic functions such as sexual arousal. If a person is in a state of deprivation, the reinforcing value of certain consequences increases and the likelihood of behaviors that result in those consequences also increases. This has important relevance for all behavior including sexual offense. The important fourth term of the contingency, motivating operations, is discussed in more detail in Chapter 5.

REFERENCES

Abel, G.G. (1989). Paraphilias. In H. I. Kaplan, & B. J. Sadock (Eds.), *Comprehensive Textbook of Psychiatry,* Vol. 2, 5th ed.; pp. 1069-1085). Baltimore, MD: Williams and Wilkins.

Abel, G.G., Becker, J.V. & Cunningham-Rathner, J. (1984). Compliance, consent and cognition between children and adults. *International Journal of Law and Psychiatry, 7,* 89-103.

Abel, G.G., & Blasingame, G. (2005). *The Abel-Blasingame assessment system for individuals with intellectual disabilities (ABID): Clinical guide.* Atlanta, GA: Abel Screening, Inc.

Arkowitz, S., & Vess, J. (2003). An evaluation of the Bumby RAPE and MOLEST scales as measures of cognitive distortions with civilly committed sexual offenders. *Sexual abuse: A Journal of Research and Treatment, 15,* 237-249.

American Psychiatric Association: *Diagnostic and Statistical Manual of Mental Disorders, (5th ed., text rev.)* (2013). Washington, DC: American Psychiatric Publishing.

Blanchard, R., Kuban, M.E., Blak, T., Klassen, P. E., Dickey, R., & Cantor, J.M. (2012). Sexual attraction to others: A comparison of two models of alloerotic responding in men. *Archives of Sexual Behavior, 41,* 13-29.

Blasingame, G.D., Abel, G.G., Jordan, A., & Wiegel, M. (2011). The utility and psychometric properties of the Abel-Blasingame assessment system for individuals with intellectual disabilities. *Journal of Mental Health Research in Intellectual Disabilities, 4,* 107-132.

Boer, D. P., Haaven, J.L., Lambrick, F., Lindsay, W. R., McVilly, K. R., Sakdalan, F. & Frize, M. (2013). *The Assessment of Risk and Manageability of Individuals with Developmental and Intellectual Limitations Who Offend – Sexually (ARMIDILO-S).* Retrieved from www.armidilo.net

Broxholme, S.L. & Lindsay, W.R. (2003). Development and preliminary evaluation of a questionnaire on cognitions related to sex offending for use with individuals who have mild intellectual disabilities. *Journal of Intellectual Disability Research, 47*(6), 472-482.

Bumby, K.M. (1996). Assessing the Cognitive Distortions of Child Molesters and Rapists: Development and Validation of the MOLEST and RAPE Scales. *Sexual Abuse: A Journal of Research and Treatment, 8,* 37-54.

Cooper, J.O., Heron, T.E., & Heward, W.L. (2007). *Applied Behavior Analysis* (2nd ed.). Upper Saddle River, NJ: Pearson Education Inc.

Fedoroff, J.P., & Moran, B. (1997). Myths and misconceptions about sex offenders. *The Canadian Journal of Human Sexuality, 6,* 263-276.

Finkelhor, D. (1984). *Child sexual abuse: new theory and research.* New York: Free Press.

Fletcher, R., Loschen, E., Stavrakaki. C. & First, M. *(Eds.) (2007). Diagnostic Manual-Intellectual Disability* (DM-ID). Kingston, NY: NADD Press.

Fredericks, B. & Nishioka-Evans, V. (1997). Functional assessment for a sex offender population. In Repp, A.C. & Horner, R.H. (Eds.), *Functional analysis of problem behavior: From effective assessment to effective support.* Belmont, CA: Wadsworth Publishing Co.

Freund, K. (1965). Diagnosing heterosexual pedophilia by means of a test for sexual interest. *Behavior Research and Therapy, 3,* 229-234.

Freund, K. & Blanchard, R. (1989). Phallometric diagnosis of pedophilia. *Journal of Consulting and Clinical Psychology, 57,* 1-6.

Friestad, C. (2012). Making sense, making good, or making meaning? Cognitive distortions as targets of change in offender treatment. *International Journal of Offender Therapy and Comparative Criminology, 56*(3), 465-482.

Gresham, F.M., Watson, T.S., & Skinner, C.H. (2001). Functional behavioral assessment: Principles, procedures, and future directions. *School Psychology Review, 30*(2), 156-172.

Griffiths, D. (2007). Sexuality and persons with intellectual disabilities. In I. Brown and M. Percy (Eds.) *A Comprehensive Guide to Intellectual and Developmental Disabilities* (pp. 571-581). Baltimore, MD: Paul H. Brookes.

Griffiths, D. & Fedoroff, J. P. (2009). Persons with intellectual disabilities who sexually offend. In F.M. Saleh, Grudzinskas, A.J., Bradford, J.M. & Brodsky, D.J. (Eds.), *Sex offenders: Identification, risk assessment, treatment and legal issue*s (pp. 353-378). Oxford, UK: Oxford University Press.

Griffiths, D., Hingsburger, D., Hoath, J., & Ioannou, S. (2013). Counterfeit deviance revisited. *Journal of Applied Research in Intellectual Disabilities, 26,* 471-480.

Griffiths, D. & Lunsky, Y. (2003*). Socio-sexual knowledge and attitude assessment tool – Revised (SSKAAT-R)*. Stoelting Company: Wood Dale, Illinois

Griffiths, D. M., Quinsey, V. L., & Hingsburger, D. (1989). *Changing inappropriate sexual behavior: A community-based approach for persons with developmental disabilities.* Baltimore, MD: Paul H. Brookes Publishing.

Hamann, S., Herman, R. A., Nolan, C. L., & Wallen, K. (2004). Men and women differ in amygdala response to visual sexual stimuli. *Nature Neuroscience, 7,* 411-416.

Hanson, R. K., & Bussière, M. T. (1998). Predicting relapse: A meta-analysis of sexual offender recidivism studies. *Journal of Consulting and Clinical Psychology, 66,* 348-362.

Hanson, R. K., Harris, A. R., Scott, T., & Helmus, L. (2007). Assessing the risk of sexual offenders on community supervision: The Dynamic Supervision Project. Ottawa, ON: Government of Canada. Retrieved from: http://www.publicsafety.gc.ca/cnt/rsrcs/pblctns/ssssng-rsk-sxl-ffndrs/index-en.aspx

Hanson, R. K., & Morton-Bourgon, K.E. (2005). The characteristics of persistent sex offenders: A meta-analysis of recidivism studies. *Journal of Consulting and Clinical Psychology, 73,* 1154-1163.

Harris, G.T., Rice, M.E., Quinsey, V.L., & Chaplin, T.C. (1996). Viewing time as a measure of sexual interest among child molesters and normal heterosexual men. *Behavior research and therapy, 34,* 389-394.

Hingsburger, D. (1996). *The ten commandments of reinforcement.* Algonquin, IL: Creative Core, New Orient Media.

Hingsburger, D., Griffiths, D. & Quinsey, V. (1991). Detecting counterfeit deviance. *Habilitative Mental Healthcare, 9,* 51-54.

Hoath, J., Lynn, L. & Miller, K. (2013) Experimental analysis of risk and recidivism. Presented at the Association for the Treatment of Sexual Abusers Conference, Chicago, IL.

Hoffmann, H., Janssen, E., & Turner, S. L. (2004). Classical conditioning of sexual arousal in women and men: Effects of varying awareness and biological relevance of the conditioned stimulus. *Archives of Sexual Behavior, 33*(1), 43-53.

Iwata, B. A., Dorsey, M. F., Slifer, K. J., Bauman, K. E., & Richman, G. S. (1994). Toward a functional analysis of self-injury. *Journal of Applied Behavior Analysis, 27,* 197–209. (Reprinted from Iwata, Dorsey, Slifer, Bauman, & Richman [Eds.] (1982), *Analysis and Intervention in Developmental Disabilities, 2,* 3–20.)

Jespersen, A. F., Lalumière, M. L., & Seto, M. C. (2009). Sexual abuse history among adult sex offenders and non-sex offenders: A meta-analysis. *Child Abuse & Neglect, 33,* 179-192.

Kalmus, E., & Beech, A.R. (2005). Forensic assessment of sexual interest: A review. *Aggression and Violent Behavior, 10*(2), 193-217.

Kolton, D.J.C., Boer, A., & Boer, D.P. (2001). A revision of the Abel and Becker Cognition Scale for intellectually disabled offenders. *Sexual Abuse, 13,* 217-220.

Lalumière, M.L., & Quinsey, V.L. (1994). The discriminability of rapists from non-sex offenders with phallometric measures: A meta-analysis. *Criminal Justice and Behavior, 21,* 150-175.

Lalumière, M.L., & Quinsey, V.L. (1998). Pavlovian conditioning of sexual interests in human males. *Archives of Sexual Behavior, 27,* 241-252.

Laws, D.R. & Osborn, C.A. (1983). How to build and operate a behavioral laboratory to evaluate and treat sexual deviance. In J.G. Greer, & I.R. Stuart (Eds.), *The sexual aggressor: Current perspectives on treatment* (pp. 293-335). New York, NY: Ban Nostrand Reinhold.

Lindsay, W. R. (2009). *The treatment of sex offenders with developmental disabilities.* Sussex, UK: Wiley-Blackwell.

Lindsay, W., Steptoe, L., & Beech, A. (2008). The Ward and Hudson pathways model of the sexual offense process applied to offenders with intellectual disability. *Sexual Abuse, 20,* 379-392.

Lindsay, W.R., Whitefield, E., & Carson, D. (2007). An assessment for attitudes consistent with sexual offending for use with offenders with intellectual disabilities. *Legal and Criminological Psychology, 12,* 55-68.

Lunsky, Y., Frijters, J., Griffiths, D.M., Watson, S.L., & Williston, S. (2007). Sexual knowledge and attitudes of men with intellectual disability who sexually offend. *Journal of Intellectual and Developmental Disability, 32,* 74–81.

Marshall, W. I., & Fernandez, Y.M. (2003). Sexual preferences: Are they useful in assessment and treatment of sexual offenders? *Aggression and Violent Behavior, 8,* 131-143.

Martin, G., & Pear, J.J. (2015). ***Behavior modification: What it is and how to do it,*** (10th ed.). New York, New York: Routledge.

Maruna, S., & Mann, R.E. (2006). A fundamental attribution error? Rethinking cognitive distortions. *Legal and Criminological Psychology, 11,* 155-177.

McCabe, M. (1999). Sexual knowledge, experience and feelings among people with disabilities. *Sexuality and Disability, 17,* 157-170.

McGuire, R.J., Carlisle, J.M., & Young, B.G. (1965). Sexual deviations as conditioned behavior: A hypothesis. *Behavior Research and Therapy, 3,* 185-190.

Michie, A.M., Lindsay, W.R., Martin, V., & Grieve, A. (2006). A test of counterfeit deviance: A comparison of sexual knowledge in groups of sex offenders with intellectual disability and controls. *Sexual Abuse: A Journal of Research and Treatment, 18,* 271-278.

Miltenberger, R.G. (2008). ***Behavior modification: Principles and procedures*** (4th ed.). Belmont, CA: Wadsworth.

Money, J. (1986). *Lovemaps: Clinical concepts of sexual/erotic health and pathology, paraphilia, and gender transposition of childhood, adolescence, and maturity.* New York: Irvington Publishers.

Murphy, W. D., Coleman, E. M., & Haynes, M. R. (1983). Treatment and evaluation issues with the mentally retarded sex offender. In J. D. Greer & I. R. Stuart (Eds.) *The sexual aggressor: Current perspectives on treatment,* pp. 22-41. New York: VanNostrand Reinhold.

Novaco, R.W., & Taylor, J.L. (2004). Assessment of anger and aggression in male offenders with developmental disabilities. *Psychological Assessment, 16*(1), 42-50.

O'Neill, R.E., Horner, R.H., Albin, R.W., Sprague, J.R., Storey, K., & Newton, J.S. (1997). *Functional assessment and program development for problem behavior: A practical handbook.* Pacific Grove, CA: Brooks/Cole.

Plaud, J.J. & Martini, R. (1999). The respondent conditioning of male sexual arousal. *Behavior Modification, 23,* 254-268.

Plaud, J.J., & Newberry, D.E. (1996). Rule-governed behavior and pedophilia. *Sexual Abuse: A Journal of Research and Treatment, 8*(2), 143-159.

Quinsey, V.L., Harris, G.T., Rice, M.E. & Cormier, C. (2015). *Violent offenders: Appraising and managing risk (3rd* Ed.). Washington, DC: American Psychological Association.

Rea, J.A., DeBriere, T., Butler, K. & Saunders, J.K. (1998). An analysis of four sex offenders arousal in the community using portable penile plethysmograph. *Sexual Abuse: A Journal of Research and Treatment, 15,* 239-255.

Reyes, J. R. (2009). Assessment of sex offenders with developmental disabilities. *Dissertation Abstracts International,* 69. (UNI No.3334500)

Reyes, J.R., Vollmer, T.R., & Hall, A. (2017). Comparison of arousal and preference assessment outcomes for sex offenders with intellectual disabilities. *Journal of Applied Behavior Analysis, 50*(1), 27-37.

Reyes, J. R., Vollmer, T. R., Whitehouse, C. M., & Jansen, G. (2009). The use of in situ assessments for sex offenders with developmental disabilities. Presented in symposium, Behavioral Assessments for Covert Behavior Problems. Association for Behavior Analysis, Phoenix, Az.

Rupp, H. A., & Wallen, K. (2008). Sex differences in response to visual sexual stimuli: A review. *Archives of Sexual Behavior, 37,* 206-218.

Schmidt, A. F., Babchishin, K. M., & Lehmann, R. J. (2016). A meta-analysis of viewing time measures of sexual interest in children. *Archives of Sexual Behavior,* 1-14.

Skinner B.F. (1957). *Verbal behavior.* New York: Appleton-Century-Crofts.

Sobsey, D. (1994). Sexual abuse of individuals with intellectual disabilities. In A. Craft (Ed.), *Practice issues in sexuality and intellectual disability* (pp. 91-112). London, UK: Routledge.

Sobsey, D. & Varnhagen, C. (1989). Sexual abuse, assault and exploitation of Canadians with disabilities. In C. Bagley & J. Thomlison (Eds.), *Child sexual abuse: Critical perspectives on prevention, intervention and treatment* (pp. 203-216). Toronto: Wall and Emerson.

Stoléru, S., Fonteille, V., Cornélis, C., Joyal, C., & Moulier, V. (2012). Functional neuroimaging studies of sexual arousal and orgasm in healthy men and women: A review and meta-analysis. *Neuroscience & Biobehavioral Reviews, 36,* 1481-1509.

Southam-Gerow, M.A. (2013). *Emotion regulation in children and adolescents: A practitioner's guide.* New York, NY, US: Guilford Press.

Talbot, T.J. & Langdon, T.E., (2006). A revised sexual knowledge tool for people with intellectual disabilities: Is sexual knowledge related to sexual offending behavior? *Journal of Intellectual Disability Research*, 50, 523-531.

Thompson, R. A. (1994). Emotion regulation: A theme in search of definition. *Monographs of the Society for Research in Child Development, 59*, 25-52.

Tough, S. & Figliolia, L. (2007, November). *Diagnosing deviance in men who are developmentally disabled.* Presentation made the 26th Annual Conference of the Association for the Treatment of Sexual Abusers, San Diego, CA.

Vaughan, M.E., & Michael, J.L. (1982). Automatic reinforcement: An important but ignored concept. *Behaviorism, 10*, 217-227.

Vollmer, T. R. (2014, June). Ethical issues for applied behavior analysts: Covert observation. *Severe and Challenging Behavior of Persons with Intellectual Disabilities or Autism: Supporting Individuals in the Community.* Dual Diagnosis Certificate Programme, Brock University, St. Catharines, ON.

Vollmer, T.R., Reyes, J.R., & Walker, S.F. (2012). Behavioral assessment and intervention for sex offenders with intellectual and developmental disabilities. In. J.K. Luiselli (Ed.), *A handbook of high-risk challenging behaviors in people with intellectual and developmental disabilities* (pp. 121-144). Baltimore, MD: Paul H. Brookes

Ward, T., & Hudson, S. M. (1998). A model of the relapse process in sexual offenders. *Journal of Interpersonal Violence, 13*, 700-725

Ward, T., Hudson, S.M., Johnston, L., & Marshall, W.L. (1997). Cognitive distortions in sex offenders: An integrative review. *Clinical Psychology Review, 17*, 479-507.

Wilson, R.J. (1998). Psychophysiological indicators of faking in the phallometric test. *Sexual Abuse, 10*, 113-126.

Wilson, R.J., & Burns, M. (2011). *Intellectual disability and problems in sexual behavior: Assessment, treatment, and promotion of healthy sexuality.* Holyoke, MA: Neari Press.

Wilson, R.J. & Miner, M.H. (2016). Measurement of male sexual arousal and interest using penile plethysmography and viewing time. In D.R. Laws & W.T. O'Donohue (Eds.), *Treatment of sex offenders: Strengths and weaknesses in assessment and intervention.* New York: Springer.

Worling, J. R. (2006). Assessing sexual arousal with adolescent males who have offended sexually: Self-report and unobtrusively measured viewing time. *Sex Abuse, 18*(4), 383-400.

Wulfert, E., Greenway, D.E., & Dougher, M.J. (1996). A logical functional analysis of reinforcement-based disorders: alcoholism and pedophilia. *Journal of Consulting and Clinical Psychology, 64*, 1140-1151.

Yates, P., Prescott, D., & Ward, T. (2010). *Applying good lives and self-regulation models to sex offender treatment: A practical guide for clinicians.* Brandon, VT: Safer Society Press.

Chapter Five

Exploring the Role of Motivating Operations in the Sexual Offending Behavior of Persons with an Intellectual Disability

Sexual offending must be understood not as a result of a univariate factor but as a result of complex and multiple factors (Ward, Polaschek, & Beech, 2005). In Chapter 4 we described how a complex interaction of operant and respondent conditioning is involved in both appropriate and deviant sexual behavior and a complete analysis of all potential biological and environmental variables is needed to assess for function or cause of sexual offending behavior. Finkelhor (1986) suggested that since sexual offending behavior is the result of multiple factors, then treatment should also examine and address all factors. Thus, simplistic approaches that have attempted to treat sexual offending by addressing only a single variable (e.g., biology) have been shown to have limited and short-lived results (see meta-analysis in Schmucker & Lösel, 2015). Wulfert, Greenway, and Dougher (1996) have posed a number of questions that must be addressed:

1. What are the different contingencies of reinforcement controlling the behavior?
2. Are there differences in the establishing operations that potentiate contingencies (in other words, are there motivational differences)?
3. Do different situations precede the offense?
4. Are their differences in the reinforcers or consequences that affect the future probability of the behavior occurring?
5. Are there deficits or excesses in other concomitant repertoires of behavior? (p. 1146)

Wulfert and colleagues (1996) further suggested that "the behavioral processes addressed in these questions stand in complex dynamic relations to one another" (p. 1147). In this chapter, the role of establishing operations (now more commonly known as motivating operations) will be explored in the context of other important factors such as those listed above and including different contingencies of reinforcement.

A BRIEF HISTORY OF MOTIVATING OPERATIONS

"A motivating operation changes how much you "want" something and how hard you will "work" to get it" (Michael, 1982, as cited in Langthorne & McGill, 2009, p. 1). As dis-

cussed in Chapter 4, when assessing causal factors of any behavior, it is important to evaluate the three-term contingency of behavior, which includes both antecedents and consequences. A "fourth term" of the contingency that must also be assessed is motivating operations, which are antecedent to the behavior. The evolution of the concept of establishing operations started with Skinner's concept of motivation or *drive* (Skinner, 1938; 1953). Skinner argued against the common practice of viewing drive as an internal causal variable and proposed that environmental variables be the focus of the analysis. In the analysis of hunger for example, rather than talking about a "hunger drive" he proposed that the relation between food deprivation and its evocative effect on behavior be the focus of the analysis. Around the same time, in a very influential text, *Principles of Psychology,* Keller and Schoenfeld (1950) first used the term "establishing operations," arguing that the term was more precise than the term "drive," in part, because they theorized that environmental conditions of deprivation, aversive stimulation, and satiation "established" a drive for humans. The behavior analytic community embraced this term because it implied that environmental conditions, not internal events, increase the occurrence of certain behaviors. Although Keller and Schoenfeld (1950) adopted the term *establishing operation* to describe how antecedent manipulations, such as food deprivation, could affect the strength of a response, Jack Michael aptly pointed out that the analysis of such events was absent which, according to Michael, left "a gap in our understanding of operant functional relations" (Michael, 1993, p. 191). To address this, Michael (1982, 1983, 1993) revised the theory of establishing operations, which he described as:

> *[an] environmental event, operation, or stimulus condition that affects an organism by momentarily altering (a) the reinforcing effectiveness of other events and (b) the frequency of occurrence of that part of the organism's repertoire relevant to those events as consequences (Michael, 1993, p. 1).*

Michael's writing on the concept of establishing operations provided behavior analysts with a useful way to describe an important class of operant controlling variables. After Michael published his seminal papers, there was a rapid increase in frequency of citations and articles pertaining to establishing operations. However, the *establishing operation* terminology had some limitations. For use as an omnibus term for all operations that have motivational effects, the term *establishing* implies only an *increase* in the effectiveness of a consequence as a reinforcer or punisher, yet many motivating variables decrease the effectiveness of consequences. For example, researchers have found that time-based presentation of attention non-contingent on behavior (non-contingent reinforcement procedures) reduces the effectiveness of attention as a reinforcer. Michael thought that introducing the complementary term *abolishing* would be inconvenient, so he suggested that establishing should be taken to mean both establishing and abolishing. It is clear how this, too, could cause confusion for individuals in the field and, perhaps, led to confusion or ignorance about the potential abolishing effects.

In response to this limitation, Laraway, Snycerski, Michael, and Poling (2003) suggested the term, *motivating operations* (MOs) be used to account for both the establishing and abolishing effects of establishing operations, and it is the term that is most commonly used in the field of behavior analysis today. Motivating operations have two effects on behavior: (1) a *value-altering effect* in which there is an increase *or* decrease in the reinforcing effectiveness of some stimulus, object, or event; and (2) a *behavior-altering effect* in which there is an increase in the current frequency of behavior that has been reinforced by some stimulus, object, or event (an evocative effect) *or* a decrease in the current frequency of behavior that has been reinforced by some stimulus, object, or event (an abative effect; see Laraway et al., 2003). It is important to note that the behavior-altering effect is not limited to changes in frequency of behavior; it can impact other dimensions of behavior including relative frequency (rate), response latency, magnitude, etc. (Michael, 2007).

THE EFFECTS OF MOTIVATING OPERATIONS

A common example used to describe motivating operations is deprivation and satiation of food or water. Deprivation of food is an establishing operation in that it creates a state of hunger, which temporarily increases the value of food as a reinforcer, and thereby also evokes behaviors that have been reinforced with food in the past (e.g., going to the fridge and getting something to eat). Conversely, going to a buffet and filling up on food is an abolishing operation that creates a state of satiation, which decreases the reinforcing value of food in that moment and has an abative effect on any behaviors that have been followed by food in the past (e.g., may be less likely to go to the fridge to grab something to eat when full; Cooper, Heron, & Heward, 2007, Laraway et al., 2003; Martin & Pear, 2015). In this example the value-altering effects are unconditioned since the reinforcing value of the food is innate and does not have to be learned. However, the behavior altering effect is learned in that certain food-seeking behaviors, such as going to the fridge, have been reinforced in the past and are therefore more likely to happen again in the future. Sexual behavior can be discussed in the same way; the value altering effect or reinforcing properties of sexual behavior are innate, but the behavior altering effects are learned. For example, physiological sensations of sexual arousal to pornography (or value-altering effect) are innate, whereas the behavior altering effect of accessing pornography online is learned. To add a level of complexity, conditioned motivating operations occur when previously neutral stimuli acquire value-altering effects through being paired with an unconditioned motivating operation, another conditioned motivating operation, or other reinforcement or punishment contingencies. We know that human behavior is complex and multiple control of behavior is common and sexual behavior is no exception (Michael, 1993).

STIMULUS CONTROL VERSUS MOTIVATING OPERATIONS

Michael (1993) made an important distinction between antecedent variables that act as a sign of the availability of reinforcement or punishment (discriminative stimuli, S^D) and antecedent variables that act on a person's "motivation" for such consequences (motivating operations). Recall that in Chapter 4 we discussed stimulus control and how a discriminative stimulus (S^D) signals the availability of a reinforcer. In other words, it is a cue that a certain behavior will pay off (S^D) or will not pay off (S^Δ). For example, a green light is an S^D for driving forward but an S^Δ for stopping (Martin & Pear, 2015). A green light on a drink machine is an S^D for putting in change (reinforced with a drink in the past for doing so), whereas an "out of order" sign or red light is an S^{Δ} for putting money in the machine (putting change in in the past has not been reinforced with a drink).

Both discriminative stimuli and motivating operations evoke behaviors, but for different reasons: discriminative stimuli have to do with the *availability* of a reinforcer, and motivating operations have to do with the *effectiveness* of a reinforcer at a particular time (i.e., how reinforcing the stimulus is at that time). We will again use food deprivation to illustrate two questions that can be asked to determine if a behavior is discriminative or motivating as described by Langthorne and McGill (2009):

(1) "Is the consequence more available or more valuable following a period of deprivation? The antecedent event is likely to be a discriminative stimulus if the reinforcer (access to food) is more available in the presence of the event. Of course, access to food is no more likely when you are food deprived, so food deprivation is not a discriminative stimulus. Rather access to food is more valuable when you are food deprived, so food deprivation is an MO." (p. 24)

(2) "An antecedent event, such as food deprivation, can only be considered a discriminative stimulus if (a) in its presence, reinforcement is available for a certain class of responses, and (b) in its absence, reinforcement is not available for that class of responses. When an individual is food deprived, reinforcement (access to food) is available for responses such as snack preparation so the requirements of (a) are met. When an individual is not food deprived, access to food remains just as available should the individual engage in snack preparation so the second part of the test fails.» (p. 24)

THE EFFECTS OF MOTIVATING OPERATIONS AND SEXUAL BEHAVIOR

Motivating operations involving sexual behaviors can be interpreted as described above. There are a number of both establishing and abolishing operations that can have a profound effect on sexual offending behaviors and for individuals with intellectual disabilities, and there are many combinations of motivating operations to consider. See Table 5.1 for further explanation of this concept with relatively straightforward examples of sexual offending behavior.

Table 5.1. ***Impact of motivating operations on sexual offending behavior***

Type of Motivating Operation	Value Altering Effect (Temporary)	Behavior Altering Effect (Temporary)
Establishing Operation		
Sexual deprivation (no or infrequent engagement in any type of sexual behavior)	Increases the reinforcing value of sexual behavior (unconditioned, innate)	Increases behaviors that have led to reinforcement from sexual behavior in the past (conditioned, learned)

Example:		
Johnny has recently been put on one-on-one supervisory watch 24 hours a day in his group home for engaging in sexually inappropriate behavior (masturbating in public). Part of his treatment plan is that he is restricted from possessing any erotic paraphernalia in his room, and he is not given privacy or opportunity to masturbate. If he attempts to masturbate, group home staff redirect him to a table activity or something else to keep his hands occupied.	Johnny sees a female on an outing one day who looks like a woman in one of the posters that used to hang in his room that he found arousing and was allowed to masturbate to in private. The reinforcing value of engaging in a sexual behavior such as masturbation is increased since Johnny is experiencing a state of sexual deprivation (temporary increase in the value of sexual behaviors).	Johnny gets very close to the female while his staff member is helping another individual tie his shoes. Johnny approaches the woman to about the same distance he used to be from the poster that hung in his room and begins masturbating (temporary increase in engagement in sexual behaviors).
Abolishing Operation		
Sexual satiation (engagement in any type of sexual behavior)	Decrease the reinforcing value of sexual behavior (conditioned, innate)	Decreases behaviors that have led to reinforcement from sexual behavior in the past (conditioned, learned)
Example: Cameron has recently been put on one-on-one supervisory watch 24 hours a day in his group home for engaging in sexually inappropriate behavior (masturbating in public). Part of his treatment plan is that he is given a time each day (or more if requested) where he can access sexually arousing stimuli and be given the opportunity to masturbate in the privacy of his bedroom. Recently, Cameron has been requesting to masturbate frequently, perhaps due to the fact that staff members are reinforcing him for engaging in the behavior in private vs. public settings.	Cameron is on an outing with the group home staff, and there is a woman in the park sunbathing topless. Typically, this would have evoked masturbation attempts. Cameron notices the woman on the outing but does not attempt to masturbate. Cameron masturbated before leaving the group home. Therefore, the reinforcing value of doing so is decreased as he is in a state of sexual satiation (temporary decrease in the value of sexual behavior).	Cameron does not make any attempt to masturbate given that he had just done so before leaving the group home and was in a state of sexual satiation (temporary decrease in sexual behaviors).

We have attempted to demonstrate that just as certain situations and stimuli can increase the reinforcing value of certain behaviors and therefore evoke those behaviors, so too can situations decrease the reinforcing value of certain behaviors and have an abolishing effect on those behaviors. In the examples with Johnny and Cameron, it is evident that depriving Johnny of privacy and a healthy sexual outlet increased his likelihood for inappropriate sexual behavior. The example scenario with Cameron illustrates how a different approach to a similar historical problematic behavior (seen in Johnny) can eliminate inappropriate sexual behavior. Sexual deprivation, as stated previously, may make sexual contact more reinforcing. In the same way, satiation of sexual activity may decrease the value of sexual contact. This can have important considerations for treatment and management of sexual offending behavior.

For Cameron in Table 5.1 above, engaging in masturbation created a condition in which, at least for a time, sexual contact was less reinforcing. Cameron was exposed to environmental stimuli, which had previously led to inappropriate sexual behavior, but since he was in a state of sexual satiation those stimuli did not have the same reinforcing value, and therefore there was an abolishing effect on his typical behavior. This example was relatively straightforward; however, other situations may have multiple complex variables to consider such as medication compliance, which can often be an issue that can affect appropriate sexual interests. Further, Baker, Blumberg, Freeman, & Wieseler (2002) argue that "an underlying psychiatric disorder can be seen as an establishing operation that changes the likelihood of problem behavior by altering the reinforcing and punishing value of consequences in an individual's environment" (Baker et al., 2002, p. 118). This affirms that complex cases, such as sexual offending behavior of individuals with intellectual disabilities require a comprehensive and thorough analysis of all variables involved.

Wulfert and colleagues (1996) suggested that "[a] predisposition for sexual arousal to children could facilitate the ontogenic conditioning of specific deviant interests and repertoires, but attention to behavioral principles is necessary to account for the broad and rather resistant repertoires of sexually deviant behavior" (p. 1147). They further note that there is a difference between individuals with preferential or situational interests (as described in Chapter 4) with regard to motivating operations. When examining the motivating operation for offending against a child, an individual who prefers sex with children may have sexual deprivation as an establishing operation. Acting on the sexual urge results in a positive reinforcement contingency in the form of sexual satisfaction (Wulfert et al., 1996). The motivation to engage in the behavior increases with the time from the last occurrence. On the other hand, persons with situational interests, who actually have greater arousal for sex with adults, are motivated by proximal establishing operations, such as a loss of job, loss of relationship, or sexual reinforcement. The deprivation related to the loss of reinforcement creates a condition where an offender is motivated to fill the reinforcement void and/or escape from discomfort. If the individual lacks the skills to deal with the discomfort in an appropriate way, and if children are present, then the situation is opportune for the offender to use children to meet the needs. The operant process at work here is negative reinforcement where pedophilic behavior results in the reduction of stress (Wulfert et al., 1996). Langevin, Hardy, Day, and Russon (1985) suggest that there is a complex psychological history that is involved with these offenders, which often results in a profile of them as inadequate or immature, possibly serving as a very distal setting event for offending behavior (Wulfert et al., 1996).

Past experiences form histories of reinforcement and punishment that impact future behavior: "Events from the individual's more remote past can also serve as an establishing function. For example, having been sexually abused as a child may increase the evocative effectiveness of children as discriminative stimuli and the reinforcing value of engaging in that behavior" (Wulfert et al., 1996, p. 1146). The most common explanation of the influence of distal factors is the abused/abuser hypothesis (Garland & Dougher, 1990; Jespersen, Lalumiere, & Seto, 2009; Money, 1986). It has been reported that individuals who have sexually offended who have also experienced or witnessed violent sexual acts in early life demonstrate increased risk of future sexual violence (Becker, Harris, & Sales, 1993). For example, Groth (1979) reported that 40% of pedophiles and 25% of persons who are accused of sexual assault had been abused as children. Hanson and Slater (1988) found an average of 28% of persons who have sexually offended had abuse histories based on prior literature, while Dhawan and Marshall (1996) found even higher rates, with 58% of persons who have sexually offended having some sexual abuse history. The rate of abuse among persons with intellectual disabilities is much higher than in the population of persons without intellectual disabilities (Sobsey, 1994).

Finkehor (1986) suggested that the sexualized behavior of some individuals who have targeted children represents a recapitulation of their own offense history. According to this theory, some individuals who sexually offend against children are re-enacting the sexual abuse they experienced as a child by engaging in sex with a child of the same age, based upon a pairing between the onset of their fantasy-driven sexual aggression and the age of their own abuse (Pithers, 1993). This relationship between the history of childhood violence and the development of sexual offending behavior has been called the traumagenic model of offense. Finkelhor and Browne (1985) suggested that the sexuality of the child is altered by the sexual abuse, including the rewards for sexual behavior, a focus on certain body parts, fear regarding sexual contact, and confusion about appropriate sexual behavior and the social mores that accompany it. In this way the individual who has experienced abuse has a different sexual learning history that may alter how sexual satisfaction is sought in the future, including who (e.g., the age, sex of individual) might set occasion for arousal or under what conditions arousal might occur, which may recapitulate their own abuse history.

Laws and Marshall (1990) proposed the theory that sexual interest in children is conditioned in the offender in the developing years. This conditioning theory is, perhaps, particularly relevant for persons with intellectual disabilities, for whom the abusive event may have been their first and only sexual contact and, in the absence of counselling or sexual education to the contrary, may replay their own learned traumagenic experience. Specific to individuals with intellectual disability, sexual abuse in childhood has been found to increase the likelihood of engaging in inappropriate sexual behavior as an adult (Lindsay, Elliot, & Astell, 2004). Experiencing abuse in childhood can be looked at as a distal antecedent to offending in adulthood. This is one important part of assessment to be targeted in treatment, among the presence of other important variables. In fact, some research suggested that not only the presence, but type of abuse, affects later offending (Lindsay, Steptoe, & Haut, 2012). Individuals who were sexually abused later engaged in topographically similar behaviors as did those who were physically abused.

MOTIVATING OPERATIONS IN CONTEXT

What conditions and what situations make sexual behavior more likely to occur? When looking at sexuality and intellectual disability, it is critical to understand the uniqueness of the culture and environment in which this population lives. The attitudes towards sexual behavior and intellectual disability are often negative. Cuskelly and Gilmore (2007) suggested that the literature has presented two conflicting stereotypes regarding the sexuality of persons with intellectual disabilities; one stereotype is that of being the eternal child and innocent, and the other is that of being oversexed and promiscuous. As mentioned earlier in this book, Griffiths (2007) noted that although these stereotypes appear conflicting, in reality they both achieve the same result, which is to place people with intellectual disabilities outside of the typical range for sexual behavior and thereby deny their inherent sexuality.

As a result, despite legislation to the contrary, such as the *Services and Supports to Promote the Social Inclusion of Persons with Developmental Disabilities Act* (Government of Ontario, 2008), individuals with intellectual disabilities are routinely denied the opportunity to date, masturbate in private, or engage in consenting sexual activity. Additionally, stigma and societal bias prevents individuals with intellectual disabilities from being exposed to the same social situations and opportunities as the typical population. Schools are informally segregated with separate classes and events for students with intellectual disability, including unequal access to sex education (Barnard-Brak, Schmidt, Chesnut, Tianlan, & Richman, 2014). Employment is often achieved in non-competitive day programs, again segregated from the typical population. And, even within the home, staff and family may prohibit sexual activity, even masturbation. Without the ability to engage in appropriate sexual behavior, this basic human need is unmet and any sexual activity, appropriate or offensive, becomes more valuable (reinforcing) and frequent. Individuals who are unable to masturbate in their homes may do so in the community. Lack of sexual opportunity may become an establishing operation that makes any sexual activity more reinforcing and more likely. For example, individuals who are not allowed to engage in appropriate relationships may seek inappropriate alternatives such as sex with minors or non-consenting and/or vulnerable individuals. Again, these situations create a condition in which sexual behaviors, through deprivation, become increasingly reinforcing and more likely. Unfortunately, inappropriate sexual behaviors, albeit maybe not deviant, are more likely to result in this case.

As discussed more fully in Chapter 2, some individuals with intellectual disability who have sexually offended may commit a sexualized crime that appears topographically rooted in sexual deviance/automatic reinforcement; however, they may commit the offense for other reasons. These persons who have sexually offended have been referred to as demonstrating "counterfeit deviance" instead of true deviance (Hingsburger, Griffiths, & Quinsey, 1991). Counterfeit deviance is important to understand as behaviors that appear with a topography similar to offenses motivated by deviant or sensory functions may be motivated by vastly different variables. Sexual offending behaviors such as these are the result of lack of privacy in the environment (structural), modeling by others, inappropriate partner selection or courtship, lack of sexual knowledge or moral training, a maladaptive learning history, medical disorders, or medication effects (Griffiths, Hingsburger, Hoath, & Ioannou, 2013; Hingsburger et al., 1991). If these variables play a role in the commission of the sexual offense then treatment needs to reflect that. As a note, caution should be used when applying the theory of counterfeit deviance; the authors suggested that in individual cases these factors may play a role and as such should be explored as part of treatment. It bears repeating that the theory never excluded the possibility of paraphilia nor did it claim that these factors were homogeneous for all offenders with intellectual disability (for further explanation see Griffiths et al., 2013).

Another way that the environment can make inappropriate sexual behavior more or less likely to occur involves the social verbal community of individuals with an intellectual disability who have sexually offended, and the desire to be accepted. If peers who support and encourage offending surround an individual, it can create a motivating operation (establishing operation) for offending behavior. The access to reinforcement in the form of acceptance from peers and further enforcing cognitive distortions temporarily increases the value of offending behaviors and may increase the frequency. In the same way, peers that discourage offending can also have an abolishing effect on the reinforcing value and frequency of sexually offensive behavior, making it less valuable and less likely to occur. Peers' verbal statements may also function as rules that exert control over the behavior of others.

The use of drugs or alcohol can also serve as motivating operations in relation to sexual offending, increasing or decreasing the reinforcing value of sexual behavior and increasing or decreasing the behaviors that lead to sexual behavior. Although the prevalence of substance abuse in the intellectual disability population of persons without sexual offense histories is low, this population is more likely to develop substance abuse issues than the non-disabled population (Chapman & Wu, 2012). In addition, people with intellectual disabilities are less likely to receive treatment and stay in treatment for substance abuse. Therefore, the impact of drugs and alcohol may be particularly relevant and is a critical aspect of assessment. Substance abuse is an acute dynamic risk factor for people with intellectual disabilities, where the presence of or an increase in substance abuse is one predictive variable for sexual offending (Lofthouse et al., 2013). Substance use may have an evocative effect on sexual offending behavior, through a simultaneous reduction in inhibition and increase in impulsivity, all of which may increase the value of offending during that altered state.

PORNOGRAPHY AS AN ESTABLISHING OPERATION

The role of pornography as an establishing operation in the development of sexual offending behavior has been both controversial and equivocal. In the 1990s, the Criminal Code of Canada defined pornography based on the level of violence and whether material was degrading or not. Currently, the Criminal Code of Canada only includes and defines child pornography in Section 163.1 (Government of Canada, 2018). In contrast, erotica typically involves sexually explicit material involving consensual adults that are neither violent nor degrading (Marshall & Barrett, 1990). However, it is important to determine what represents an arousing image for an individual. For example, a person with sexual arousal to children may find an image of a child in a bathing suit in a catalog or an advertisement for diapers depicting children being changed to be erotic. These images were not intended to induce sexual feelings or imagery but may have that effect on particular individuals and, of course, should be avoided.

Pornography has been examined as a potential antecedent to sexual offense, although a causal relationship has never been demonstrated (Diamond, 2009; Kingston, Fedoroff, Firestone, Curry, & Bradford, 2008). The role of pornography as it relates to the development of sexual offending behavior has been explored in terms of classical and operant conditioning (Laws and Marshall, 1990). According to conditioning theory, masturbation to orgasm while viewing pornographic images results in shifting of sexual response in a deviant (e.g., violent) direction, which may be increased over time as the individual habituates to the nature of the images and, as such, seeks out more intense content (Seto, Maric, & Barbaree, 2001). This theory lies behind the rationale for the use of behavioral approaches such as covert sensitization in treatment of sexual offending behavior (e.g., Quinsey & Earls, 1990). Empirically, the effects of violent and nonviolent pornography have typically shown differential effects for various types of pornography (e.g., Donnerstein & Linz, 1998). However, Gunter (2002) has suggested that even nonaggressive pornography may be associated with increased risk for sexual aggression.

Ramasubramanian and Oliver (2003) suggested that meta-analyses on the topic of pornography have typically reported that increased acceptance of violence and aggression against women has been shown to be associated with exposure to pornography (both violent and non-violent). For example, in a meta-analytic review of the exposure to pornography on aggressive behavior, Allen, Dalessio, and Brezgel (1995) concluded that viewing nude pictures reduced aggression, however pornography involving nonviolent and violent sexual activity increased aggression, with violent sexual activity resulting in the greatest effect on aggression. Further, Vega and Malamuth (2007) found that high pornography use was significantly associated with the prediction of sexual aggression. Other researchers (e.g., Diamond, 2009) have found no strong association between sexual violence and pornography. However, Vega and Malamuth (2007) further added that the predictive validity of this finding was mitigated by other risk characteristics, such as those already predisposed to sexual aggression. For example, Seto and colleagues (2001), conducted a review of the existing empirical evidence to the link between pornography and sexual offending and concluded that:

> *there is little support for a direct causal link between pornography use and sexual aggression...[they] argue that individuals who are already predisposed to sexually offend are the most likely to show an effect of pornography exposure and are the most likely to show the strongest effects. Men who are not predisposed are unlikely to show an effect; if there actually is an effect, it is likely to be transient because these men would not normally expose themselves to violent pornography. (p. 46).*

A meta-analysis conducted by Kingston and Malamuth (2011) provides a perspective on the current problem with pornography data and inferring that its use increases risk. They argue that most of the data on pornography use is aggregate, meaning it is collected using multiple measures and then summarized to make broad statements about individuals, without accounting for individual differences. In their meta-analysis, they found that individual differences have an impact on the effects of pornography, yet these differences are not accounted for in most of the research. They posit that studies done at the individual level have shown that people who view pornography do not commit acts of violence. Also, some studies do show an increased risk of inappropriate behavior due to pornography, but only if the individual has additional risk factors (Kingston & Malamuth, 2011).

These findings present an important question about the use of pornography as a potential abolishing operation to produce an abative effect on sexual offending. Relatedly, using a reversal design with high experimental control, Reyes, Vollmer and Hall (2011) showed that pre-session masturbation lowered arousal levels to deviant stimuli in one individual; however, further replications are needed.

Given the equivocal nature of the research regarding pornography, the use of violent and perhaps even nonviolent media with individuals who have demonstrated a predisposition to sexual offending may be counterproductive. However, the use of stand-alone nude images has not been shown to have deleterious effects and as such may serve a therapeutic role in some cases. Indeed, we are aware of programs that provide clients in advanced stages of treatment with specially chosen erotic media (colloquially referred to as "sexy pictures") to assist in shaping and maintaining appropriate masturbatory fantasies (see Wilson & Burns, 2011). Therefore, rather than blanketing all pornography as a contributing factor for all individuals, its use in treatment should be done on an individual basis, determined from a thorough assessment and evaluation of individual risk factors.

SUMMARY

Motivating operations (with both establishing and abolishing effects) can have profound effects on any behavior including those that are sexual offending in nature. When assessing individuals with an intellectual disability, it is critical to examine the historical context and current environment in which the behavior occurs. Internal factors, such as the automatic reinforcing value of sexual behavior, and external factors, such as lack of opportunity for appropriate sexual activity, can increase the likelihood of offending and should be addressed accordingly. A benefit of considering motivation in terms of environmental rather than internal influences (e.g., desire) is that clinicians may be able to predict the behavior of clients in treatment and identify possible causes of the behavior in order to more adequately intervene when sexual behaviors are deviant in nature.

REFERENCES

Allen, M., Dalessio, D. & Brezgel, K. (1995). A meta-analysis summarizing the effects of pornography: Aggression after exposure. *Human Communications Research, 22,* 258-283.

Baker, D. J., Blumberg, E. R., Freeman, R., & Wieseler, N. A. (2002). Can psychiatric disorders be seen as establishing operations? Integrating applied behavior analysis and psychiatry. *Mental Health Aspects of Developmental Disabilities, 5,* 118-124.

Barnard-Brak, L., Schmidt, M., Chesnut, S., Tianlan, W., & Richman, D. (2014). Predictors of access to sex education for children with intellectual disabilities in public schools. *Intellectual & Developmental Disabilities, 52,* 85-97. doi:10.1352/1934-9556-52.2.85

Becker, J. V., Harris, C. D., & Sales, B. D. (1993). Juveniles who commit sexual offenses: A critical review of research. In D. Hall (Ed.), *Sexual Aggression: Issues in Etiology, Assessment, and Treatment* (pp. 275-228). New York, NY: Taylor and Francis.

Chapman, S. L. C, & Wu, L. (2012). Substance abuse among individuals with intellectual disabilities. *Research in Developmental Disabilities, 33*, 1147-1156.

Cooper, J. O., Heron, T. E., & Heward, W. L. (2007). *Applied behavior analysis* (2nd ed.). Upper Saddle River, NJ: Pearson Education Inc.

Cuskelly, M., & Gilmore, L. (2007). Attitudes to Sexuality Questionnaire (Individuals with an Intellectual Disability): Scale development and community norms. *Journal of Intellectual and Developmental Disability, 32*, 214-221.

Dhawan, S., & Marshall, W. L. (1996). Sexual abuse histories of sexual offenders. *Sexual Abuse: A Journal of Research and Treatment, 8*, 7-15.

Diamond, M. (2009). Pornography, public acceptance and sex related crime: A review. *International Journal of Law and Psychiatry, 32*(5), 304-314.

Donnerstein, E. & Linz, D. (1998). Mass media, violence and the male viewer. In M. E. Oden and J. Clay-Warner (Eds.), *Confronting Rape and Sexual Assault* (pp 181–198). Wilmington, DE: SR Books/Scholarly Resources.

Finkelhor, D. (1986). *Child sexual abuse: New theory and research.* New York: Free Press.

Finkelhor, D. & Browne, A. (1985). The traumatic impact of child sexual abuse: A conceptualization. *American Journal of Orthopsychiatry, 55*, 530-541

Garland, R. J., & Dougher, M. J. (1990). The abused/abuser hypothesis of child sexual abuse: A critical review of theory and research. In *Pedophilia* (pp. 488-509). Springer, New York, NY.

Government of Canada. (2018, January 30). *Criminal Code.* Retrieved from: http://laws-lois.justice.gc.ca/eng/acts/C-46/FullText.html.

Government of Ontario (2008). *Services and Supports to Promote the Social Inclusion of Persons with Developmental Disabilities Act*, c. 14. Retrieved from: https://www.ontario.ca/laws/statute/08s14.

Griffiths, D. (2007). Sexuality and persons with intellectual disabilities. In I. Brown and M. Percy (Eds.) *A comprehensive guide to intellectual and developmental disabilities* (pp. 571-581). Baltimore, MD: Paul H. Brookes.

Griffiths, D., Hingsburger, D., Hoath, J., & Ioannou, S. (2013). 'Counterfeit deviance' revisited. *Journal of Applied Research in Intellectual Disabilities, 26*, 471-480.

Groth, N. (1979). Sexual trauma in the life histories of rapist and child molesters. *Victimology: An International Journal, 4*(1), 10-16.

Gunter, G. (2002). *Media sex: What are the issues?* Mahwah, NJ: Lawrence Erlbaum Associates.

Hanson, R. K., & Slater, S. (1988). Sexual victimization in the history of sexual abusers: A review. *Annals of Sex Research, 1*, 485-499.

Hingsburger, D., Griffiths, D., & Quinsey, V. (1991). Detecting counterfeit deviance: differentiating sexual deviance from sexual inappropriateness. *The Habilitative Mental Healthcare Newsletter, 10*, 51-54.

Jespersen, A. F., Lalumière, M. L., & Seto, M. C. (2009). Sexual abuse history among adult sex offenders and non-sex offenders: A meta-analysis. *Child Abuse & Neglect, 33*(3), 179-192.

Keller, F. S., & Schoenfeld, W. N. (1950). *Principles of psychology: A systematic text in the science of behavior.* New York: Appleton-Century-Crofts.

Kingston, D. A., Fedoroff, P., Firestone, P., Curry, S., & Bradford, J. M. (2008). Pornography use and sexual aggression: The impact of frequency and type of pornography use on recidivism among sexual offenders. *Aggressive Behavior: Official Journal of the International Society for Research on Aggression, 34*(4), 341-351.

Kingston, D. A., & Malamuth, N.M. (2011). Problems with aggregate data and the importance of individual differences in the study of pornography and sexual aggression: Comment on Diamond, Jozifkova, and Weiss (2010). *Archives of Sexual Behavior,* 40, 1045-1048.

Langevin, R., Handy, L., Day, D. & Russon, A. (1985). Are incestuous fathers pedophilic, aggressive and alcoholic? In R. Langevin (Ed.), *Erotic preference, gender identify and aggression* (pp. 161-180). Hillsdale, NJ: Erlbaum.

Langthorne, P., & McGill, P. (2009). A tutorial on the concept of the motivating operation and its importance to application. *Behavior Analysis in Practice, 2,* 22–31.

Laraway, S., Snycerski, S., Michael, J., & Poling, A. (2003). Motivating operations and terms to describe them: Some further refinements. *Journal of Applied Behavior Analysis, 36,* 407-414.

Laws, D. R., & Marshall, W. L. (1990). A conditioning theory of the etiology and maintenance of deviant sexual preference and behavior. In W. L. Marshall, D. R. Laws, & H. E. Barbaree (Eds.), *Handbook of sexual assault: Issues, theories, and treatment of the offender* (pp. 209-229). New York: Plenum Press.

Lindsay, W. R., Elliot, S. F., & Astell, A. (2004). Predictors of sexual offense recidivism in offenders with intellectual disabilities. *Journal of Applied Research in Intellectual Disabilities, 17,* 299-305.

Lindsay, W., Steptoe, L., & Haut, F. (2012). Brief report: The sexual and physical abuse histories of offenders with intellectual disability. *Journal of Intellectual Disability Research, 56,* 326-331.

Lofthouse, R. E., Lindsay, W. R., Totsika, V., Hastings, R. P., Boer, D. P., & Haaven, J. L. (2013). Prospective dynamic assessment of risk of sexual reoffending in individuals with an intellectual disability and a history of sexual offending behavior. *Journal of Applied Research in Intellectual Disabilities, 26,* 394-403.

Marshall, W. L., & Barrett, S. (1990). *Criminal neglect: Why sex offenders go free.* Toronto: Doubleday.

Martin, G. L. & Pear, J. J. (2015). ***Behavior modification: what it is and how to do it*** (10th ed.). New York, NY: Routledge.

Michael, J. (1982). Distinguishing between discriminative and motivational functions of stimuli. *Journal of Experimental Analysis of Behavior, 37,* 149-155.

Michael, J. (1983). Evocative and repertoire-altering effects of an environmental event. *The Analysis of Verbal Behavior, 2,* 19-21.

Michael, J. (1993). Establishing operations. *The Behavior Analyst, 16,* 191-206.

Michael J. (2007). Motivating operations. In J.O Cooper T. E. Heron, & W. L. Heward (Eds). *Applied Behavior Analysis* (2nd ed., pp. 374–391). NJ: Merrill Prentice Hall; 2007.

Money, J. (1986). *Lovemaps: Clinical concepts of sexual/erotic health and pathology, paraphilia, and gender transposition of childhood, adolescence, and maturity.* Ardent Media.

Pithers, W. D. (1993). Treatment of rapists: Reinterpretation of early outcome data and exploratory constructs to enhance therapeutic efficacy. In D. Hall (Ed.), *Sexual aggression: Issues in etiology, assessment, and treatment* (pp. 167-196). New York, NY: Taylor and Francis.

Quinsey, V. L., & Earls, C. M. (1990). The modification of sexual preferences. In W. L. Marshall, D. R. Barbaree, & H. E. Barbaree (Eds.), *Handbook of sexual assault: Issues, theories, and treatment of the offender* (pp. 279-295). New York: Plenum Press.

Ramasubramanian, S, & Oliver, M. B. (2003). Portrayals of sexual violence in popular Hindi films, 1997–1999. *Sex Roles, 48,*327–336.

Reyes, J. R., Vollmer, T. R., & Hall, A. (2011). The influence of presession factors in the assessment of deviant arousal. *Journal of Applied Behavior Analysis, 44,* 707-717.

Schmucker, M., & Lösel, F. (2015). The effects of sexual offender treatment on recidivism: An international meta-analysis of sound quality evaluations. *Journal of Experimental Criminology, 11*(4), 597-630.

Seto, M. C., Maric, A., Barbaree, H. E. (2001). The role of pornography in the etiology of sexual aggression. *Aggression and Violent Behavior, 6,* 35-53.

Skinner, B. F. (1938). *The behavior of organisms: An experimental analysis.* New York: Appleton-Century-Crofts.

Skinner, B. F. (1953). *Science and human behavior.* New York: The Macmillan Company.

Sobsey, D. (1994). *Violence and abuse of persons with intellectual disabilities.* Baltimore MD: Paul H. Brookes.

Vega, V. & Malamuth, N. M. (2007). Predicting sexual aggression: the role of pornography in the context of general and specific risk factors *Aggressive Behavior, 33,* 104-117

Ward, T., Polatchik, D. & Beech, A. T. (2005). *Theories of sexual offending.* Cichester, UK: John Wiley & Sons.

Wilson, R. J. & Burns, M. (2011). *Intellectual disability and problems in sexual behavior: Assessment, treatment, and promotion of healthy sexuality.* Holyoke, MA: NEARI press.

Wulfert, E., Greenway, D. E., & Dougher, M. J. (1996). A logical functional analysis of reinforcement-based disorders: alcoholism and pedophilia. *Journal of Consulting and Clinical Psychology, 64,* 1140-1151.

Chapter Six

Exploring the Functions of Sexual Offending Behavior in Persons with an Intellectual Disability

At face value, sex offending behavior, either in the form of rape against an adult or child molestation, makes little sense. The issue of arousal becomes even more confusing when the more unusual aberrant sexual behavior such as voyeurism, sexual sadism, or exhibitionism is explored. However, from a behavioral perspective what appears to be senseless or bizarre sexual behavior to the observer may be because the reinforcement history of that offender is simply unknown. (McGuire, 2001, p. 129)

All behavior serves a function, including sexual offending behavior. "Functional assessment of problem behavior is a *process* that involves a lot of highly discriminated, professional expertise. More precisely, it is a process by which the variables influencing problem behavior are identified" (Hanley, 2012, p. 54). The functional assessment process allows practitioners to gather information about the antecedent and consequence variables that are functionally-related to the behavior to identify an effective treatment for the problem behavior (Miltenberger, 1997). In isolating these variables, clinicians have used four basic functions to describe why behavior occurs. These functions are either socially mediated (access to a tangible, attention from others, escape from demands) or non-socially mediated (pain reduction/sensory stimulation) (Carr, 1977; Iwata, Dorsey, Slifer, Bauman, & Richman, 1982). Functional replacement requires an understanding of which of these function(s) reinforces and motivates the behavior and then finding a more appropriate replacement behavior that serves the same function. To do so, an analysis is conducted to determine the situation in which the behavior is most likely to occur based on which function (attention, tangible, escape, or sensory) is maintaining it. However, can a functional assessment be conducted on sexual offending behavior? Can a function be properly assessed and analyzed with behaviors that are so dangerous and harmful?

Sexual offending behavior may be perceived to be the result of "inappropriately reinforced responding" in which the individual has found that some goal, such as social attention or sexual satisfaction, can be gained by engaging in a sexually inappropriate behavior (McGuire, 2001, p. 129). Sexual offending behavior can be maintained by both positive and negative reinforcement. Alternatively, if a sexual offense results in the removal of a discomfort, such as loneliness or feelings of loss or rage, then the behavior will also be negatively reinforced. McGuire (2001) further notes, however, that secondary reinforcement can also play a role. "Secondary reinforcement postulates that a neutral stimulus, such as infliction of pain, accompanying primary rewards, such as orgasm, would acquire a conditioned reward value of its own right" (p. 132). For example, an individual engaging in an assault may see fear or humiliation in the victim. This can positively reinforce the act of forced sexual contact in the future. The sexual satisfaction and the reaction of the victim can combine to strengthen the behavior and the likelihood of it occurring again in the future.

Classic research studies involving persons with intellectual disabilities demonstrated that behaviors serve four basic functions: attention (Lovaas, Frietag, Gold, & Kassorla, 1965), escape or avoidance (Carr, 1977), access to tangibles (Durand & Crimmins, 1988) and automatic reinforcement (Rincover, Cook, Peoples, & Packard, 1979). More recent research in ABA has shown that these contingencies can operate on their own or simultaneously (Hanley, Jin, Vanselow, & Hanratty, 2014). For example, does the behavior serve to bring about attention in order to gain tangible reinforcement, social reward, or access to a desired activity? Does the behavior serve to escape an undesired task/activity in order to access automatic reinforcement?

Although reported to be successful, previous behavioral approaches to the treatment of inappropriate sexual behavior by persons with intellectual disabilities relied on treatment interventions without knowledge of the function the behavior served (Fyffe, Kahng, Fittro, & Russell 2004). They cite as examples Provinale and Lutzker (1980) who employed restitutional overcorrection and differential reinforcement and LeBlanc, Hagopian, and Maglieri (2000) who used a token economy and response cost procedure. Moreover, Haynes and O'Brien (1990) noted that despite best practice guidelines and ethical standards, many behavior analysts do not base intervention decisions on a functional analysis. In other words, many clinicians who approach these behaviors in practice are not basing their treatments on an evidence-based process. This appears to be more often the case when dealing with sexualized offending behaviors. As a result, behavior analysts may be providing intervention without accurately identifying the function of the behavior. A lack of identification of function presents significant concern regarding the efficacy of the treatments being employed and equal concern for the ethics in using treatments that are subjective and based in opinion instead of data. Additionally, researchers note that in the treatment of other severe and challenging behaviors, any behavioral treatment is more effective and less restrictive if based on behavioral function (Kahng, Iwata, & Lewin, 2002). This practice is not only likely to lead to ineffective intervention but may indeed reinforce the behavior that the intervention intends to reduce.

Different individuals who sexually offend are motivated differently; they do not all commit sexual assaults for the same reasons, nor are they reinforced in similar manners (McGuire, 2001). Hazelwood and Harpold (1986) suggested that strategies that may be effective in reducing offenses for one individual may have the opposite effects on another and may actually lead to strengthening of their motivation to offend.

Fredericks and Nishioka-Evans (1999) noted that "very little research has extended functional assessment procedures to the issue of sex offenders" (p. 280) yet explain that the current methodology employed in sexual violence prevention conforms to the techniques employed to conduct functional assessments. These techniques include self-report data from the individual and observations of others, in addition to the use of plethysmography as an objective measure of arousal.

Some behavioral researchers have demonstrated that they were able to employ functional assessment to demonstrate the function of sexualized offending behavior in persons with intellectual disabilities. Fyffe and colleagues (2004) conducted a functional analysis of the inappropriate sexual behavior of a nine-year old boy with traumatic brain damage to determine a functionally based treatment strategy. They found that the behavior served the function of gaining attention; the therapeutic approach employed was communication training and extinction. Similarly, Wright, Herzog, and Seymour (1992) identified that a man with Down's syndrome, who touched staff in a sexualized way, exposed his genitalia, and made sexually suggestive comments, did so to both gain access to attention, as well as to escape from a task. It is also pertinent, however, to assess for idiosyncrasies when determining functions of behavior. In particular, is there something specific about the type of reward desired or the unpleasant situation that the person seeks to escape or avoid? Is attention from a specific individual more reinforcing? Is the behavior designed to escape boredom, avoid a certain unpleasant situation or task, or reduce an internal discomfort or distress such as anxiety or anger?

A behavior analyst would expand the assessment of function to determine if this is indeed the case or if the behavior serves more than one function. Sexual behavior typically results in two immediate responses: attention and distance from the individual. These behaviors are naturally reinforced heavily and quickly in the environment if the function is based in either attention or escape. A case presentation by Hoath and Boutsis (2010) described an individual who was grabbing female staff's genitals. The immediate response was attention from staff, removal from the area, and redirection. When the data were further analyzed, it became clear that escape from aversive situations was the motivating contingency. Treatment involved teaching functional communication that enabled the individual to escape from these situations; the result was a nearly 70% decrease in the behavior almost immediately. Cases like this highlight the need for a thorough assessment and function-based treatment, regardless of topography.

FUNCTIONAL BEHAVIORAL ASSESSMENT

Functional behavioral assessment (FBA) often includes a combination of indirect measures (interviews, questionnaires, etc.), descriptive/direct measures (direct observation without manipulation, antecedent, behavior, consequence data, etc.), and functional analysis (direct observation with the manipulation of environmental events) (Hanley, 2012; Iwata, Vollmer & Zarcone, 1990; Iwata et al., 1982).

> *A functional analysis aims to identify: (1) the environmental context in which the sexual offending behavior occurs, (2) the frequency that the sexual offending behavior occurs, (3) the immediate and delayed consequences to the offender of his sex offending behavior, both positive and negative, and finally (4) access to appropriate reinforcing variables in the offender's current lifestyle (McGuire, 2001, p. 142).*

Although functional assessment/analysis is standard practice in ABA for evaluating variables associated with challenging behaviors in persons with intellectual disabilities, it appears unlikely that this approach, as traditionally applied, has been employed typically to evaluate sexualized offending behavior. However, application of a functional analysis can lead to defining and prioritization of areas for individualized treatment (McGuire, 2001).

Some authors, such as Iwata and Dozier (2008) and Hanley et al. (2014), have developed methods to modify functional analysis to accommodate for these challenges. Hanley (2012), in discussing other challenging behavior, suggests a three-stage assessment including a structured, open-ended interview, a brief observation of the problem behavior to identify putative factors that may be influencing the behavior, and a targeted functional analysis founded on the outcomes of the indirect and direct assessments to test the contingencies maintaining problem behavior. A functional analysis involves "identification of relevant, controllable and causal functional relations that apply to particular behaviors of an individual" (Haynes et al., 1993, p. 191; Iwata et al., 1982). The assessment results should lead to a case formulation based on the relationship between the behavioral features and those events that are associated with the behavior.

Direct Observation Methods

Direct observation methods, in which the person is observed, and the antecedents and consequences related to the behavior are recorded over time, pose unique challenges for observing sexualized offending behavior due to the low frequency, covertness, and potential for harm to others (Vollmer, Reyes & Walker, 2012). Assessing the function of sexual offending behavior through direct observation raises both practical and ethical challenges; sexual offending behaviors are typically high intensity, low frequency behaviors by nature with significant impact and immediate consequences. These behaviors are extremely difficult to predict and are far too dangerous to be evoked for the purposes of direct assessment. In fact, any indicators that offending may occur should result in an immediate response from caregivers to prevent the behavior from occurring. When it does occur, it often occurs in private and given the highly reinforcing nature of the behavior, individuals who have sexually offended typically go to great lengths to conceal it. This means that typical methods, such as direct observation to conduct a functional assessment, are difficult although there are some exceptions in the literature as noted above (See Fyffe et al., 2004 and Wright et al., 1992).

Because persons who have sexually offended are often not in settings where the behavior can be observed or where there is little or no opportunity to observe the individual in natural circumstances with potentially vulnerable persons, the therapist must rely more on indirect functional assessment or experimental methods. As a result, behavioral analysts may need to be creative in assessing the function of these behaviors. Smith and Churchill (2002) evaluated the value of examining the function of precursor behaviors that are associated with a specific dangerous behavior as a method of functional assessment. Najdowski, Wallace, Ellsworth, MacAleese, and Cleveland, (2008) identified that there was functional similarity between the strength of precursor behaviors and severity of problem behaviors, such as those that are sexually inappropriate. In these cases, conducting a functional analysis may be unethical, and therefore the identification of the function of precursor behaviors may serve as a basis for development of functional based treatment where typical functional analysis would be avoided.

However, the use of these methods should be subject to careful clinical and ethical review to ensure they are justifiable and properly conducted (Griffiths, Ioannou, & Hoath, 2017). Hanley (2012) has suggested that in both the use of precursor analyses (Smith & Churchill, 2002) and covert observations, there is an element of inference that needs to be applied to determine behavioral function but adds to the power of the analysis when combined with file review, indirect measures (interviews), phallometric measures (both in controlled laboratory conditions and *in situ* with portable PPG; Chapter 4), sexual interest assessments, and conducting covert probes (Vollmer et al., 2012) .

Indirect Functional Assessment

Indirect functional assessment methods involve gathering information from past incidences, reviewing evaluation reports, and conducting behavioral interviews/questionnaires with the individual and others who know them best. The Functional Assessment Interview (FAI; O'Neill et al., 1997) is an effective and commonly used tool for persons with challenging behaviors and can also be used to gather more information on inappropriate sexual behavior. The indirect method of assessment also poses some unique challenges. The indirect functional assessment is used to generate objective information about the behavior and the antecedents and consequences related to that behavior based on past experiences. Therefore, it should not be relied upon alone and must be combined with direct methods of assessment, such as observing precursor behaviors.

Fredericks and Nishioka-Evans (1999) suggested that a comprehensive assessment of sexual violence potential includes a social and family history and a review of medical, clinical, and psychiatric reports, as well as a behavioral history. Unfortunately, experience has shown that reports written about sexualized behavior often lack sufficient detail to provide clear and objective hypotheses regarding the behavior. The descriptions provided rarely provide clear indications of antecedent conditions or consequences that surrounded the behavior. Additionally, reports of this nature are often prone to either positive or negative bias due to the nature of the offense and as such are lacking objectivity.

Garnering information from others who are familiar with the individual's history, in particular the index offense and any other incidence, is critical to this assessment. Factors such as the age and gender of persons harmed, the relationship of those individuals to the person engaging in sexual abuse, the details and specific nature of the offense, potential motivating operations at work, or the influence of drugs or alcohol are critical sources of information.

Fredericks and Nishioka-Evans (1999) further suggested that the history should include familial history and distal events, such as abuse and previous sexual interactions. Family and staff often serve as valuable sources of information that has been garnered through their own observations or through natural conversations. For example, they may have noted precursor behaviors that have preceded previous incidents (e.g., incessant talking about sexual things or an increase in pornography use) or at-risk behaviors that have been noted (e.g., a person with interest in children staring at youngsters through the window while masturbating).

In addition, information from the individual provides important data for the functional assessment (Fredericks & Nishioka-Evans, 1999). Unfortunately, the validity of these interviews can be hampered by both the secretive nature of the behaviors and the threat of punishment, as well as challenges due to communication skills, expression of feelings, and in providing details such as time. The therapist can seek information from the person about the offenses, the onset of offending, sexual preferences, and specific circumstances surrounding the offense. Fredericks and Nishioka-Evans (1999) suggested that through this process a therapist can evaluate the cognitive 'private' elements related to the offense such as thinking errors, fantasies underlying the offense and apparently unrelated stressors that may have been present around the time of the offense. Lindsay (2009) suggested that a key factor to examine is the individual's knowledge of the mores and laws of society and an understanding regarding which are applicable to the individual and have real consequences.

When conducting behavioral interviews to understand function, it is important to ask *what, when, and how* questions and avoid asking *why* questions (Cooper, Heron, & Heward, 2007). Asking an individual why they molested a child can evoke frustration and a negative response, because the individual likely does not know the reason behind their behavior. Similarly, asking caregivers why they think the individual sexually assaulted a woman will evoke responses that are characteristic to the individual (e.g., because they are a predator, because they are impulsive, etc.). These responses imply traits inherent in the person that cannot be altered, rather than describing the behavior, the contingencies, and the environmental circumstances in which they occur and do not occur.

Unfortunately, many of the interventions for persons who engage in sexualized offending behavior have been based on indirect evaluations only, which poses a potential risk of failing to identify the appropriate stimulus conditions, motivational factors, or other possible constellations of factors.

Experimental Methods

Experimental methods, in which antecedents or consequence variables are manipulated to influence the sexual behavior, are further fraught with ethical challenges. As with other severe behaviors such as self-injurious behavior, it is difficult and potentially unethical to set up conditions to evoke the sexual offending behavior. A typical assumption is that a sexually offensive behavior always serves the function of satisfying a sexual urge, which may include arousal in the presence of children or arousal to aspects of coercion or violence.

It would be too simplistic to say that sexual behavior in general is motivated solely by sexual arousal. There may be an obvious sensory component that is reinforcing, but what are the specific features that made it arousing? Were the features that made it reinforcing deviant (reinforced by age inappropriate or nonconsenting acts) in nature? Are there functional and appropriate replacement behaviors?

Sexually gratifying behaviors, although motivated by their physical and sensory properties, may still have complex variables that interact to make them strongly reinforcing. For example, the features of the person being abused, physical or otherwise, may be relevant. The nature of the behavior, whether it was contact (e.g., assault) or non-contact (e.g., voyeurism), may have specific relevance. Another factor that may be relevant to the reinforcing nature of the offense is the abused person's response. An example of this is exhibitionism. In these cases, a person exposes his or her genitals to another person and receives a major response from the latter.

It is critical that the function of the behavior be determined so that an appropriate replacement or compensatory skill can be provided. Assessing sexual preference (as discussed in Chapter 4) can provide insight into the potential function of a behavior, primarily by determining the likelihood that the behavior is automatically or sensorally reinforced. Being able to establish whether or not a particular abused person falls within the individual's preference and victim type indicates whether or not the behavior was functionally reinforced on its own, influenced by environmental factors or establishing operations or possibly counterfeit deviance. For example, the function of a sexual offending behavior of some individuals with an intellectual disability may not be motivated by the elements of offense (violence, humiliation, etc.), but by the natural reinforcement elements of social contact and relationships. Thus, the function is to serve to gain attention, but the means is inappropriate. Numerous methods to assess sexual arousal and preference were discussed in Chapter 4, and each has their own ethical and practical considerations (see Wilson, 2016; Wilson & Miner, 2016).

In Chapter 5 on motivating operations, we noted that there may be many proximal establishing operations that have also been linked to re-offense. Proximal establishing operations are apparently unrelated events that have occurred in close proximity to the most recent offense that serve to make it more likely that another offense might occur. These include such factors as loss of job, onset of sexual problems, isolation, or deprivation. These events may secondarily affect desired social reinforcement and self-worth and may increase the sensitivity of the triggering effect while moderating whether the individual will act on the triggering effect. Additionally, it may indicate that the behavior serves multiple functions. This does not mean that the individual is not being reinforced by the sexual contact but that the function of the behavior may be serving multiple functions: for example, sexual and reduction or alleviation of emotional discomfort. In fact, drive states have previously been linked with sexual behavior (Ariely & Loewenstein, 2006; Loewenstein, 1996), and sex as a coping skill has been identified as a dynamic risk factor (Cortoni & Marshall, 2001; Hanson, Harris, Scott & Helmus, 2007). These previously mentioned variables create a situation where sexual activity can be used to alleviate the negative emotions and impact.

LOGICAL FUNCTIONAL ASSESSMENT

Here, we will be commenting on various contributing factors that may be underlying the function of behavior. Behaviors can be multiply controlled, in that there is the function and then the maintaining contingencies. By looking beyond the function to the underlying contributing variables, we are examining behaviors *in a context* and, as such, conducting a holistic assessment is required for this population.

Sexual arousal as a sensory function will allow us to understand some persons who have sexually offended; however, "non-sexual reinforcers also need to be explored to better conceptualize the offending behavior" (McGuire, 2001, p. 142). For example, examining if there are any distinctive patterns to the assaults is important. "The sexual assaults may only occur under acute emotional episodes, such as recent rejections, separations, unanticipated social isolation, or where more related to emotional states of anger and rage" (McGuire, p. 142). Thus, the function joins together with the motivating operations to present a complex functional relationship.

This premise is founded on the understanding that there may be additional functions that contribute to or trigger the sexual offending behavior. An example would be an individual who is motivated sexually to offend against a child or other non-consenting person, but who is actively seeking to control the sexual urges. These individuals are described as following an avoidant pathway to offending (Ward, Hudson & Keenan, 1998). The avoidant individual, although attempting not to offend, may ultimately do so because of a lack of skill. Deficits in social and anger management skills or a lack of socio-sexual knowledge about age, the law, consent, and privacy are components of most sexual violence treatment programs. The premise is that persons who have sexually offended require self-regulation skills to effectively handle socio-sexual situations, or they may lack self-control to handle emotions (e.g., anger, impulsivity) when in the presence of arousing stimuli (Ward & Gannon, 2006). Another area that has been identified is a lack of empathy for persons who are victimized; this skill deficit condition may relate to a misunderstanding or lack of appreciation of the impact of the behavior on others (Wastell, Cairns, & Haywood, 2009). Although sexual gratification is a motivating force behind the offenses in these avoidant cases, it is the lack of skill that provides failure of the individual's attempts to not offend. Thus, doing a proper comprehensive assessment for function not only tells us the contingencies that are maintaining the offending behavior, but the various risk factors (setting events), skill deficits, and motivating operations that contribute to the complexity of offending behavior.

SELF-REGULATION AND PATHWAYS

The Self-Regulation or Pathways Model (see Ward, Hudson & Keenan, 1998; Yates, Prescott, & Ward, 2010), as described in Chapter 3, is a theory of sexual offending behavior that emerged from re-evaluating the previously popular relapse prevention model (see Laws, Hudson, & Ward, 2000). Instead of the previous single assumed pattern of offending, which is that all offenders actively seek to offend, it posits four distinct pathways to sexual offending, with numerous variable factors differentiating individual motivations and methods as described in Chapter 4.

The self-regulation approach has many similarities to functional behavior theories. The four basic functions are attention, tangible, escape, and sensory; these motivate and reinforce behaviors, and finding appropriate replacements that serve the same function is a cornerstone of ABA. Essentially, the function relates to the need the behavior is fulfilling; as in, what purpose did the target behavior serve? Sexual offending behavior is often seen as motivated purely by physiological desires; however as we have noted, it is not always so simple, and, as with any behavior, there may be multiple functional contributors. This is similar to self-regulation as each of the four pathways correspond to the different goals and desired outcomes of the behavior and the means in which they attempt to obtain it. The Self-Regulation/Pathways model asks what the function and motivating contingencies are that maintain a behavior, as well as the ways by which those functions are obtained; the problem is often the means by which a goal is obtained and not the goal itself. This theory would then look to find an appropriate way of obtaining the goal, building in a functional replacement.

The four self-regulation pathways included in the model are a means of describing the functions behind problematic sexual behavior and the inappropriate means of obtaining typically appropriate goals. These pathways are based on whether the goal is to engage in or avoid offending, and the means by which they obtain that goal. This perspective is unique from previous theories in that it expands upon the motivations for behavior (no longer assuming all persons who have sexually offended want to avoid re-offense), describes why the goals may be appropriate, and that the means of obtaining them are the concern.

Behavior can either be approach-based, which means an individual's behavior is in line with an offense, or avoidant-based, which means the individual's behavior is attempting to prevent offense. The choice of behavior relates to what strategies individuals used to obtain their goal. Approach-based individuals can be explicit, using planning to offend, or automatic, putting themselves in risky situations and reacting more impulsively. Avoidant-based goals are looked at in the same way, with individuals being avoidant-active in that they actively avoid re-offense and have strategies to that effect, or they are avoidant-passive and may want to avoid offending but use no strategies or methods to do so.

Other factors that need to be assessed because they may also serve to provide insight into the function served by the behavior are distal establishing operations. Distal establishing operations are events that have occurred in the distant past but may retain influence on current behavior and determine if an offense is more or less likely to occur. Historical events, such as past abuse, which is often overlooked with persons with intellectual disabilities, have been reported to be correlated to sexual offenses (see Laws & Marshall, 1990). These factors have been found to play a role potentially in proximal establishing operations or even triggers. For example, it has been observed that some individuals with intellectual disabilities who were sexually abused as children, direct their sexual advances to children of the same age and gender, and in a manner similar to their own abuse (Laws & Marshall, 1990). Laws and Marshall (1990) proposed a theory that sexual interest in children is conditioned during the individual's developing years. This conditioning theory is, perhaps, particularly relevant for persons with intellectual disabilities, for whom the abusive event may have been their initial and possibly repeated sexual contact and, in the absence of counselling or sexual education to the contrary, may replay their own learned traumagenic experience. As noted earlier, some research suggests that not only the presence but type of abuse affects later offending (Lindsay, Law, Quinn, Smart, & Smith, 2001). Individuals who were sexually abused later engaged in topographically similar behaviors as did those who were physically abused.

Other distal factors may relate to a lack of experience in areas such as moral or legal instruction or a harboring of cognitive distortions relative to sexuality that may relate to inappropriate sexual histories (e.g., institutionalization or abuse). Cognitive distortions are important to assess and may be difficult to treat. These are deep-seated beliefs that some researchers assert may contribute to pro-offending behaviors or that may lead to more hostile world perspectives, reducing victim empathy and making offending behaviors more likely (Helmus, Hanson, Babchishin, & Mann, 2013).

GOOD LIVES MODEL

The Good Lives Model (GLM; Ward & Stewart, 2003; Yates, Prescott, & Ward, 2010) is an individualized assessment and treatment model that is complementary to Self-Regulation/Pathways. GLM is a strength-based system that assesses individuals holistically, as well as important life goals, known in GLM parlance as primary goods (see Peel Behavioral Service & Wilson, 2017). Essentially, it is important to assess what is important to clients and how they achieve these primary goods? In terms of treatment for sexual violence, the Good Lives Model is used to find functional replacements and competing reinforcers to limit the need for and desire to engage in sexual offending behaviors. The theory is behavioral in nature and the assessment process involves isolating the goals in the individual's life that they value, as well as any needs that are currently unmet. Essentially, the model looks at what motivates and reinforces individuals and whether the means of attaining reinforcement are appropriate. The goals are not often the issue; rather the means of attaining the goals are problematic. Often, there are multiple reinforcers at play in offending behavior, which can include intimacy and physical sensations. Even if there are no appropriate replacements for these behaviors, if the behavior is violent or intrinsically deviant and the reinforcing properties cannot be replicated safely, adherence to GLM constructs can be used to provide the individual with a life worth having. Essentially, building natural and contrived reinforcements for the individual provides competing reinforcers to offending behaviors. These goods are often incompatible with offending and the legal consequences within and this can be used to motivate the individual to manage risk.

Treatment using the Good Lives approach (Ward & Marshall, 2004) can include teaching functionally specific replacement behaviors or creating a wider range of positive behaviors and interactions that can be reinforced to enhance quality of life. A Good Lives assessment would involve identifying what life goals the person may have that have been missed or sought inappropriately; life goals can include areas that may be pursued to enrich the person's life and to provide valuable sources of positive reinforcement valued by the person and, as such, worth defending. During a Good Lives assessment, the clinician will identify flaws in the client's Good Lives plan. These flaws can include how the individual achieves their goals, as well as lack of scope in the number of goals or incompatible goals. Treatment focuses on two aspects: finding solutions for the flaws in goals and in building a number of pro-social goods to create a life worth keeping. A lack of scope refers to an individual with very few valued goals. Individuals in this situation may find that offending is one of the only reinforcing activities remaining in someone's life, and, therefore, it is difficult to establish competing goals. Inappropriate means often refers directly to the offending behavior itself, as the goal behind the behavior may be prosocial (e.g., sexual relationship), but the means of achieving the goal is antisocial or criminal (e.g., coercive sexual behavior). Incompatibility refers to two or more goals that are competing or mutually exclusive; treatment involves highlighting these incompatibilities as they relate to offending. This is critical for motivation, in that it is important to identify conflict between sexual offending behaviors and other life goals. Sexual offending behaviors typically result in a number of sanctions that limit freedom and employment opportunities, among other consequences, and ultimately have a dramatic impact on social supports. Offending is incompatible with many other valued goals, and this conflict needs to be highlighted in treatment, especially if client motivation is poor.

More functionally based goals found in the Good Lives plan can shed light on the motivating causes and functions of the offending. The behavior may be motivated by a goal that is achieved by inappropriate means; for instance, the goal of happiness (seeking pleasure and contentment in one's life) can be achieved through coercive or deviant sexual activity. The goal of pleasure is not inherently flawed, but the means of attaining it are. If the goal can be shaped to something more appropriate – through skill building and opportunities – then the inappropriate and antisocial behaviors used to attain that goal should decrease. If the goal is prosocial, but was being sought through inappropriate means, then a functional replacement can be sought by changing the means of attaining that goal.

Sexual behavior can be linked to a number of goals. It may serve to bring physical pleasure, be a release from anger, or be a means of releasing stress or anxiety. Some of these goals appear more internal and difficult to quantify and describe than the traditional functions; however, these goals can have an impact on behavior and assessing their influence is worth the effort. The goal of emotional regulation may be implicated in the behavior, and research has suggested this may play a factor in offending to the extent that it is recognized as a dynamic risk factor for re-offense (Hanson et al., 2007). The key is in providing the individual with the skills required to self-manage and return to a preferred state in a more pro-social way. This can include dialectical behavior or cognitive behavioral techniques depending on functioning level. Some individuals can learn Dialectical Behavior Therapy techniques (DBT; Linehan, 1993), such as Soles of the Feet (Singh, Wahler, Adkins & Myers, 2003) to maintain stability. DBT works on managing emotional and cognitive responses to alter maladaptive behavior patterns. In Soles of the Feet, focus is shifted to different parts of the body as a means of recognizing physiological changes and reclaiming balance. For other individuals, speaking with a therapist or engaging in shared problem-solving may be necessary. All strategies must be modified and individualized for the clients with intellectual disabilities, as many individuals in this population may have difficulty with abstract concepts or techniques.

Sexual behavior is sometimes motivated or reinforced by a desire for power and control. Good Lives theory incorporates the need for control and recognizes it as an essential good – autonomy. Autonomy is defined as having control and a sense of independence; this can be demonstrated by having a job, living on your own, and being self-sustaining. These are appropriate means of attaining that good but given the lives often typical of individuals with intellectual disabilities, it is difficult or potentially impossible to achieve these goals as the struggle for greater decision-making authority is a longstanding one (Jenkinson, 1993). Individuals with an intellectual disability (including those who offend) are rarely in competitive employment and typically live in residential settings with support staff controlling the majority of their decisions. This leaves little opportunity for independence and freedom, which may create a need that manifests in less appropriate ways. As such "(control issues) and agency (self-esteem) may be imported to the sexual domain and subjugated to the overriding end of sexual satisfaction" (Ward & Gannon, 2006). Acts of coercion and force during sexual offending can serve to provide a sense of power that is otherwise absent from the individual's life (i.e., when individuals are tightly controlled, sometimes the only decision they have left is the decision to act out in defiance of that control). The sense of control may be more localized and less global, and sexual control may be specifically reinforcing. Individuals who target children may feel a sense of accomplishment in tricking or manipulating those they victimize by establishing a position of trust. For individuals who use physical force in their offending, this serves a similar role in providing a sense of authority and power. As stated according to Good Lives theory, the goals of autonomy and independence are not inappropriate, but the means of attaining these goals may be harmful and include elements of deviance.

SUMMARY

The purpose of a functional analysis of sex offending is to both eliminate (not just reduce) sexual offending behavior and to also provide appropriate alternative behaviors (that either replace or compensate for the offending behavior). "If the offender is not taught appropriate behavior to engage in for reinforcements, there will be an eventual return to previous behavior" (McGuire, 2001, p, 142).

In the chapters that follow, intervention approaches will be explored to develop treatment that addresses the function of the behavior. Function-based treatment focuses on the specific goals outlined in the assessment, whether the individual is approach or avoidant-based. If the function of the behavior is approach-based and the individual is motivated to re-offend, then this must be addressed. In the approach-based pathways, the function is the offending itself; this means that motivation to remain offense-free must be addressed or functionally replaced. In these cases, the Good Lives Model is invaluable in targeting motivation. Otherwise, the means of achieving the goal (i.e., sexual pleasure) can often be appropriately replaced. Through skill building and embedding social opportunities, appropriate and consenting intimate relationships can be fostered. If the topography and reinforcing properties are more deviant in nature, as assessed through sexual preference/interest measures, then the issue becomes more complex, and risk management – rather than internal motivation – may be required to ensure community safety.

The means of attaining any particular life goal may also be targeted. If motivation to remain offense-free is present, then treatment is focused on skill building. In this scenario, the individual wants to change his previous behavior patterns but finds the process difficult. Numerous areas need to be targeted, depending on the individual's history and typical pathway to offending. Avoidant-based individuals are either passive or active, relating to what strategies they previously used (or didn't use) to avoid re-offense. Avoidant individuals either have no strategies to avoid re-offense (passive) or have strategies that are poorly used or ineffective (active). Treatment should focus on filling those gaps, providing knowledge and skills to avoid re-offense based on an assessment of the deficits present.

REFERENCES

Ariely, D., & Loewenstein, G. (2006). The heat of the moment: The effect of sexual arousal on sexual decision making. *Journal of Behavioral Decision Making, 19*(2), 87-98.

Carr, E. G. (1977). The motivation of self-injurious behavior: A review of some hypotheses. *Psychological Bulletin, 84*, 800-816.

Cooper, J. O., Heron, T. E., & Heward, W. L. (2007). *Applied behavior analysis*, (2nd ed.). Upper Saddle River, NJ: Pearson Education Inc.

Cortoni, F., & Marshall, W. L. (2001). Sex as a coping strategy and its relationship to juvenile sexual history and intimacy in sexual offenders. *Sexual Abuse: A Journal of Research and Treatment, 13*(1), 27-43.

Durand, V. M, & Crimmins, D.B. (1988). Identifying the variables maintaining self-injurious behavior. *Journal of Autism and Developmental Disorders, 18*, 99-117.

Fredericks, B. & Nishioka-Evans, V. (1999). Functional assessment for a sex offender population. In A. C. Repp & R. H. Horner (Eds.), *Functional analysis of problem behavior: From effective assessment to effective support* (pp. 279-305). Belmont, CA: Wadsworth Publishing Co.

Fyffe, C. E., Kahng, S., Fittro, E., & Russell, D. (2004). Functional analysis and treatment of inappropriate sexual behavior. *Journal of Applied Behavior Analysis, 37*, 401-404.

Griffiths, D., Ioannou, S. & Hoath, J. (2017). Sexuality and people who have developmental disabilities: From myth to emerging practices. In M. Wehmeyer, I. Brown, M. Percy, K.A. Shogren, W.L.A. Fung (Eds.), *A Comprehensive Guide to Intellectual and Developmental Disabilities.* (pp. 596-608). Baltimore, MD: Paul H. Brookes.

Hanley, G. P. (2012). Functional assessment of problem behavior: Dispelling myths, overcoming implementation obstacles, and developing new lore. *Behavior Analysis in Practice*, 5, 54-72.

Hanley, G. P., Jin, C. S., Vanselow, N. R., & Hanratty, L. A. (2014). Producing meaningful improvements in problem behavior of children with autism via synthesized analyses and treatments. *Journal of Applied Behavior Analysis, 47*(1), 16-36.

Hanson, R. K., Harris, A.J., Scott, T. L., & Helmus, L. (2007). *Assessing the risk of sexual offenders on community supervision: The Dynamic Supervision Project* (Vol. 5, No. 6). Ottawa, ON: Public Safety Canada.

Haynes, S. N., & O'Brien, W. H. (1990). Functional analysis in behavior therapy. *Clinical Psychology Review, 10*(6), 649-668.

Haynes, S. N., Uchigakiuchi, P. Meyer, K., Orimoto, L., Blaine, D., & Obrien, W.H. (1993). Functional analytic causal modes and the design of treatment programs: Concepts and clinical applications with childhood behavior problems. *European Journal of Psychological Assessment, 9*, 189-205.

Hazelwood R. R. & Harpold, J. A. (1986). Rape: The dance of providing confrontational advice. *FBI Law Enforcement Bulletin*, 55, 1-5.

Helmus, L., Hanson, K. R., Babchishin, K. M., & Mann, R. E. (2013). Attitudes supportive of sexual offending predict recidivism. *Trauma, Violence, & Abuse, 14*(1), 34-53.

Hoath, J., & Boutsis, E. (2010). ABA and sexually acting out behavior in individuals with intellectual disabilities: assessment and treatment. Presented at the *Association for the Treatment of Sexual Abusers Conference*, Phoenix, AZ.

Iwata, B. A., & Dozier, C. L. (2008). Clinical application of functional analysis methodology. *Behavior Analysis in Practice, 1*(1), 3-9.

Iwata, B. A., Dorsey, M. F., Slifer, K. J., Bauman, K. E., & Richman, G. S. (1982). Toward a functional analysis of self-injury. *Analysis and Intervention in Developmental Disabilities, 2*(1), 3-20.

Iwata, B. A., Vollmer, T. R., & Zarcone, J. R. (1990). The experimental (functional) analysis of behavior disorders: *Methodology, applications, and limitations, 27*(2), 215-241

Jenkinson, J. C. (1993). Who shall decide? The relevance of theory and research to decision-making by people with an intellectual disability. *Disability, Handicap & Society, 8*(4), 361-375.

Kahng, S., Iwata, B. A., & Lewin, A. B. (2002). Behavioral treatment of self-injury, 1964 to 2000. *American Journal on Mental Retardation, 107*(3), 212-221.

Laws, D. R., Hudson, S. M. & Ward T. (2000). *Remaking relapse prevention with sex offenders: A sourcebook.* Thousand Oaks, CA: Sage.

Laws, D. R. & Marshall, W. L. (1990). A conditioning theory of the etiology and maintenance of deviant sexual preference and behavior. In W. L. Marshall, D. LR. Laws and H. E. Barbaree (Eds.), *Handbook of sexual assault: Issues, theories and treatment of the offender* (pp. 209-229). New York: Plenum Press.

Leblanc, L. A., Hagopian, L. P., & Maglieri, K. A. (2000). Use of a token economy to eliminate excessive inappropriate social behavior in an adult with developmental disabilities. *Behavioral Interventions, 15*(2), 135-143.

Lindsay, W. R. (2009). *The treatment of sex offenders with developmental disabilities: A practice workbook.* Chichester, UK: Wiley-Blackwell.

Lindsay, W. R., Law, J., Quinn, K., Smart, N., & Smith, A. H. W. (2001). A comparison of physical and sexual abuse: Histories of sexual and non-sexual offenders with intellectual disability. *Child Abuse and Neglect, 25*(7), 989-995.

Linehan, M. M. (1993). *Cognitive behavioral treatment of borderline personality disorder.* New York: Guilford

Loewenstein, G. (1996). Out of control: Visceral influences on behavior. *Organizational behavior and human decision processes, 65*(3), 272-292.

Lovaas, O. I., Frietag, G., Gold, V. J.., & Kassorla, J. C. (1965). Experimental studies in childhood schizophrenia. *Journal of Experimental Child Psychology, 2,* 67-84.

McGuire, T. J. (2001). Sex offending: a behavioral analysis perspective. *Advances in Psychology Research, 6,* 129-155.

Miltenberger, R. (1997). *Behavior modification: principles and practice.* Pacific Grove, CA: Brooks/Cole.

Najdowski, A., Wallace, M., Ellsworth, C., MacAleese, A., & Cleveland, I. (2008). Functional analyses and treatment of precursor behavior. *Journal of Applied Behavior Analysis, 41,* 97-105.

O'Neill, R. E., Horner, R. H., Albin, R. W., Sprague, J. R., Storey, K., & Newton, J. S. (1997). *Functional assessment and program development for problem behavior.* Pacific Grove, CA: Brooks/Cole Publishing

Peel Behavioral Service & Wilson, R.J. (2017). *Passport to independence.* Holyoke, MA: NEARI Press.

Provinale, R. ., & Lutzker, J. R. (1980). Elimination of assaultive and inappropriate sexual behavior by reinforcement and social restitution. *Mental Retardation, 18,* 27-30.

Rincover, A., Cook, R., Peoples, A., & Packard, D. (1979). Sensory extinction and sensory reinforcement principles for programming multiple adaptive behavior change. *Journal of Applied Behavior Analysis, 12,* 221–233.

Singh, N. N., Wahler, R. G., Adkins, A. D., Myers, R. E., & Mindfulness Research Group. (2003). Soles of the feet: A mindfulness-based self-control intervention for aggression by an individual with mild mental retardation and mental illness. *Research in Developmental Disabilities, 24*(3), 158-169.

Smith, R. G., & Churchill, R. M. (2002). Identification of environmental determinants of behavior disorders through functional analysis of precursor behaviors. *Journal of Applied Behavior Analysis, 35*(2), 125-136.

Vollmer, T. R., Reyes, J. R., & Walker, S. F. (2012). Behavioral assessment and intervention for sex offenders with intellectual and developmental disabilities. In. J.K. Luiselli (Ed.), *A handbook of high-risk challenging behaviors in people with intellectual and developmental disabilities (pp. 121-144).* Baltimore, MD: Paul H. Brookes.

Ward, T. & Gannon, T. A. (2006). Rehabilitation, etiology, and self-regulation: The comprehensive good lives model of treatment for sexual offenders. *Aggression and Violent Behavior, 11,* 77–94.

Ward, T., Hudson, S. M., & Keenan, T. (1998). A self-regulation model of the sexual offense process. *Sexual Abuse: A Journal of Research and Treatment, 10,* 141-157.

Ward, T., & Hudson, S. M. (1998). A model of the relapse process in sexual offenders. *Journal of Interpersonal Violence, 13*(6), 700-725.

Ward, T., & Marshall, W. L. (2004). Good lives, etiology, and the rehabilitation of sex offenders: A bridging theory. *Journal of Sexual Aggression, 10,* 153 – 169

Ward, T., & Stewart, C.A. (2003). The treatment of sexual offenders: Risk management and good lives. *Professional Psychology: Research and Practice, 34,* 353-360.

Wastell, C. A., Cairns, D., & Haywood, H. (2009). Empathy training, sex offenders and re-offending. *Journal of Sexual Aggression, 15*(2), 149-159.

Wilson, R. J. (2016). The use of phallometric testing in the diagnosis, treatment, and risk management of male adults who have sexually offended. In L. Craig & M. Rettenberger (Eds.), *The Wiley handbook on the theories, assessment & treatment of sexual offending: Volume 2* (pp. 823-849). Chichester, UK: Wiley-Blackwell

Wilson, R. J. & Miner, M. H. (2016). Measurement of male sexual arousal and interest using penile plethysmography and viewing time. In D.R. Laws & W.T. O'Donohue (Eds.), *Treatment of sex offenders: Strengths and weaknesses in assessment and intervention.* New York: Springer.

Wright, D., Herzog. G., & Seymour, J. (1992). Treatment of a constellation of inappropriate sexual and social behaviors in a 20-year old man with Down syndrome. *Sexuality and Disability, 10,* 57-61.

Yates, P. M., Prescott, D. S., & Ward, T. (2010). *Applying the good lives and self-regulation models to sex offender treatment: A practical guide for clinicians.* Brandon, VT: Safer Society Press.

Chapter Seven

Combining Assessment Components into an Integrated Treatment Plan

Behavior analysts have known since the 1960s (Ayllon & Azrin, 1968) that inappropriate behaviors can be reduced by rewarding appropriate behaviors or providing the individual with access to reinforcement for an alternative appropriate behavior that serves the same function as an inappropriate or challenging behavior (Azrin & Holz, 1966). Since the 1980s these principles have become standard in any program designed to reduce an inappropriate behavior, except in the area of sexually inappropriate behavior.

As noted in Chapter One, there are seven characteristics of ABA that need to be built into any program (Baer, Wolf, & Risley,1968). To recap, first, it must be *applied* to a behavior that has social significance or direct relevance to the individual. Second, *behavioral* approaches are systematic and must be measured precisely. Third, the analysis must demonstrate that the program (or specific variables) account for the occurrence and non-occurrence of the behavior. Fourth, it must be *technological*, meaning that the program must be operationally defined to limit confusion and ensure consistency. Fifth, it must be based on *conceptual systems* by describing procedures in the same terms as they were derived from the science of behavior. Sixth is that it must show *effectiveness* by demonstrating change in a socially significant behavior that is sufficient to be meaningful or has practical value to the individual(s). Seventh, the behavior must have *generalized* outcomes, which will occur in all applicable environments and in the presence of multiple people.

In preceding chapters, we have demonstrated how current standards of practice can be used to determine the factors that might influence the commission of a sexual offense and how those could be applied to an integrated treatment package (e.g., function, antecedents and consequences, and motivating operations) that uses such knowledge to establish a program of prevention and intervention.

As we have mentioned earlier, one of the first caveats when treating this type of problem is prevention. Unlike other inappropriate behaviors, there is a zero tolerance for even one sexual offense (Lindsay, 2015), with "no more victims" being a familiar societal refrain. A reduction in the behavior, even significantly, is not considered to be acceptable in society or clinically. Therefore, with sexual offending behavior the goal is to eliminate the possibility of a re-offense entirely through a combination of treatment and prevention strategies.

In order to demonstrate how to pull integrated treatment together, we will revisit the cases we introduced at the beginning of the book. A comprehensive treatment package for any individual who has offended would include multiple elements that respond to the assessment findings. They would include teaching alternative and coping skills to compensate for or modify the inappropriate behavior, such as education about and establishing known consequences, adjusting the antecedents that were associated with the offense, and modifying the motivating operations to establish a non-offense pattern.

However, first and foremost, the initial focus is on ensuring that there is no future re-offense, which means establishing environmental supports to protect both the individual and potentially vulnerable persons. When the treatment effects have been demonstrated and maintained under conditions where protection is assured, then generalization to all settings where the individual will frequent, with different people and involving multiple scenarios, must be trained for and assessed.

Let's begin with the Case of Jerry.

THE CASE OF JERRY

Jerry is a 21-year-old male, diagnosed with mild intellectual disability, oppositional defiant disorder, and attention deficit hyperactivity disorder. He is the eldest son in his family. Jerry's family did not have a lot of money, so he often had to find ways to keep himself busy. His father believed that men were the head of the household, so Jerry had to learn on his own how to be a man, just like his dad did.

Jerry has a long history of engaging in sexual assault; the first was when he was 16 and he fondled a 5-year-old girl in his neighbourhood. There were no charges, as the family dealt with the assault internally. When Jerry was 17, he invited a 7-year-old neighborhood boy into his family home to watch movies in the basement. Jerry's parents were upstairs and believed it was okay for him to invite a boy into the basement because "Jerry is like a child himself." Jerry rubbed himself on top of the boy with their clothes on; the boy told his parents and police arrived at Jerry's house. Jerry's parents minimized the assault and placed blame on the boys' parents for not keeping track of their son. No charges were laid with the agreement that Jerry would leave the neighborhood.

When Jerry was 19 he was placed in a secure group home an hour from his parent's house, with 24/7 staffing. There were four other male residents, aged 19-23. At this home, Jerry would enter his peers' bedrooms at night and rub up against them or fondle them on top of their clothes, without their consent. This occurred against all four males in the home, on numerous occasions. Eventually, Jerry was removed from the group home and placed temporarily in the psychiatric unit of a hospital. No charges were laid, and a behavior analyst was brought in for assessment and to help with determining an appropriate placement for Jerry.

Question for the reader: What were your first impressions of Jerry and what would need to be done?

Initial assessment by a behavior analyst consisted of reviewing historical files, interviewing staff at the group home, interviewing Jerry, conducting an environmental assessment, and completing a socio-sexual knowledge assessment, and an assessment of age discrimination. The ARMIDILO-S (Boer et al., 2013), an assessment of dynamic risk potential, was conducted to determine Jerry's risk of sexual re-offense.

Through reviewing Jerry's files, documentation showed that he underwent phallometric testing at age 18 (see a depiction of his test results in Figure 7.2 and 7.3 below) and he displayed arousal for forced sex, female and male prepubescents, and female adults.

***Figure 7.1:* Jerry's Phallometric Test Results of Age-Gender Preference**

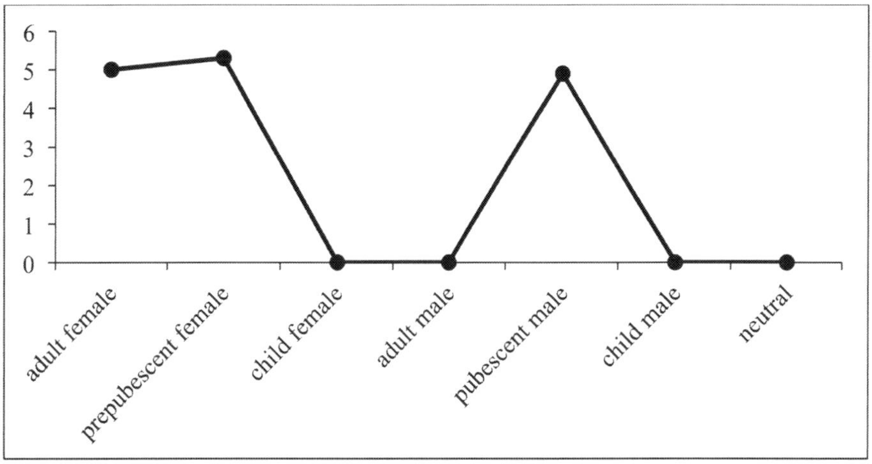

***Figure 7.2:* Jerry's Phallometric Test Results for Interest in Violence**

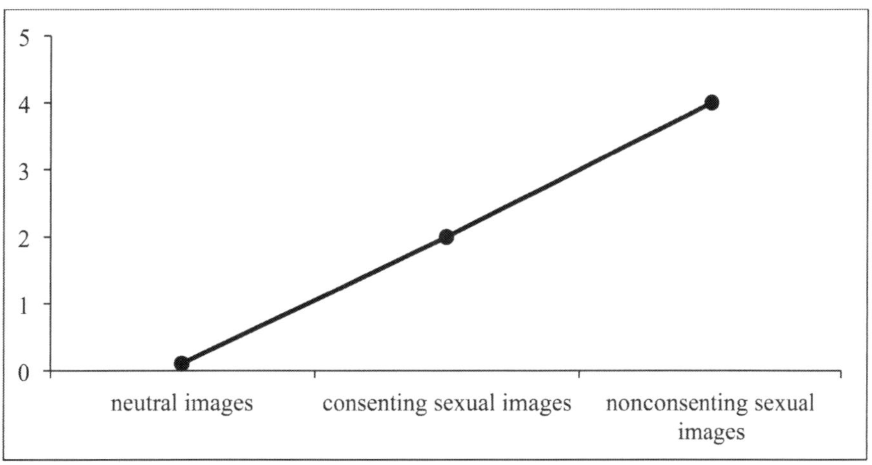

In the previous graphs, Figure 7.2 shows that Jerry demonstrated sexual arousal to both female adults and prepubescents, as well as male prepubescents. Figure 7.3 shows that his arousal to nonconsenting sexual stimuli is stronger than his arousal to consenting sexual stimuli.

In conducting an environmental assessment of the group home where the most recent offenses occurred, the behavior analyst documented that there were two overnight asleep staff on the main floor, all four bedrooms were on the upper floor, there were no locks or alarms on the bedroom doors, and the overall set up of the home was vacant and bare. For example, the living room consisted of just a television with a couple of channels. The staff reported that due to risk of property destruction, the home did not permit many items intended for entertainment in the main areas of the home or in the individual's bedrooms.

The behavior analyst interviewed the staff at the secured group home. To gather information on setting events and antecedents, the behavior analyst asked what was occurring before Jerry entered into his peers' bedrooms. The staff said all the individuals were in their bedrooms having "quiet time," and the two staff members on shift were asleep on the main floor. In speaking to Jerry, the behavior analyst asked him what happened after he entered each peer's bedroom. Jerry responded that staff didn't wake up, it felt good, and that it gave him something to do and ended his "boredom." It was determined that although there was a definite sensory reinforcement component, deprivation from attention and engagement served as motivating operations for entering his peers' bedrooms. Jerry also reported that when he told staff he was bored and had nothing to do, they ignored him. Entering peers' bedrooms continued to occur due to the automatic and negative reinforcement contingencies.

Jerry never received any socio-sexual education due to his family's cultural beliefs against receiving this type of education. Because Jerry never received any socio-sexual education, the behavior analyst administered the SSKAAT-R (Griffiths & Lunsky, 2003). The results of the SSKAAT-R showed that Jerry had very limited socio-sexual knowledge in all areas including intimacy, anatomy, consent, and acts against the law. An age discrimination test showed that Jerry was able to correctly differentiate different age groups (children, pre-teens, teens, adults).

Table 7.1: ***Summary of Socio-Sexual Knowledge and Attitudes Assessment Tool-Revised***

SSKAAT-R	
Sub-tests	**T-Score**
Anatomy	48
Men's Bodies	50
Intimacy	33
Pregnancy, Childbirth, Childrearing	21
Birth Control & STDs	30
Healthy Social-Sexual Boundaries	28

Note: A T-score of 50 represents the average for the standardization sample.

In Figure 7.3, the record form from the SSKAAT-R shows that Jerry's overall scores (except Men's Bodies) are much lower than other individuals who present with the same intellectual functioning.

The circled scores indicate Jerry's raw scores on each section. The squared scores indicate the expected scores from other individuals within Jerry's level of intellectual disability. In relation to others in his functioning level, Jerry falls well below the normative scores across all categories, most notably in Intimacy, Pregnancy, Birth Control, and Healthy Boundaries. Thus, Jerry requires teaching that focuses extensively on these categories, including some focus on anatomy and men's bodies (even though he scored okay in the latter categories, there was still room for improvement where education would be beneficial).

Figure 7.3: **Record Form of Jerry's SSKAAT-R Results**[1]

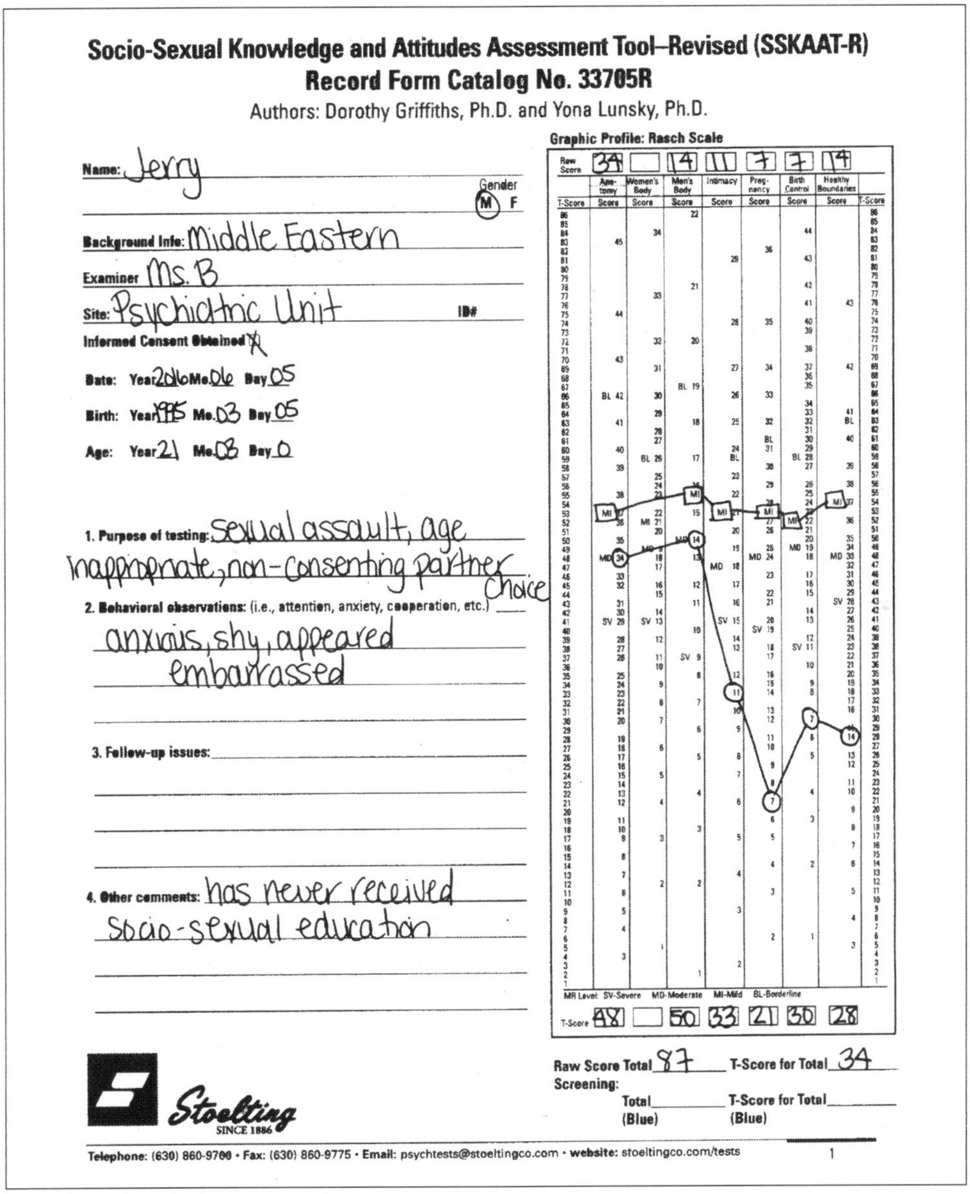

Socio-Sexual Knowledge and Attitudes Assessment Tool–Revised (SSKAAT-R)
Record Form Catalog No. 33705R
Authors: Dorothy Griffiths, Ph.D. and Yona Lunsky, Ph.D.

Name: Jerry
Gender (M) F
Background Info: Middle Eastern
Examiner Ms. B
Site: Psychiatric Unit ID#
Informed Consent Obtained X
Date: Year 2016 Mo. 06 Day 05
Birth: Year 1995 Mo. 03 Day 05
Age: Year 21 Mo. 03 Day 0

1. Purpose of testing: Sexual assault, age inappropriate, non-consenting partner choice
2. Behavioral observations: (i.e., attention, anxiety, cooperation, etc.) anxious, shy, appeared embarrassed
3. Follow-up issues:
4. Other comments: has never received socio-sexual education

Graphic Profile: Rasch Scale

	Anatomy	Women's Body	Men's Body	Intimacy	Pregnancy	Birth Control	Healthy Boundaries
Raw Score	34		14	11	7	7	14
T-Score	48		50	33	21	30	28

MR Level: SV-Severe MD-Moderate MI-Mild BL-Borderline

Raw Score Total 87 T-Score for Total 34
Screening:
Total (Blue) T-Score for Total (Blue)

Stoelting SINCE 1886

Telephone: (630) 860-9700 • Fax: (630) 860-9775 • Email: psychtests@stoeltingco.com • website: stoeltingco.com/tests 1

[1] *The above material was reproduced from the SSKAAT-R (Catalog Number 33705), available from Stoelting Co., 620 Wheat Lane, Wood Dale, IL 60191, or from StoeltingCo.com Copyright 2003, Stoelting Co., 620 Wheat Lane, Wood Dale, IL 60191. All rights reserved.*

An antecedent and setting event analysis revealed that prior to the sexual assaults, Jerry was in a barren environment with very few activities and opportunities for pro-social engagement with others. There was an absence of direct staff supervision, as two staff members were asleep on a separate floor of the house, and all four bedrooms were in close proximity to each other on the same floor of the house.

There were various potential functions of Jerry's behavior, depending on the offense. Reviewing documents about his first offense against a five-year old girl points to a sensory function, due to his self-reported arousal prior to the offense and the onset of puberty. His sexual assaults against four male peers had a number of components involved. Looking at it from the perspective of automatic reinforcement contingency, this offense lines up with phallometric results showing arousal to forced sex; however, there was a discrepancy in that the test results did now show a sexual preference for male adults. Other factors involved – aside from seeking sexual gratification – might include boredom, lack of engagement, and an attempt to gain staff attention. From a preliminary analysis, the function appears to be dual: sensory (automatic) reinforcement and access to social attention in which the maintaining consequence included both positive and negative reinforcement through gaining sexual gratification and termination of the environment lacking in stimulation.

Examining maintaining consequences to Jerry's behavior from a more distal analysis, there was no potential for a punishing consequence, as Jerry never received charges or jail time for his actions. However, it was noted that Jerry's house mates stopped talking to him and wanting to be near him, and most of the staff felt uncomfortable and fearful interacting with Jerry. Jerry also had to leave the home and was placed in a hospital setting.

For Jerry, the depictions in Table 7.4 below illustrate the hypothesized functions of his behavior.

Table 7.2: ***Summary of Jerry's Sexual Incidents***

Incident	Setting Events	Antecedents	Behavior	Consequences
1	Jerry was aroused, he had just started puberty, and he received no socio-sexual education due to family cultural dynamics.	Jerry was not properly supervised and was often left alone with barrier-free access to children.	Jerry fondled a five-year old girl in his neigh-bor-hood.	The assault was sexually stimulating and his behavior was dismissed as if it never happened. Jerry did not face any negative repercussions or added restrictions.
2	Jerry was going through puberty, he had no socio-sexual education, and was expected to 'fend for himself' due to family cultural dynamics.	Jerry was allowed to invite a neighborhood boy over, encouraged by family to play with him, and left alone in a separate room with the boy.	Jerry rubbed on top of the seven-year old boy while left alone in the basement playing games.	The assault was sexually stimulating, it was accepted by his parents where blame was placed on the boy's parents rather than Jerry's actions. Jerry was able to avoid legal implications by agreeing to leave the neighborhood.

3	Jerry was living in a barren environment with excess free time, lack of structure, and no social engagement. He still had not received any socio-sexual education.	Jerry was not properly supervised. He was left alone without anything to do on a separate floor of the house where other vulnerable individuals were in close proximity. Jerry was not given opportunities to develop pro-social relationships, he was left alone with nothing to do.	Jerry repeatedly entered four male peers' bedrooms at night time when staff were asleep on a separate floor and fondled them on top of their clothes. The male peers did not fight against him as they were afraid.	The assaults were sexually stimulating. Jerry was able to end his boredom. He was never reprimanded or prevented from fondling his peers after the first incident. After many successful assaults with no negative repercussions, Jerry was removed from the home and placed in psychiatric ward.

Lastly, the results of the ARMIDILO-S dynamic risk assessment showed Jerry was in the moderate-high risk category of re-offending. This pointed to a need for solid risk management strategies until Jerry's risk could be reduced and re-evaluated.

Developing an Integrated Treatment Plan for Jerry

The behavior analyst's treatment plan covered many areas.

Risk Management

From both an ethical standpoint and to improve adherence and treatment integrity (as well as maintain treatment responsivity – see Bonta & Andrews, 2017), it is important to include the individual in the development of their treatment plans, including risk management aspects. Therefore, the behavior analyst worked with Jerry to create a personalized safety plan. The contents of this safety plan included Jerry's triggers (people/places/situations that are unsafe and can lead to an offense), positive strategies that he can use to stay safe, and identification of people in his support team he can talk to and access for help. Part of this plan focused on environmental changes to reduce the opportunity for Jerry to offend. First, Jerry received eyes-on, 1:1 supervision at all times. In finding a place for Jerry to live, it was determined that door alarms on bedroom doors would be beneficial and that an overnight awake staff would be available to monitor any attempts Jerry might make to leave his bedroom at night. It was determined that Jerry's bedroom should not be in close proximity to other individuals' bedrooms. These strategies were put in place in hope that extinction of the sexual offenses would occur. That is, the goal was eliminating any probability of Jerry entering a peer's bedroom and offending, so as to not receive reinforcement for the inappropriate behavior. At the same time, replacement behaviors and skill teaching would need to occur, with ongoing review of the need for restrictions as Jerry demonstrated the use of his skills.

Altering the Value of the Behavior (creating an abolishing operation for inappropriate behavior)

Jerry engages in sexually assaultive behaviors to, in part, escape boredom. That is, the value of offending increases, and behaviors that increase the probability of offending are most problematic, when he is bored. Therefore, non-contingent reinforcement, or providing reinforcement for no specific behavior may serve as an effective strategy. As well, making Jerry's environment more engaging and rich with activities would ensure that he has preferred items and activities available in his bedroom and in the common areas of a future home.

Teaching Functional Replacement and Coping Skills

A comprehensive behavior replacement plan should include both proximal and distal replacement skills. Since Jerry has never had any socio-sexual education and showed significant gaps in knowledge, he should receive teaching in areas of consent, boundaries, acts against the law, and how to start and maintain healthy relationships. According to phallometric testing results and Jerry's self-report, he demonstrated deviant sexual arousal to prepubescent children as well as forced sex. He also showed arousal to adult women – an appropriate target group. Therefore, treatment should consist of building opportunities for Jerry to access relationships with consenting adults. Based on his sexual behavior with his male peers, potential relationships with adult males would also be explored in treatment.

Due to the severity of the assaultive behavior and the need to quickly eliminate it, Jerry created his own punishment contingency with the guidance of the behavior analyst, in which he would lose an outing to the community if he demonstrated any precursor assaultive behaviors (as identified in his treatment plan). Jerry really enjoyed outings in the community and losing these as a consequence is reasonable to ensure Jerry is practicing his treatment skills rather than inappropriate sexual behavior in order to access the community. Losing an outing due to risky sexual behaviors also ensures both Jerry's and the community's safety, while he works on developing positive skills and treatment goals.

Generalization and Maintenance

For replacement behaviors to generalize, Jerry must be in an environment that provides more reinforcement with less effort, and more activities and privileges to lose by engaging in sexually assaultive behavior. If future sexual assaults were to occur, Jerry should face natural consequences by being charged and having to go through the justice system. Jerry must have a healthy sexual outlet (such as masturbation), an environment that promotes and encourages healthy sexual expression, and access to purposeful and meaningful activities that are individualized.

Jerry's offenses present as Approach-Automatic. He does not stalk or plan his offenses; rather, he responds to opportunity and circumstances when they occur. He also demonstrates arousal to images of age-appropriate partners and situations that do not involve violence. This provides an opportunity for the therapist to teach Jerry self-control strategies regarding his attraction to age-inappropriate partners and arousal that involves violence, while fostering interest in sexual behaviors, even if only self-stimulatory, involving age-appropriate and consenting relationships.

THE CASE OF PORTER

You may recall that Porter is 21 years old. He has been assessed as having mild intellectual disability. He lives in a large multi-bed setting. The staff reported that he was placed there by his family for "sexual reasons." Porter was reported to have engaged in three known episodes of sexually offensive behavior within this setting. Staff described him as a "sexual predator." His last incident involved Sally, a person who was new to the facility. She and Porter had no relationship prior to the offense. Sally had limited cognitive abilities and would not be deemed to have the capacity to consent to sexual activities. Her family want Porter charged as a sexual offender and the staff agreed, given his history of sexual offending. Porter was put on 1-1 staffing 24/7 following this event.

Question for the reader: What were your first impressions of Porter and what would need to be done?

When investigating the antecedents to the offense, the behavior analyst discovered that Porter's alleged attack on Sally happened in the day program attached to the facility. He had been on 24-hour watch by the staff because of his previous history, but, as can happen on such a watch, staff can become distracted by another client or may be lackadaisical in their watch, to the extent that Porter had the chance to wander off. He was found with Sally in the bathroom. Sally's clothes were in disarray, and her panties were down at her ankles. After they were found, Porter was forcibly removed from the day program and placed in a private room in the residence with staff watching outside his room. Sally was quickly dressed and taken back to her day program station as if nothing had happened. Sally's parents were contacted, and they subsequently called their lawyer. They wanted the residence to be sued for their failure to provide their daughter with a safe environment and to expedite her move to another environment.

Question for the reader: How does this new information change your perspective of Porter's situation?

The behavior analyst wanted to understand more about the function of the behavior and any potential motivating operations that might have been involved and thought that an examination of the reports regarding previous incidents might be helpful. A full file review was conducted on how the facility had handled Porter's past offenses. The behavior analyst reviewed all previous incidents to examine the grounds for his label as a sexual predator. The incident involving Sally certainly made him look like someone who was overtly seeking vulnerable individuals who he could sexually assault, and the therapist wanted to determine if this was a pattern. In the index offense, Porter did not know Sally, as she was new to the facility. He was only free from staff observation for a short period, so the event seemed opportunistic. However, the file history of the previous events painted a different picture.

He had been placed in the facility at age 16 because his parents became concerned that he was becoming interested in girls. He had done nothing inappropriate in the community, but the family became concerned when he expressed interest in dating one of the young women in his class at school. Thus, discussion with the family revealed that the impression staff reported that Porter was placed because of sexual reasons was only partially correct. The parents were concerned about his burgeoning sexuality, but not because he had been inappropriate.

As well, the three situations that had occurred previously in the facility were critically different than had been previously reported. The first incident was with a woman named Paula, who lived in the same residence as Porter. The two of them appeared to be mutually attracted to one another and spent time together doing a variety of things, such as watching TV, eating at the same table, going for walks, playing card games, etc. The relationship began to strengthen. They were often seen holding hands and, on occasion, hugging on the couch in the TV room. At one point they were found in the TV room with the door closed, engaged in heavy petting. Although she was clothed, her shirt was unbuttoned, and her bra was unhooked. Because of the policy of the setting – *no sexual contact allowed* – she was moved to another residence, and he was sent to a sex education class. Porter and Paula never saw each other again. Staff members were told to watch Porter in the residence for any inappropriate behavior.

The second incident occurred approximately two years later. At his day program, Porter became attracted to a young woman named Jane. Jane was also attracted to Porter. As with Paula, they became close and spent as much time together as possible at the day program during lunch and breaks and social events that occurred at the program. Their relationship had been going on for many months when, at a Christmas party, they were found in the shipping area having sexual intercourse. Jane was moved to another day program, and Porter was sent to a social skills program, because it was determined that it was not appropriate to have sexual contact at work. Staff members were also alerted to watch him at the day program for any sexually inappropriate behavior.

The third incident occurred in the community at an integrated leisure program a year later. Porter became infatuated with Alice, who also was attracted to him. Over many months they built a relationship. After months of flirting, they were found in the cloak room engaged in sexual contact. Porter was restricted from the community setting and placed on a one-to-one watch following this incident.

Table 7.3: ***Summary of Porter's Sexual Incidents***

Incident	Setting Events	Antecedents	Behavior	Consequences
Age 21 at time of index offense.	Porter had been on 1-1 watch in all settings for two years.	Porter was in the workshop and 1-1 staff attention was diverted.	Porter was found engaging in sexual activity in the washroom with Sally, an individual with whom he had no previous relationship and who would have been unable to legally provide consent.	A staff found them and took Porter to a separate room. 1-1 watch was reinstated and staff believed that charges should be laid because he was deemed to be a repeat offender based upon earlier offense history and the supposition that the family had placed him for predatory reasons.

Age 19	Porter had been on staff alert to watch him in his residential and day program. He had developed a mutual social relationship with Alice, another attendee at the program, over several months.	Porter was at Leisure Program in the community and it was "free time."	Alice and Porter were found in the closet engaging in sexual activity.	Porter was placed on 1-1 watch at all times and restricted from community activities.
Age 18	Porter developed a relationship with Jane at his day program. They engaged in open mutual attraction for many months.	Porter was at a Christmas Party and all staff was engaged with others at the party.	Porter and Jane went into the shipping area and engaged in sexual intercourse.	A staff member found them in the shipping room and separated them immediately. Jane was removed to another day program. Porter was sent to social skills training because it was inappropriate to have sex at work, and staff at the day program were advised to place him on staff alert at all times in the day program because of his offending history.
Age 16	Porter developed a relationship with Paula, who also lived in his residence. They spent time together and showed open affection.	Porter was alone in the TV room with Paula.	Porter closed the door to the TV room and engaged in heavy petting with Paula. Staff found the two of them with their clothes in disarray but deemed that no sexual intercourse had occurred.	The staff members immediately separated them. Paula was moved to a different residence to eliminate their contact. Porter was sent for sex education, in which assessments showed he learned that all sexual contact was considered bad. Staff members in the residence were told to keep him on staff-alert (to watch at all times).

At 16	Porter was at school in the community and living with his parents.	Porter was with his parents and saw a female classmate in the mall.	Porter voiced interest in dating the young girl from his school.	His parents told him he was not allowed to date and subsequently placed him in a residential program where no sexual activity was allowed.

Question for the reader: Does your view of Porter change now that you know his history?

Lastly, the behavior analyst was interested in understanding Porter's level of understanding of socio-sexual matters, especially his understanding of issues of consent. Porter's sexual knowledge was assessed using the SSKAAT-R (Griffiths & Lunsky, 2003 – as described in Chapter 4). Although records showed he had received sex education following the first incident, the education he had received was very basic. Moreover, the message they had given him in his sex education class was that sex is bad and that he should not have sex. When he saw the picture in the SSKAAT-R depicting rape, he identified that the woman was in distress and that it was wrong to hurt her. However, he also identified many of the sexual scenes, even those as consenting were wrong, just as he had learned. The assessment explored his perceptions of where it is okay to have sex. He had been taught it was wrong to have sex at work, but he could not identify where it was okay to have sex, except to say in a private place.

The challenge for Porter was that his world had no privacy. As is the case for many persons with intellectual disabilities who live in multi-bed settings, Porter was living in a setting that did not provide any privacy for sexual behavior nor was it sanctioned by those operating the facility. The assessment showed that he had developed perceptions that he could never have a relationship or be married because he was a person with an intellectual disability living in a facility.

Question for the reader: Does this alter your perceptions of the potential function of the behavior?

Developing an Integrated Treatment Package for Porter

Risk Management

Porter's current setting had attempted to provide protection by placing Porter on a 1-to-1 watch at all times. This approach failed. It is extremely difficult to have someone monitored 24/7. Staff become distracted by another client in need or are increasingly lackadaisical or lacking in vigilance if there have been no incidents over a period of time. Therefore, although supervision geared to risk factors is vital, this type of approach alone will not stop someone from offending. Sexual drive is natural, and prohibition of that natural drive is often futile, if not abusive. In order to ensure that Porter does not re-offend, any supervision must be paired with two elements. First, he needs to have another means to serve the function of sexual satisfaction, but in a way that is appropriate. Unfortunately, in his current setting, Porter's options are limited. Secondly, he needs to learn self-regulation of his sexual urges, and, to do so, he needs education about methods for self-management and understanding of the potential consequences of dysregulation.

Teaching alternative coping skills

Porter had received sex education following his first offense, but the education he received was geared toward teaching him what not to do, rather than what he could do. The reality was that in the incidents leading up to the situation with Sally, his relationships had been mutual, consenting, and long term. The behavior analyst suggested that Porter required sex education that was more complete; however, he also needed to learn that appropriate sexual behavior with another must be age-appropriate, consenting, and private. If not within these parameters, he needed to learn that the behavior would be inappropriate, illegal, and could result in charges being laid.

An important element in understanding the implications of Porter's behavior is making him aware of what he has to lose if another offense occurs, and, perhaps, more importantly in his case, he needs to establish a life with elements that would establish this as a reality. A lot of individuals who have offended have already had so many positive elements in their lives taken away or restricted that they virtually have nothing left to lose. In some cases, jail is not seen as a great punishment. Therefore, the key to the success of any strategy for self-control is ensuring that the effort put forward to not offend results in sustaining a quality of life worth having. For Porter, it is important to utilize a Good Lives Model approach to establish valued "goods" in his daily life and to establish goals to achieve that *good life* as motivation to prevent future offenses.

In the current environment in which Porter lived, the policy against any sexual contact meant that he needed to learn an appropriate way to gain sexual satisfaction. When an appropriate partnered relationship was not available, or allowed, such as in his current setting, Porter needed to learn to use self-stimulation and could have been provided with non-pornographic erotica if needed, such as a poster in his room. Additionally, he needed to be afforded sufficient privacy to engage in that act.

Corrective and Remedial Consequences

Porter was confused by the education he received after his first offense. The message he received in his sex education was simply that all sex was bad; however, his own experience with his first girlfriend was not bad, in fact it was good. He was therefore left with two different impressions – leading to cognitive dissonance (two competing understandings, which often accentuates anxiety and confusion for persons with intellectual disabilities). Until the incident with Sally, his own experience of sex had been reinforcing. Also, following the index offense against Sally, he was told that it was wrong because she did not give consent. However, even though his prior sexual interactions had been consenting, he was punished for those interactions. Even his sexual contact with Sally was not forced; an interview with Sally revealed that she said she thought Porter was now her boyfriend, and it appeared that although not legally consensual because of her cognitive understanding, she had assented to the act. Thus, although the act was illegal he did not attempt to force or hurt her in the sexual content, and he was not motivated by non-consensual sex. Lastly, Porter had attempted to be private in his sexual contacts by engaging in contact in the TV room with a closed door, in a shipping area when everyone was in the main room at a party, and in a clothes closet. However, each time he was punished by having his love interests removed, being sent to therapy, and being given sanctions on his freedom in various settings eventually leading to 24/7 supervision.

Porter's earlier sexual behaviors would be deemed as appropriate in other living environments, but in his current setting all sexual behavior was punished. As such, both appropriate and inappropriate (non-consensual) relationships were dealt with in the same fashion. In all cases his partner was removed from the environment, and he lost freedom by receiving increased supervision. Thus, the consequences for both appropriate and inappropriate behavior were the same – the only thing that changed was that Porter learned from the first two consensual contacts that when he developed a relationship before having sex, there was a greater probability of being caught than if he engaged in a quick sexual act with whoever the opportunity afforded him, even if she was legally unable to give consent. Therefore, the consequences for these different behaviors needed to be differentiated.

Question for the reader: What would you recommend in this case?

The obvious goal for intervention for Porter is to reduce his sexually inappropriate behavior to zero, wherein sexually inappropriate behavior is defined as any sexual contact that involves an age-inappropriate partner, is not consensual, and lacks privacy. The concept of no tolerance for any re-offense sets a socially valid benchmark for this type of behavior, and anything but zero would be deemed a failure. The key to building confidence that treatment effects are taking place is through accurate data collection. However, just knowing he has not offended is insufficient; especially when he is living in a controlled setting with constant supervision that tells us little about the efficacy of Porter's treatment package beyond highly controlled settings. It is also important to examine his behavior when the presence of possible victims and the frequency of appropriate sexual knowledge and behaviors.

As with other behavior problems, it is insufficient to merely set absence of the behavior as the primary goal. An equally important goal is establishing and measuring the acquisition of new coping skills and knowledge. For example, recording Porter's use of private time requested for personal stimulation would give an indication that he is developing alternative behaviors to access appropriate sexual outlets. Also, in Porter's case there had been no indication in his file as to what specifically he had been taught about socio-sexual matters and how much of what he had been taught had actually been learned. As part of his integrated program, it is important to directly measure both his knowledge and his ability to apply that knowledge.

Generalization and Maintenance

Lastly, in order for Porter to be able to generalize what he has learned in the educational programs, he needs to be in an environment that will support appropriate (age-appropriate, consenting, and private) relationships. Although this may not be immediately possible, this should be a goal that is put in place and worked toward as part of his long-term plan. However, in preparation for this, Porter needs to show that he has understanding of what is appropriate and that consequences are both appropriate and consistent. Generalization and maintenance are unlikely unless he is placed in an environment that can promote and respect healthy and appropriate sexual relationships.

Question for the reader: How would you approach Porter compared to Jerry?

Porter represents a case that could fall into the counterfeit deviance category. Porter had no desire to engage in forced or nonconsenting sexual activity, as shown by his earlier courtships and relationships with Paula and Jane. His socio-sexual assessment showed that he felt that forcing sexual contact with another was wrong. However, his sexual interaction with Alice was nonconsenting because Alice did not have the capacity to understand the implications of the act. However, he did not force her in any way, and, in fact, she was assenting, believing that this meant they were boyfriend and girlfriend.

To a large extent, the agency supporting Porter had created a no-win situation for him. He had been taught that all sexual activity was bad. However, his experience was that it was not bad – leading to conflicting rule formation and potentially cognitive dissonance and confusion. He had been told that relationships had to be consenting and mutual, but when he engaged in them he was punished, and he lost the affiliation of the person for whom he cared – exacerbating that dissonance. The agency had created an environment in which the only way he could be sexually involved with another person was to attempt to secret himself away with a willing/assenting, although nonconsenting partner with the hope that for the brief time that his supervision was diverted he might be able to engage in sexual contact and not get caught. Had Porter lived and worked in a different setting, where his relationships with Paula and Jane had been respected, do you think he would have sexually offended?

THE CASE OF SCOTT

Scott is a 25-year-old man with high functioning cognitive challenges and because of his abilities was seen as a "junior staff" in his day program. One of the individuals at day program indicated to staff that Scott had touched his genitals; however, staff were adamant that these behaviors were an accident and there was no way Scott knew what he was doing. This behavior continued on an ongoing basis and day program staff members were reluctant to notify the residence as they feared that Scott would be unfairly restricted. Eventually the police had been called; however the police officer failed to press charges claiming that people with disabilities and people like Scott "don't know what they're doing." His residential staff were eventually informed of the behavior and supervision was enhanced in the home. However, some residential staff members agreed with the day program staff that this "accident" at work was unintentional and so they failed to be consistent in their supervision. At one point, a residential staff member witnessed Scott holding down another client and engaging in anal penetration during which the other individual showed obvious discomfort and resistance. Police were called again and this time he was arrested and charged. When the police arrived, Scott appeared angry and confused as to why he was being arrested.

Even though he was arrested, the prosecutor was very reluctant to press charges. She felt that Scott was a "confused child," and it would be unfair to charge someone with a disability. He was, however, eventually charged with Sexual Assault, but the charges were immediately diverted, and he was charged instead with simple Assault. Scott received no prison time and was put on probation with no conditions, other than the establishment of a treatment protocol. The judge himself addressed Scott and told him he was "a fine young man who is the victim of a misunderstanding. He needs support and compassion, not a sentence."

Question for the reader: What were your first impressions of Scott and what would need to be done?

A behavior analyst was called in to assess the situation and to determine the risk that Scott posed to others. As part of a typical assessment, historical variables were obtained. His early history was largely unremarkable. Scott had a typical upbringing in a small town located outside a large city. His parents, Nathan and Rachel, are still married and involved in his life. Scott did not have a notable childhood and there were very few behavior problems. Because of his high level of functioning (IQ = 68), he was able to integrate reasonably well into the mainstream school system. He received very little early intervention, with the exception of some tutoring in middle school. He experienced boundaries issues in his early teens, but these were addressed swiftly by the school and education was deemed successful and discontinued. When he was 18 years old, he moved to supported living in a city several hours from home.

Scott fit in well with the group home environment. He was initially placed with same-age peers and appeared to adjust to the situation. Soon, Scott began trying to take on extra "chores" and aligned himself closely with staff. This is when he began to refer to himself as a "junior staff" and tried to direct and order the other residents. Unfortunately, the staff members encouraged this behavior, which created a power dynamic within the house. After two years, that home was shut down, and he was moved to another residence within the same agency. This residence was significantly different, in that he was housed with much lower functioning and older individuals who were more vulnerable. At his new residence, Scott continued to present his role as "junior staff." At this time, he also began working in the day program of the agency, doing piece-meal work for a company making train brakes. Scott became bored and sought competitive employment. Given his level of functioning, and with staff support, he got a job at a local coffee shop of which he was quite proud. Within a year, however, Scott requested a move back to the day program. This was timely as he began to receive complaints from his supervisor for inappropriate comments about some customers and attempts to hug them in the restaurant.

Scott returned to the day program, and although the work was not challenging for him he enjoyed it and seemed content. Here as well, Scott began working his way into a "supervisory" position; he was eventually able to help plan the shifts and jobs of the other members and could assign them special projects that he oversaw. This continued for nearly two years, and staff noted no difficulties with Scott, but his arrival seemed to disrupt the other residents. Many of the individuals in the home appeared fearful of Scott and began exhibiting new behaviors themselves. The majority of these individuals were nonverbal and staff had a very difficult time understanding the issues they were facing.

It was at this time that one of the individuals at the day program indicated to staff that Scott had touched his genitals and, as mentioned earlier, it was initially handled as accidental rather than sexual touching. Staff believed that Scott did not know that his behavior had been sexual. However, the behavior continued. Even so, the staff at the day program protected Scott by not telling his residence because they felt he might be punished.

Over time it appeared the behaviors were not occurring since Scott had learned to hide the behavior by only assaulting individuals who were non-verbal. He would assign vulnerable males to special tasks that he would oversee and during which he would isolate them and take sexual advantage of them.

On one occasion the staff became aware of an incident and notified the authorities, but police refused to press charges; the responding officers said they had met people with disabilities, and people like Scott "don't know what they're doing." Staff members at the residence were also notified, and they became concerned that the behavior may have also been happening at the residence. Just as in the day program, Scott had taken on a number of extra responsibilities, including doing the laundry for other residents. His helpful tasks allowed him to have unsupervised time with the other members.

Staff began providing supervision as they were able, but many of the team agreed with the day program that this behavior was likely accidental and only occurred at the day program. This resulted in a very uneven and inconsistent amount of supervision, with some staff refusing to watch him around other residents, ostensibly as a means of proving his innocence.

While grabbing the laundry one day, a staff member caught Scott holding down a house-member in his own bedroom as he was anally penetrating the individual. Though non-verbal, it was clear that this was not consensual, and staff immediately intervened. The supervisor was notified, and staff called the police to report the crime. Throughout the follow-up investigation, Scott maintained his innocence and feigned confusion. He did so even when the police arrived; Scott was surprised and very angry when he was arrested and charged with Sexual Assault, later reduced to Assault. Even for this assault charge, he virtually received no deterrent consequences with the exception that he must participate in a treatment program and was placed on probation.

As part of the post-incident evaluation, Scott was administered the SSKAAT-R (Griffiths & Lunsky, 2003). As shown in Table 7.1 below, he demonstrated a high degree of socio-sexual knowledge, greater than even many in the typical population as he had received education through his supporting agency. As part of his agency's new policies, which anticipated provincial-wide changes, Scott was provided with the opportunity to receive education in relationships and social skills, abuse prevention, and personal boundaries. Scott was quite eager and took advantage of each course, expanding his knowledge significantly over time.

Table 7.4: ***Summary of Socio-Sexual Knowledge and Attitudes Assessment Tool-Revised***

SSKAAT-R	
Sub-tests	**T-Score**
Anatomy	83
Men's Bodies	56
Intimacy	63
Pregnancy, Childbirth, Childrearing	49
Birth Control & STDs	63
Healthy Social-Sexual Boundaries	58

Note: A T-score of 50 represents the average for the standardization sample.

Figure 7.4, the Record Form from the SSKAAT-R, shows that Scott's overall score is higher than other individuals who present with the same intellectual functioning.

Figure 7.4. **Record Form of Scott's SSKAAT-R Results**[2]

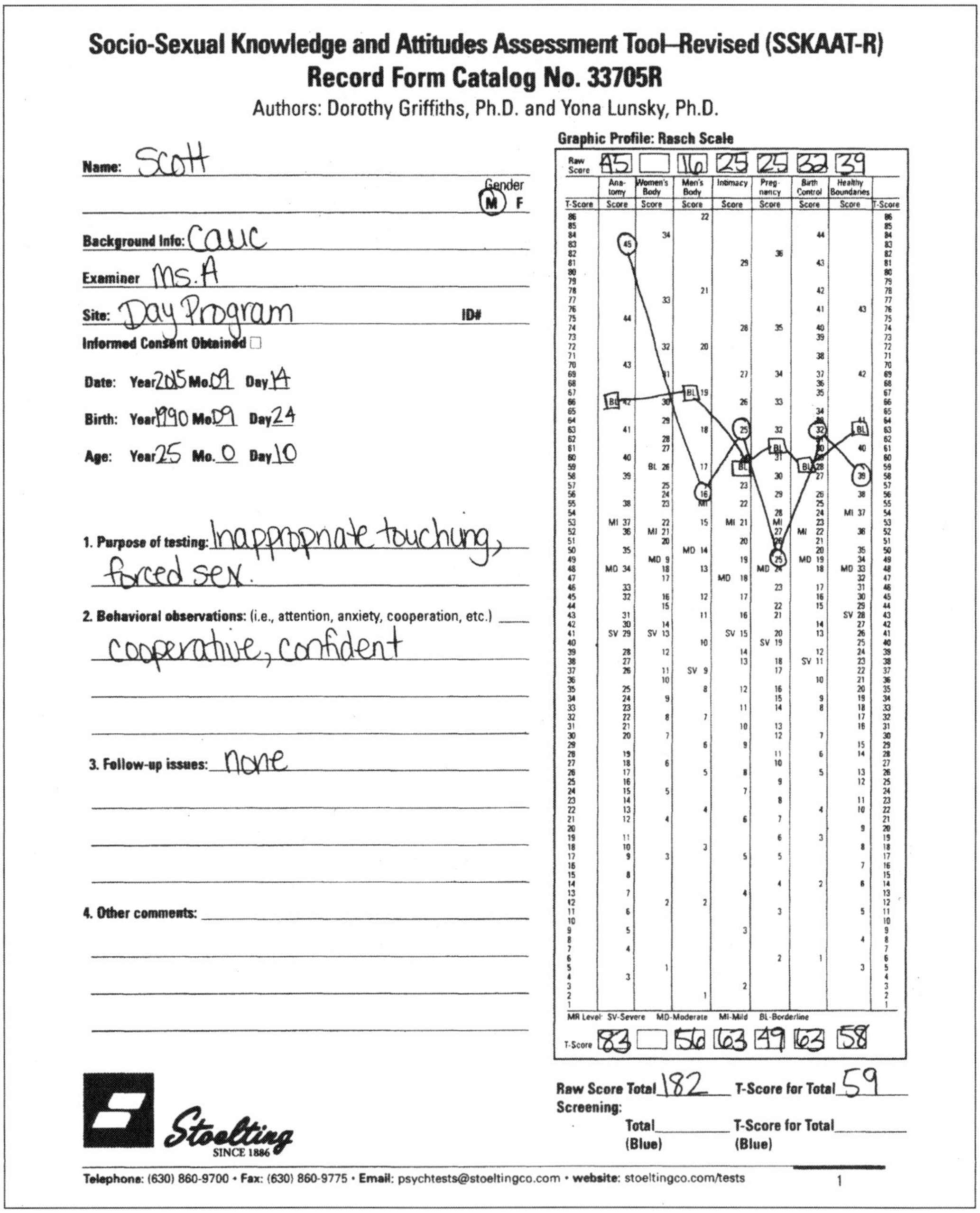
Socio-Sexual Knowledge and Attitudes Assessment Tool–Revised (SSKAAT-R)
Record Form Catalog No. 33705R
Authors: Dorothy Griffiths, Ph.D. and Yona Lunsky, Ph.D.

Name: Scott
Gender (M) F
Background Info: Cauc
Examiner Ms. A
Site: Day Program ID#
Informed Consent Obtained ☐
Date: Year 2015 Mo. 09 Day 14
Birth: Year 1990 Mo. 09 Day 24
Age: Year 25 Mo. 0 Day 10

1. Purpose of testing: Inappropriate touching, forced sex.

2. Behavioral observations: (i.e., attention, anxiety, cooperation, etc.) cooperative, confident

3. Follow-up issues: none

4. Other comments:

Graphic Profile: Rasch Scale

	Anatomy	Women's Body	Men's Body	Intimacy	Pregnancy	Birth Control	Healthy Boundaries
Raw Score	45		16	25	25	32	39
T-Score	83		56	63	49	63	58

MR Level: SV-Severe MD-Moderate MI-Mild BL-Borderline

Raw Score Total 182 T-Score for Total 59
Screening:
Total ______ T-Score for Total ______
(Blue) (Blue)

Stoelting SINCE 1886

Telephone: (630) 860-9700 • Fax: (630) 860-9775 • Email: psychtests@stoeltingco.com • website: stoeltingco.com/tests

1

[2]*The above material was reproduced from the SSKAAT-R (Catalog Number 33705), available from Stoelting Co., 620 Wheat Lane, Wood Dale, IL 60191, or from StoeltingCo.com Copyright 2003, Stoelting Co., 620 Wheat Lane, Wood Dale, IL 60191. All rights reserved.*

In the figure above, the circled scores indicate Scott's raw scores on each section. The squared scores indicate the expected scores from other individual's in Scott's level of intellectual disability. In examining the chart, it is noted that he had a high score on anatomy that was far superior to the norm compared to those with similar functioning levels. The chart allows clinicians to see how Scott is functioning in different categories compared to others, which identifies where work is needed. In relation to others, the focus of teaching for Scott should target Men's Bodies, Pregnancy, and Healthy Boundaries.

Scott understood physical and emotional boundaries quite well. He also knew that boundaries change over time and over the course of a relationship. He could describe what consent is and some means by which to obtain it. However, there were some issues in regard to cognitive distortions. Scott felt that consent could be obtained non-verbally and that if his victims did not want to have sex they should have fought back harder. Scott also stated that although boundaries can change over time, it is his decision when and how they change. Scott opined that his offenses caused no impact to those he victimized and suggested that they had likely already forgotten the incident.

Although Scott did not initially want to discuss his offenses with the therapist, over time he revealed that he had a strong interest in coercive sex, having no interest in pursuing consensual relationships. He identified himself as homosexual. Scott was able and willing to describe, in great detail, the joy (and arousal) he received forcing another male to have sex and then ejaculating. Scott was highly motivated to re-offend and asked why this was an issue: If what he did was wrong, why was he not in jail? Why would the judge treat him so well?

The therapist concluded that Scott's offending tended to follow a consistent pattern. Scott was highly sexual and could be described as hyper-aroused. Unfortunately, given the nature of the group home in which he resided, he did not always have the opportunity to masturbate. This created a situation in which sexual activity was highly reinforcing and extremely motivating. Scott would often find ways of accessing Wi-Fi in order to watch pornography on his phone before work.

Because of the restrictive nature of his residence regarding masturbation, Scott would often go to day program extremely aroused and with no chance for appropriate sexual behavior. Scott's orchestration of situations at the day program in which he could isolate the other individuals and "supervise" them, may have been partly related to this high arousal that had not been satisfied. In that state he was faced with supervision of individuals who were vulnerable to his advances, and this would exacerbate his arousal. He would then isolate individuals he could potentially victimize. The lack of supervision had allowed him to offend, and he would ensure the individuals he targeted were non-verbal. Scott would offend and then continue his day at work. The immediate consequences for his behavior were unfortunately positive; he often achieved ejaculation, and there were no sanctions imposed. His behavior, initiated by his arousal, was maintained and reinforced by the very powerful primary reinforcer of sexual gratification, with the inappropriate element of coercion.

A list of Scott's sexual incidents is outlined in Table 7.5 below.

Table 7.5: ***Summary of Scott's Sexual Incidents***

Incident	Setting Events	Antecedents	Behavior	Consequences
1	Aroused in the morning, unable to masturbate at home due to time.	Isolated from other staff and no supervision. No task and nothing to do.	Touched genitals of female "peer" over pants.	Sexual excitement and ejaculation. Reported as very reinforcing. No aversive consequences.
2	Reported to staff that he wanted to stay in his room all day. Staff took him to day program.	Supervising two "peers" cleaning work area. Sent one individual to another area.	Undressed (pants) female "peer" and fondled privates.	Sexual excitement but caught by staff. Stopped immediately and said that he was helping her dress. Not reported to authorities.
3	Ate breakfast at residence and planned the day.	On a day trip to the mall, offered to accompany male member to the family washroom.	Locked door, restrained individual, and possibly assaulted him.	Both individuals left the washroom without incident. Victim was nonverbal but indicated to staff later that night what Scott restrained and hurt him. Not reported to authorities as victim was thought to be unreliable.
4	Uneventful weekend day at residence. Watched movies.	Staff left Scott to supervise individuals while they picked up another resident.	Followed co-resident into bedroom. Unknown what occurred.	Staff arrived at home and found Scott leaving co-resident's room. Staff could get very few details due to limited communication.
5	Generally happy and productive during day.	Staff members were in basement having a team meeting. Scott was "supervising" other residents.	Held co-resident down. Victim was undressed and struggling when staff intervened. Scott was anally penetrating victim.	Staff removed Scott and notified police. He was arrested later that night.

Developing an Integrated Treatment Plan for Scott

Risk Management

The motivating and maintaining contingencies would need to be altered to reduce the risk, opportunity, and reinforcing properties of the offending behavior. Several immediate changes were made. First and foremost, victim access and lack of supervision, which were the immediate antecedents to his behavior, were altered. Scott was provided 1:1 eyes-on supervision at all times and was never allowed to be alone with any other client, at home or in the community. Given Scott's motivation to re-offend, it was critical to provide external risk management until Scott learned new skills and secured reinforcement for more appropriate sexual behavior other than re-offense.

To reduce his arousal at times of greatest risk, he was provided a private place and some erotica prior to going to work or to any community activity so that he could masturbate, thereby reducing his urges. As well, given his perceived sexual hyper-arousal, the therapist suggested a meeting be scheduled for Scott with a forensic specialist to determine what biological contributors may be present. His blood work revealed extremely high testosterone levels and the psychiatrist suggested that he would be a good candidate for sex drive reducing medication. Scott consented to a trial of Lupron (an anti-androgen), and he showed improvement over time; he noted that he felt more control and fewer urges for sexual offending behavior when in the community.

Scott's sexual offending and coercive thoughts or fantasies were automatically reinforcing. The coercive nature of his assaults was arousing to him, and the subsequent sexual gratification of the offenses made the behaviors highly reinforcing. Unfortunately, this raised a challenge from a behavioral perspective. There was no obvious functional replacement for this behavior; there are appropriate means of attaining sexual gratification, but the coercive nature of the behavior is not so easily replaced.

The replacement behavior to be effective, must be as or more reinforcing and easier to obtain. Although the therapist could not replicate all the reinforcing properties, attempts were made to provide appropriate sexual expression easier to obtain and with fewer aversive consequences. Although masturbation may not serve the same sensory function as an intimate relationship, Scott had no desire to engage in a relationship of any kind, which was fortuitous. However, there were current barriers to even appropriate sexual expression in his residential environment, in that Scott shared a bedroom with another individual. To address this, the environment was restructured so Scott had his own room and access to privacy at all times. As noted above his schedule was altered to give him private time in the morning before work and before going to potentially risky situations. This provided easy access to sexual gratification without any harm or aversive consequences. He had free access to this whenever he wanted and could view approved erotica if he wanted (with clinical discussion and development of a media protocol prior to providing him with erotica – see Wilson & Burns, 2011).

Teaching Replacement and Coping Skills

Scott's motivation to offend was extremely high and his desire to avoid recidivism was very low. A functionally- equivalent replacement behavior may be insufficient to sustain long lasting change so a Good Lives Plan was created for Scott that highlighted the positive aspects of his life and laid out future goals. The idea is that Scott will have a good life and would want to avoid re-offense to protect it. Scott's parents were an invaluable resource in supporting the positive and appropriate goals, making them both realistic and highly motivating. Since Scott's behavior was also driven by an element of control, it was important to provide him opportunities to have control over positive elements of his life.

Scott had sufficient knowledge to understand the impact of his actions and how he orchestrated them. A good lives/self-regulation assessment (Yates, Prescott, & Ward, 2010) showed the explicit and planned nature of his offenses; Scott possessed intact self-regulation and was able to manage his behavior, should he choose to do so. However, he had not previously been motivated to use these skills to avoid offending. As his motivation increased, Scott was taught the skills and strategies to avoid re-offense from the earliest stage. Scott had to learn what his risk areas were and how to manage his sexual arousal in the community. He was taught how to rely on external supports, such as staff and family in situations. Once he began regaining some independence, there were no further inappropriate targets or heightened risk.

Corrective and Remedial Consequences

Along with teaching functional skills and replacement behaviors, it is important for individuals who have offended to learn within their treatment that there are real-life consequences to offending, which might include removal from home and community or prison sentencing and what that experience would entail (such as the loss of friends and family). Lindsay (2009) has emphasized that many offenders, because of the nature of their past experiences, may not have had appropriate or accurate exposure to information about the real-life consequences that could befall them as a result of an offense.

As an Approach-Explicit Offender, whose offenses were motivated by issues of control, it was important to ensure two things. First, that Scott was educated about the consequences that would follow if he re-offended. He had previously little/if any sanctions following an offense, however, future offenses would be met with the typical consequences that befall an offender; he would be arrested, tried, and likely receive jail time. It was important that he become acutely aware of how his life would change if this happened and what he would lose about his present life that would really be missed by him should this occur. Second, since Scott liked to be in control, the focus on treatment was to give Scott control over positive things in his life, while making him aware that a re-offense would result in other people taking control of his life. Getting Scott involved in helping to design a positive path that he could control to stay out of jail was an important part of his treatment. He needed to see the deterrence of the real and possible long-term aversive consequences as more powerful than the potential positive but fleeting consequences of a re-offense.

In pursuit of this development, a person-centred plan was proposed in which Scott would work with those individuals on his treatment team and in his life to create a plan in which his primary goal could be met. Although he openly admitted a preference for non-consensual sex, he also did not want to go to jail. A cost benefit analysis was conducted with him to show him all that he would lose if he re-offended. A treatment and supervision contract was then put in place that he would self manage under supervision and monitoring. One of the contingencies that was discussed with him was the potential use of an anti-androgen hormone to reduce his sexual impulses under high risk situations. Scott agreed to the use of this. (This will be discussed in Chapter 10).

Question for the reader: How would you approach Scott compared to Porter or Jerry?

Since Scott presented as an Approach-Explicit Offender, risk management was of paramount importance in his treatment and risk management program. Although building a good life in which he can experience control over positive aspects of his life and feel successful is an important element in creating competing contingencies, the focus must always remain on keeping safety first for him and for those individuals with whom he interacts, especially those who are most vulnerable.

SUMMARY

These cases are meant to be illustrative; however, they cannot fully represent the complexity of all the past and present circumstances that can be involved in the development of a sexual offense. They provide exemplars that can serve as a basis for application of the assessment principles in this section as they could also be applied to other cases. These cases illustrate the need to go beyond simply targeting the absence of the deviant behavior, to developing strengths and elements that will aid in resiliency and adherence. As we have said previously, if treatment fails to provide the individual with a strong motivation and reinforcement history for alternative behaviors, then it is unlikely the individual will maintain and generalize the new knowledge and skills because there is nothing worth protecting. The focus of programming must also look at prevention of any possible offenses. Unlike many other behavioral programs, there is no latitude for even one relapse. The target must be a zero rate of offending behavior. In other words, the offending behaviors must be placed on extinction, in which there is no reinforcement provided for these behaviors, and, instead, there is ample reinforcement available for more appropriate, functionally equivalent behaviors. As previously mentioned, due to the seriousness of offensive sexual behaviors, a punishment procedure, such as response cost, may also be considered in addition to reinforcement.

Lastly, it is important to realize that the therapist is part of a team that may include other professionals, such as psychiatrists and social service workers, who add important elements to the holistic understanding of the individual. Working collaboratively with open lines of communication is critical to successful outcomes with this population. The family and the primary support workers who are with the individual 24/7 represent the foundation for any success. Their participation and belief in the program are critical to ensure adherence to the program protocols and to provide the ongoing environment to support change.

REFERENCES

Ayllon, T. & Azrin, N. (1968). *The token economy: A motivational system for therapy and rehabilitation.* New York: Appleton-Century-Crofts.

Azrin, N. & Holz, W. C. (1966). Punishment. In W. K. Honig (Ed.) *Operant behavior: Areas of research and application* (pp. 380-447). New York: Appleton-Century-Crofts.

Baer, D. M., Wolf, M. M., & Risley, T. R. (1968). Some current dimensions of applied behavior analysis. *Journal of Applied Behavior Analysis, 1*, 91-97.

Boer, D. P., Haaven, J. L., Lambrick, F., Lindsay, W. R., McVilly, K. R., Sakdalan, F., & Frize, M. (2013). *The Assessment of Risk and Manageability of Individuals with Developmental and Intellectual Limitations Who Offend – Sexually (ARMIDILO-S)*. Retrieved from www.armidilo.net.

Bonta, J. & Andrews, D.A. (2017). *The psychology of criminal conduct* (6th ed.). Cincinnati, OH: Anderson.

Griffiths, D. & Lunsky, Y. (2003). *Socio-sexual knowledge and attitude assessment tool- revised (SSKAAT-R)*. Wood Dale, IL: Stoelting Company.

Lindsay, W. R. (2009). *The treatment of sex offenders with developmental disabilities*. West Sussex, UK: Wiley-Blackwell.

Lindsay, W. R. (2015, June). *Assessment and treatment of sexual offending behavior in persons with developmental disabilities and autism*. St. Catharines, ON: International Dual Diagnosis Certificate Program, Brock University.

Wilson, R. J., & Burns, M. (2011). *Intellectual disability and problems in sexual behavior: Assessment, treatment, and promotion of healthy sexuality*. Holyoke, MA: NEARI Press.

Yates, P. M., Prescott, D., & Ward, T. (2010). *Applying the good lives model and self-regulation models to sex offender treatment: A practical guide for clinicians*. Brandon, VT: Safer Society.

PART III:

TREATMENT

Chapter Eight

Setting the Stage for Success in Treating Sexual Offending Behavior

Setting the stage for success is the foundation for effective and long-term treatment outcomes. It involves creating an environment in which the individual can thrive and maintain a safe and healthy lifestyle by providing opportunities for desirable behavior and minimizing opportunities for undesirable (offending) behavior. All behavior occurs within a specific context with many complex variables that contribute to the occurrence of behavior. The variables that contribute to sexual offending behavior in individuals with intellectual disabilities need to be carefully considered to ensure that the individual has the best chance of success. This chapter will discuss some environments, where individuals with intellectual disabilities have lived, as it provides important considerations for assessing and treating the sexual offending behavior of the individual.

Setting the stage for success may seem like an intuitively simple concept, yet when it comes to persons with intellectual disabilities who have sexually offended, conditions often do not ensure that effective support and intervention can occur. Based on the authors' clinical experience, the factors that influence the offending pattern are often skewed in the following disadvantageous directions:

- Environments sometimes allow access to children and other vulnerable individuals or provide access to negative influences such as other individuals with similar problems, drugs, alcohol, and/or pornography;
- Staff may not be fully or appropriately trained to effectively support clients, have attitudes antithetical to treatment goals, or provide supervision that does not consider protection of the community and others to reduce risk;
- Environments often focus solely on management of risks and negative behaviors rather than providing opportunities for prosocial and positive development;
- Punitive and prohibitive approaches are often used without regard for habilitative strategies to encourage development of skills such as self-regulation that might allow access to less restrictive opportunities;
- Sometimes through isolation, or negative attitudes towards the offender, there is a lack of positive social relationships to provide motivation for engaging in prosocial behavior (i.e., non-offending); and
- Often, a person with an intellectual disability who has offended is not provided opportunities to create a better future.

Conditions such as these may increase risk for re-offense, because the individual does not access opportunities to receive reinforcement for alternative, more appropriate behaviors. Therefore, when setting the stage for success it is important to not only eliminate conditions associated with offending but to provide conditions that will promote non-offending. For individuals with sexual offending behavior and intellectual disabilities, there are complex variables that contribute to the behavior. Those factors and contributing variables need to be carefully considered and planned for to ensure the individual has the best chance of success.

Figure 8.1 **Factors Associated with High and Low Offense**

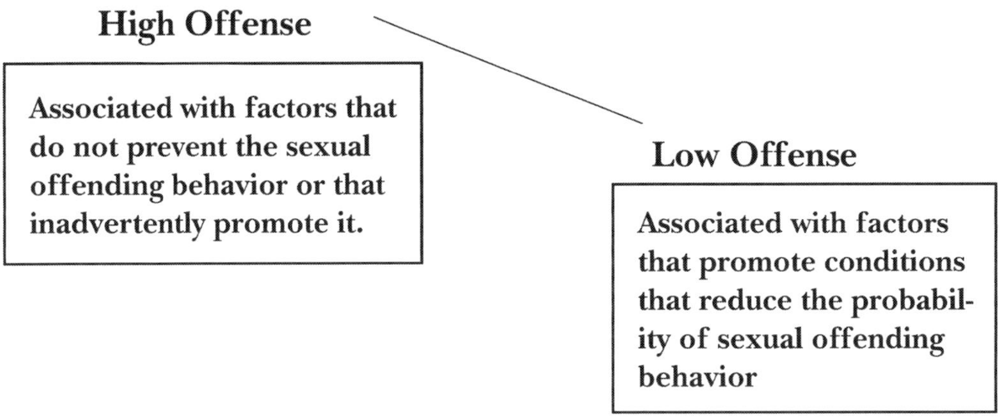

As shown in Figure 8.1, a high probability of offense may be associated with environments that either inadvertently set conditions that make re-offenses more likely to occur (e.g., allowing access to persons at risk for victimization or negative social influences) or fail to promote conditions that would prevent an offense (e.g., appropriate supervision). Low probability of re-offense is associated with environments that set conditions that make offending less likely to occur (e.g., adequate supervision) and minimize risk (e.g., restricting access to potentially vulnerable persons while simultaneously providing prosocial conditions for development and growth). Some factors may be common to all offenders, such as issues of supervision, although some may be specific to the individual and are determined during the individual's functional behavior assessment (i.e., antecedents and consequences to the behavior).

KEY FACTORS IN SETTING THE STAGE FOR SUCCESS

As shown in Figure 8.2, setting the stage for success involves four areas: (1) establishing an environment that creates conditions under which the offending behavior is less likely to occur, and appropriate, alternative, prosocial behaviors are taught, and reinforced; (2) selecting and training staff members to ensure that appropriate supervision, therapeutic interactions, and support are provided; (3) developing an individualized plan of activities and programming to provide skill building opportunities and access to reinforcement; and (4) providing opportunities for social relationships and conditions that promote motivation for appropriate engagement instead of offending behavior.

Figure 8.2 **Setting the Stage for Success**

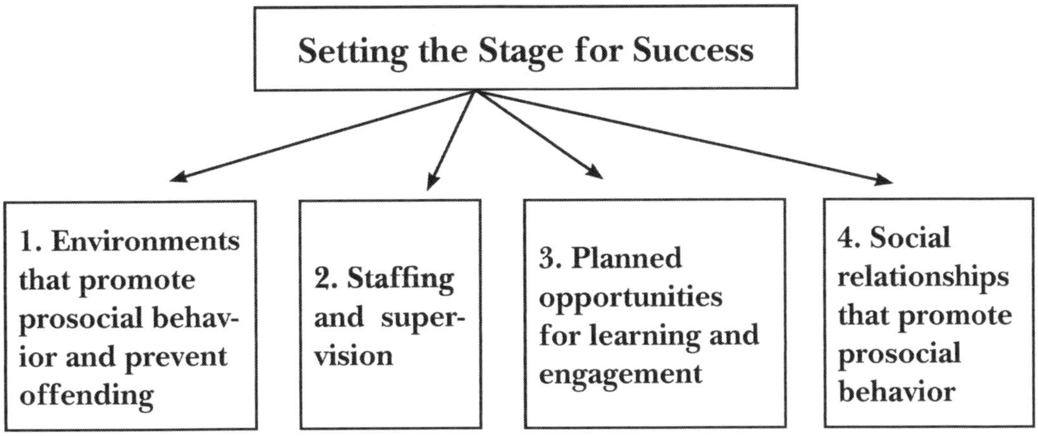

1. Environments That Promote Prosocial Behavior And Prevent Sexual Offending

The role of the environment in the development of challenging behavior in persons with intellectual disability (e.g., Gardner, Graeber & Cole, 1996; Martens & Witt, 1988) and treatment (e.g., Griffiths, Gardner, & Nugent, 1998) has been elaborated in the literature; however, until recently there has been less emphasis on the environmental supports needed for persons with intellectual disabilities who have sexually offended with some exceptions (Griffiths, Quinsey, & Hingsburger, 1989; Haaven, Little, & Petre-Miller, 1990). Griffiths et al. (1989) recommended that an habilitatively appropriate environment should be as normalized as possible in that "it promotes learning and use of those skills and behaviors that result in an enriched life-space for the individual" (p. 100). Griffiths and Fedoroff (2008) noted, however, that individuals with intellectual disabilities who have sexually offended are typically exposed to physical conditions that are not normative and that offer limited, if any, habilitatively appropriate programming. Griffiths et al. (1998) suggested that conditions that fail to provide habilitatively appropriate conditions combine with the pre-existing challenges in coping, social, and related skills to produce an increased vulnerability to the possibility of re-offense.

Selecting and Establishing an Habilitiative Environment

Individuals with intellectual disabilities who have offended live in a variety of settings: institutions, prisons or civil commitment centers, hospital or psychiatric facilities, community treatment centers or group homes, or their family homes. Each of these settings has specific variables that can contribute to the likelihood of positive treatment outcomes. A common discussion is whether treatment for individuals with intellectual disabilities should occur in the community or institution considering manageability of risk in each environment (Boer, Tough, & Haaven, 2004). Since the latter part of the last century, models for each have been successfully applied (e.g., Griffiths et al., 1989; Haaven et al., 1990). Wherever the location, a client's manageability depends on ensuring risk factors are known and ameliorated.

The habiliatively appropriate environment is more than a place in which basic needs are met; it provides opportunities, supports, and interactions suited to the needs and goals of the individual (Griffiths et al., 1998). The environment can contribute to the offending behavior if not carefully considered. First, it may contain conditions that could trigger or contribute to the offending problem, enhance the criminogenic factors that are associated with the behavior, or inadvertently allow the behaviors to be reinforced. Second, an environment that is not supportive of the individual can be detrimental to the therapeutic objectives. "It is easy to understand why persons who live in environments that are overcrowded, lacking in privacy, unstimulating, lacking in positive interactions, and in some cases, even physically or psychologically abusive, may develop challenging behaviors as attempts to cope with these conditions" (Griffiths et al., 1998, p. 105).

Regardless of where an individual who offended resides (e.g., treatment center, family home, or otherwise), the therapeutic quality of the environment is perhaps the most important element of setting the stage for success. The environment includes factors such as location, expectations, opportunity for prosocial activities, and risk reduction, all of which need to be tailored to an individual's risks and needs. The goal is to create a situation with the lowest possible risk to the community and the highest quality of life for the individual.

An habilitatively appropriate environment rests on three elements: physical elements, social characteristics, and structural factors.

Physical Elements

The location of the environments in which a person resides and frequents should be assessed to minimize, if not eliminate, potential risk. Proximity to a desired target person is obviously a significant risk factor for any individual with a history of sexual offending. Individuals who are vulnerable to abuse and those who could be potential targets should not reside with potential abusers. This is particularly important to consider given data suggesting that persons with disabilities are much more likely to be abused in care centers than neurotypical individuals (Sobsey & Doe, 1991). However, pragmatics and practicality too often interfere in the process and are used as administrative reasons for clustering of individuals in settings where this risk may be imminent. It is crucial, ethically, clinically, and legally, that every step is taken to ensure that vulnerable residents do not live with those likely to take advantage of them. Sadly, this also includes staff, which speaks to the need for heightened screening in hiring practices.

The neighboring community and places visited in the community should also be assessed for appropriateness. For some individuals, the sight of potentially vulnerable persons could increase the likelihood of sexually inappropriate conduct. For individuals who have offended against children, living in close proximity to a school or park where there are a lot of children could be problematic. Let's consider the case of Dan:

> *Dan offended against a child, ten years previously. He had been living in a highly-supervised treatment program and had done well in learning coping strategies. He had not offended in years, so the agency that supported him decided, without discussion with Dan's treatment team, to move him into a less restrictive neighborhood. An open bed came up in one of the group homes; it was located next door to a primary school. Because it had been a long time*

> *since Dan had offended, this was not considered problematic. He had been at the new home for only a week when the staff members observed that he was spending a lot of time in his bedroom at the back of the house. One lunch time, when he had not come out to have his meal, a staff member found him masturbating while standing at the bedroom window watching the children playing in the schoolyard. The staff became concerned and alerted the supervisor. They asked that he be moved to a different location. A new plan was put in place to relocate him and in the meantime, they frosted windows to obstruct his view of the playground.*

The goal is always to provide people with the most independent and autonomous lives possible without posing risk to themselves or others. As such, any decision about placement and opportunities for social engagement must be weighed against the potential risks to the community. An individual's level of security and external support must be balanced against the risks they pose, their ability to manage behavior (and, often, obtain necessary services to assist in managing behavior), and their willingness to do so. *Dan may well have been able to move to a less restrictive environment, but a home overlooking a school yard was a very poor choice and one that could have eventually led to a re-offense.*

The key to selecting the right environment for a particular client depends on evaluating the nature of the risk, the degree of self-management, and the motivation to offend or to abstain from offense. Individuals with offense histories who represent lower levels of risk, who have learned and demonstrated application of self-management strategies, and who are motivated to not offend, may be sustained in environments that are less restrictive, while still providing shelter from stimuli and conditions that are associated with offending. However, individuals who are at high-risk for re-offense, show little evidence of self-management, or are motivated to offend may require environments that not only ensure there is no access to stimuli or conditions for re-offense, but higher levels of restriction and supervision. The following example illustrates this:

> *A number of years ago one of the authors was supporting an individual who had a lengthy and violent offense history. After years of treatment, he stated very clearly that he would offend again if given the opportunity. He demonstrated no evidence that he would attempt to deter re-offending if the opportunity arose; however, he did not want to go to jail. This individual was aware that he would re-offend if given the chance and so he volunteered to enter a treatment home. This setting would provide him with an environment that would allow his behaviors to be managed. This treatment home, for all intents and purposes, was a secure facility within the community. Although treatment would probably not result in his movement to a less restrictive environment, this home provided him with the security needed to prevent re-offense. His home was equipped with automatic locks and alarm systems to prevent elopement or access to vulnerable persons in the neighborhood.*

The level of security illustrated in the example above can be extremely valuable and necessary if the client's risk to offend is sufficiently high. It is, however, extremely costly and difficult to maintain; additional and supplementary funding may be necessary to ensure the appropriate external supports are in place. For other persons whose risk profiles are less problematic, this level of security and risk management is unnecessary and intrusive. As we noted earlier, the Risk-Need-Responsivity model (Bonta & Andrews, 2017) decrees that the environment must be carefully tailored to the needs and risks associated with each individual, rather than employ a 'cookie-cutter' template.

The environment in which the person lives is of primary consideration and, ideally, is individualized. Antecedent strategies should be considered first; for instance, minimizing exposure and access to potentially vulnerable persons can reduce risk (Hanson, Harris, Scott, & Helmus, 2007).

Using knowledge of the conditions that are associated with problem behavior and the conditions associated with non-problem behavior has been used with other challenging behaviors to set the stage for success. For example, Touchette, MacDonald, and Langer (1985) worked with persons with intellectual disabilities who engaged in serious high-risk self-injurious behavior that typically would have been treated using punitive approaches or managed using intrusive strategies (e.g., restraint or seclusion). As a student of Skinner, Touchette and his associates were influenced by the importance and value of understanding the stimuli influencing the behavior and a focus on positive reinforcement rather than punishment to change behavior. He and his associates conducted careful analysis of the variables that were associated with high-risk conditions for self-injury and the conditions that were associated with no risk or low risk for self-injury using a scatter plot method of data collection, which demonstrated the correlation between specific behaviors and certain times of day, interactions, and activities. Using those data, they then developed a systematic plan to build a schedule for the individual that was enriched with all the activities and interactions that were problem-free conditions. They also eliminated, to whatever extent possible, those conditions that were associated with the problem behavior. Without using punishment or behavior management approaches such as restraint, they created an environment in which they demonstrated a reduction in self-injurious behaviors to what they termed a "zero baseline." By eliminating or reducing the risk and conditions associated with the problem behavior, they could then move forward with treatment in a proactive way to provide positive therapeutic and educative changes. Therapeutic approaches, especially those that include teaching alternative and compensatory skills, are vital for this final goal to be achieved. However, the foundation for this begins with setting the stage for success by providing conditions in which the person is set up to achieve the desired goals. This idea can be also applied to our work with individuals who have offended.

The layout of the individual's home can be tailored in advance to minimize risk. For some, the sight of potentially vulnerable persons could be a concern and could cause sexual behaviors. Frosted windows, blinds, and other forms of obstruction can be utilized. Depending on the individual's risk and motivation, homes may have automatic locks and alarm systems. This is typically meant to prevent elopement or access to vulnerable persons in the neighborhood. This level of security can be extremely valuable and necessary if the client's risk is sufficient. As noted above, however, such measures are costly and will likely require additional funding.

For some clients, this level of security and risk management is unnecessary and intrusive. As stated, the environment must be tailored to the individual. At all times, independence and autonomy must be weighed against the potential risks to the community.

It is a practical reality that most persons with an intellectual disability will not have a driver's license and will have to find alternate transportation. Transportation challenges will mean the residence needs to be within walking or public transit distance from all essentials, such as visits to the probation officer or habilitative opportunities such as a job. In the process of commuting, the potential risk of coming into contact with a potential target must be addressed. For example, if the individual has offended against children, locations such as public pools, parks, and school will be off-limits, and the individual may be required to live a certain distance away from them. Sometimes these decisions are program-based; however, some are imposed as conditions of probation. Ensuring safety is not just determining locations the person can or cannot access but may also include issues of supervision while in the community, a topic to be discussed later in this chapter.

Social Characteristics

Social characteristics involve positive relationships, stability, and meaningful activities in which to engage to attain personal goals. Staff represent an important element in creating the social characteristics of the setting. Although staffing attitudes, levels, and training will be discussed as a separate section of this chapter, some of the more social characteristics of staffing involve ensuring a positive interactional atmosphere, where there is access to a relatively high amount of positive feedback and interaction, in relation to any corrective feedback or discipline. It also involves ensuring staff spend most their time interacting with the individuals in proactive ways, whether teaching skills or enjoying leisure or recreational time, to set an atmosphere of positivity and role models for positive social interaction.

Other residents of the home also play an important role in creating the social characteristics of the setting. Unfortunately, individuals with intellectual disabilities who have committed a sex offense will often be congregated with other individuals who have committed offenses. While this may create a positive therapeutic milieu, it can often run the risk of creating situations where prosocial behaviors are not being modelled by others and where potential of abuse by other residents/peers can occur. Issues of emotional and personal safety within the setting are of paramount importance to the therapeutic process; trust cannot occur in an environment where personal boundaries are repeatedly violated. Additionally, where possible social compatibility, such as levels of functioning and potential for prosocial engagement in activities should be considered when selecting potential housemates; however, practicality often interferes with this latter element.

Structural Factors

Structuring an habilitatively appropriate program involves setting clear expectations, specifying contingencies, strengthening social motivation, problem-solving and choice-making, and decreasing aversive conditions (Griffiths et al., 1998). For most of us, the expectations to live in society have become internalized from our life-long learning experiences, however as Lindsay (2009) suggested some individuals with intellectual disabilities, by virtue of their experiences in combination with their disability, may have not acquired the internalized self-management, and some may even be unaware that they are violating set expectations. In creating a therapeutically habilitative setting, it is important to establish clear, explicit, and consistent expectations for all interactions and engagement in daily routines.

As Griffiths et al. (1998, p.119) noted, "Well defined and explicitly represented standards of conduct are critical features of the habilitative environment." By setting well defined expectations, both staff and those supported are aware of the behavioral standards that will bring about rewards in both human interaction and access to desired activities, as well as the avoidance of any sanctions that may result from a breach of expected behavior.

In addition to establishing standards of conduct, the habilitative environment also provides known contingencies that will be applied if breaches in accepted behavior occur. Educative approaches to teaching using a pleasant but matter-of-fact manner can often be helpful when establishing the standards of conduct. Adherence to the expectations should receive ample social reward, which can include access to desired reinforcement: *"Wow, since you are first to get your chores done, I guess you get to have more time in the games room. Nicely done."* This can create enhanced sensitivity to the contingencies involved in meeting expectations and further sets up the groundwork for enhanced social motivation and personal choice for their own behavior.

Setting realistic and consistent contingencies for both appropriate and inappropriate behavior emphasizes the standards of behavior that are considered acceptable. Unless the person has learned standards of conduct or inhibitory controls, the response may be impulsive and without awareness of the implications of the behavior. In the habilitatively appropriate environment, minor infractions may receive reminders or redirection until an expectation has been established; however, disruptive or persistently inappropriate behavior may require the person to be sanctioned in some way. Although certain set sanctions may be established for repeated behaviors, the nature of those sanctions would be determined by assessing the function to ensure that the person is able to learn to take responsibility for meeting the expectations but not reinforced inadvertently.

A gap exists in the literature to guide those in clinical settings to know how to assess, intervene, and impact dynamic variables (Ioannou, 2013). Boer, McVilly, and Lambrick (2007) attempted to address this gap when noting the value of examining environmental variables pertinent to persons with intellectual disabilities and sexual behavior problems when evaluating and managing risk. They identified that persons with disabilities who offended are dependent on external structures and supports and that these structures and supports affect recidivism. In their exploration of a broader framework for assessing dynamic risk factors, which typically included antisocial attitudes and substance abuse, they added environmental dynamic factors that would allow for enhanced risk management. The product of their work was the *Assessment of Risk and Manageability of Intellectually Disabled Individuals who Offend Sexually* (ARMIDILO-S; Boer et al., 2007, 2013).

The ARMIDILO-S examined environmental variables such as "staff attitudes towards individuals with intellectual disability, communication amongst supervisory staff, client knowledge by staff, supervision consistency, environmental consistency, victim availability and access, availability of intoxicants, social support changes, and use of structured daily activity plans" (Boer et al., 2007, p. 2). Blacker, Beech, Wilcox, and Boer (2011) examined the predictive value of the ARMIDILO-S compared to three other risk assessments (RRASOR, SVR-20, RM2000-V) comparing 44 mainstream individuals who had sexually offended to 44 individuals who had sexually offended who also had an intellectual disability. They demonstrated that the ARMIDILO-S provided the best predictive validity for sexual re-offenses among people with intellectual disabilities (Blacker et al., 2011). Unfortunately, their research did not have sufficient data from the files to complete the environmental subsections and to date lacks empirical validation as it is still in the construction phase (Blacker et al., 2011).

Stability plays another important part in setting the stage for success. Too often in our social service system staffing is a constantly changing factor in the lives of the persons being supported. While there is some inevitability in this dilemma, staff who work with clients who have offended may require additional incentives in the form of opportunities for personal development to remain engaged and committed to a type of social service work that can pose unique demands. Some of these opportunities can be tied into the expectations of a structured program.

Enhancing social motivation for prosocial behavior is at the heart of an habilitatively appropriate environment. At the core of behavioral change is providing access to opportunities to gain natural sources of motivation and to teach the person to value personal accomplishment and ownership over the choices that determine their future life.

As described in Chapter 6, the Good Lives Model (Ward & Gannon, 2006; Yates, Prescott, & Ward, 2010) proposed that treatment and rehabilitation for persons who have offended should ensure that there is opportunity to attain various goals that are important to the person's quality of life. This is critically important for setting the stage for success as the individual must receive enough reinforcement across aspects of their life to make offending unnecessary or at least less important than the loss of other life qualities.

Some of the common ways in which these goals can be achieved are through activities of daily living, as well as recreational and vocational opportunities. Individuals with intellectual disabilities often have underdeveloped skills in daily living and community-based domains (Belva & Matson, 2013); this is likely a result of the dependent cultures in which they are raised and skill deficits associated with their disability. They grow up with many tasks (making meals, doing laundry, handling financial matters) being done for them by a care provider; initially out of necessity and later out of convenience. However, as opportunities for community participation and independence grow, these skills may need to be taught. These areas may represent growth enhancing opportunities that can lead to independence and may foster interests for an individual to pursue.

Recreational and leisure interests should also be fostered to identify areas where the person may find personal enjoyment. Each person will be different in what is valued, be it music, cooking, physical activities, movies, etc. However, in the habilitative environment, people should be exposed to a range of opportunities to determine what recreational or leisure choices might be personally satisfying and would enhance their quality of life and purpose.

Similarly, there should be opportunities for each person to explore options for employment or volunteer work that could earn money and/or personal gratification. Although as with all opportunities risk must be considered, for many individuals employment can reduce risk of re-offense (Kruttschnitt, Uggen, & Shelton, 2000). Employment can keep an individual busy and supervised during the majority of the day. It can also offer a sense of pride and accomplishment—something worth protecting. Additionally, as with daily skills and recreational options, employment skills may need to be taught to allow the person to be successful. There are curricula that can provide the education required, such as James Stanfield's Job Smart series (www.stanfield.com), but staff should be creative in finding opportunities to nurture and practice these skills.

2. Staffing and Supervision

Staffing has been shown to be a critical factor in determining therapeutic success for persons with intellectual disabilities who have engaged in offensive conduct (Ioannou, 2013). The quality of the staffing is dependent on attitudes, training, level of supervision, and consistency.

Staff Attitudes

Staff attitudes towards sexuality and towards individuals who have sexually offended are important to examine. The expectations and biases of the staff should be assessed prior to their hiring to work with clients with intellectual disabilities who have offended:

> *Literature in the area of sexual expression of handicapped persons residing in many different settings reveals that supervision continues to be restrictive and suppressive, even when other facets of the persons' lives are fairly normalized. Direct contact-workers have been shown to be primarily responsible for establishing unwritten policy about the sexual behaviors allowed in clients in residential settings. (Bratlinger, 1983, p. 21).*

In response to this observation, Bratlinger (1983) developed the *Sexuality and the Mentally Retarded Attitude Inventory* (SMRAI). Evaluation of this measure showed that it was effective in assessing the attitudes that people held about the sexuality of persons with intellectual disability. Bratlinger suggested that this scale might be helpful for agencies that are making decisions about placement of persons with intellectual disabilities, as well as determining which direct care workers might be most suitable to provide an environment that would encourage appropriate adaptive sexual behaviors. Whether using a formalized scale or a thorough interview process, assessment of staff attitudes when hiring for positions to work with individuals who offended is critically important.

Fedoroff and Richards (2010) suggested that staff often hold beliefs that the persons with intellectual disabilities who have offended will be unable to respond to treatment or learn the skills necessary to live less restrictive lives. They noted that in addition to this being prevalent among staff, it can also be exhibited within an entire system. When this occurs, the system creates highly intrusive and restrictive contingencies, such as 24/7 supervision without timelines for review or change. The justification for these contingencies is often based on the premise that they are keeping the individual and the community safe. While risks may have been managed, this type of approach focused largely on containment does not set up staff expectations for improvement in the client's behavior. Moreover, it can set the occasion for the individual to be treated in a particularly negative way that does not support habilitative progress. Fedoroff and Richards suggested that this approach excludes the individual from the process and, as such, denies the person the opportunity to prove that they can be trusted. Respectful relationships exhibited by staff form the foundation for the development of a culture of prosociality that serves as a model for the persons with whom they work. Further, respectful interactions allow for the promotion of increased social motivation, decreased aversive elements, and, within the confines of the known expectations, encourages the development of choice and prosocial problem-solving.

Staff Training

Although hiring staff who have positive and respectful attitudes is paramount, to ensure the best support in a successful environment, staff should be trained and provided with clinical support in a variety of areas as described in Table 8.1: Modules of Staff Training. They should be fully aware of the environment and any modifications made to it. Staff should be familiar with the individuals' histories, behaviors, offenses, and any legal restrictions. Importantly, all staff must be well versed in the behavior support plan and be able to implement it. To this end, audits and regular trainings may be necessary to ensure staff members have the knowledge and skills to follow through with all behavior protocols. More specific training should be explored as needed and focus on areas such as data collection, safe management of dangerous behaviors, and appropriate boundaries with clients.

In line with the discussion above, all staff members need training and guidance in how to provide respectful and consistent interactions with the individuals they support. Training should be both global and specific. Global training refers to provision of the knowledge and skills necessary to work with individuals with intellectual disabilities who have offended; specific training refers to the knowledge and skills to work with a particular client with an intellectual disability.

Table 8.1: ***Staff Training***

	Modules of Training
Global Training	• Through performance and competency based (or behavioral skills) training • Basic ABA principles and general data collection • Risk management • Training on the treatment approach; for example, Self-Regulation and Good Lives models • Static and dynamic risk assessments • Healthy sexuality • Trauma and using trauma-informed care in a support role • Knowledge of police and probation and how to have a collaborative relationship • Crisis prevention • Training on how to manage and respond to dangerous behaviors within a rights-based context

Specific Training	• Individual risk factors and methods to reduce risk through stimulus control (e.g., access) • Training specific to their diagnoses (i.e., mental health/genetic disorders) and how this impacts behavior • Habilitative goals for the individual and methods used to develop new skills. • Individualized Self-Regulation and Good Lives models and their application in a support role • Individualized risk assessment training • The conditions and requirements of specific police or court orders (e.g., probation order, sex offender registry) • Data collection specific to the individual's tracking sheets

Reid, Parsons, and Green (2012) developed a guidebook for supervisors using evidence-based strategies to enhance staff performance to promote quality of work. They further note that "successful supervision involves working with staff in ways that are acceptable to staff and promote enjoyment in their work" (p. 6). This latter point is a critical issue to promote staff satisfaction and retention.

Staff should be fully versed in the individual's program, including teaching goals and method of instruction, rhythm of the day, expectations and restrictions, and corrective and remedial consequences. Reid et al. (2012) noted that the first step in a protocol for evidence-based supervision is to make sure that the desired outcomes for each individual have been identified. Step 2 involves specifying the role of staff in attaining those goals, and Step 3 involves training the staff to perform the skills. The goal would be to create a seamless flow throughout the program day and integrate therapeutic opportunities into the natural interactions of the day.

However, successful supervision does not stop there. Reid et al. (2012) suggested that the supervision protocol also include monitoring staff performance, supporting performance of staff who have shown proficiency, correcting staff performance that is not consistent with the plan, and evaluating both staff performance and the outcomes of the individuals on an ongoing basis. Training for staff should be based on a behavioral skills training approach that includes teaching through instruction, modelling, rehearsal, and feedback. The nature of the training should be both competency and performance based. It is insufficient to simply tell staff what to do or have them read the treatment program. Staff must be trained to use the protocols and desired approaches to reach a criterion in both global skills and the specifics of the person's program, including the daily routines, expectations, teaching approaches, and strategies.

One of the key areas that must be included in staff training relates to managing potential risks for a re-offense. Staff members need to be trained such that if an individual who offended is found to resume old patterns or fantasies and engaging in inappropriate or antisocial behavior, this is a clear warning signs that the individual who offended is not managing well and is lapsing into behaviors that are precursors to re-offense. Quinsey, Book, and Skilling (2004) followed a sample of 58 individuals with an intellectual disability and offense histories following their transition to community settings and found that ratings of inappropriate and anti-social behavior were the best predictors of subsequent inappropriate violent or sexual behavior. Therefore, staff members need training on the types of precursor behaviors that might signal that greater supervision or enhanced treatment may be needed. More specifically, Proulx, Perreault, and Ouimet (1999) found that among a group of individuals who had histories of sexual offenses against prepubescent children, frequent sexual fantasizing and masturbation to images of children had occurred prior to their sexual offenses. Inappropriate sexual fantasizing was often an immediate precursor to re-offending (Proulx et al., 1999). This finding illustrates the value of training all staff members who support clients to be familiar with a preferred type of person to victimize, grooming behavior, and the risk factors associated with each client (Boer et al., 2004). Of course, the clients also need to understand the role that these fantasies, precursors, and risk factors play in their potential for re-offense. An individual who can identify his own risk factors through open and ongoing discussion amongst the people who work with him is more likely to monitor these factors regularly and effectively and is less likely to lie about high-risk situations that they encounter (Boer et al., 2004). Well trained, informed, and dedicated staff allow the opportunity for individuals to grow their skills and better manage risk.

Boer and colleagues (2004) also recommended that staff be aware of conditions that may represent risk situations related to sexual re-offending, such as accessing pornography and pictures of children and watching television depicting potentially vulnerable persons. These behaviors require an immediate response by the supporting staff to interrupt an extremely high-risk pattern of behavior (Griffiths et al., 1989). Changes in either attitudes or behaviors related to supervision or treatment, such as refusal to attend treatment sessions or monitor their risk factors, can be an indication that a lapse is occurring. It may mean that the individual has encountered a potentially vulnerable person who is being targeted, or he has relapsed and is attempting to avoid punishment. It is critical that an open and trusting relationship with the staff support team has been established so that the individual at risk can feel comfortable reporting a lapse in behavior.

Effective staff training is not defined by just content, but by how it is taught and how staff supervisors follow-up to ensure that the direct care staff are adhering to the protocols and programs. Use of the behavior skills training (BST) approach (Miltenberger, 2004) has been demonstrated to be effective in teaching staff to implement programs and protocols, such as functional analysis (Ward-Horner & Sturmey, 2012), and has been adopted for training supports and caregivers in a variety of areas. This model utilizes a four-step process of instructions, modeling, rehearsal, and feedback. Instructions are provided to the trainee and then modelled by the trainer. The trainee then practices or rehearses these skills under supervision, and immediate feedback is provided. As noted above, this process continues until a desired level of fluency and competency has been reached. Research has shown it can be superior to other techniques (Nosik, Williams, Garrido, & Lee, 2013) and use of the feedback portion specifically shows marked improvement in skill acquisition.

Consistency

One of the prominent factors in programmatic success has been shown to be consistency, which encompasses consistency in staff, routine, and supervision (Boer et al., 2004). Griffiths and Fedoroff (2008, p. 368) suggested that:

> *Clear socially constructed expectations and standards of conduct function as guides for appropriate actions for both the individual and the care providers. Often individuals with disabilities have received inconsistent or poorly defined expectations; these conditions do not establish conditions for the development of prosocial inhibitions to impulses or stimulation present at the moment. As a result, the individual does not learn to be concerned over the immediate or long-term consequences that may result.*

Boer and colleagues (2004) identified that individuals with intellectual disability who have offended tend to manipulate and exploit any inconsistencies between staff members. Inconsistency in staffing can provide a dynamic risk to re-offense. When discussing consistency, there are three main areas: consistency in staff members, consistency in routines and consistency in expectations.

Inconsistency can be caused by a lack of training for each staff member who works with a particular client, by a staff member, unintentionally or intentionally, not following the same approach as prescribed and used by others, or when a new staff member, without sufficient training or supervision, begins to work with the individual who offended. Ioannou (2013) suggested that inconsistency can arise if a staff member treats an individual who offended as if they are a child or a favorite. These biases can result in harmful consequences when other clients identify that differential treatment is being applied to various peers. It further disadvantages other staff members by negatively influencing their relationship with the favored individual. Consistency among care providers shifts the emphasis in interactions from "testing the limits of each staff" to developing more constructive interactions (Griffiths & Fedoroff, 2008, p. 368). Boer et al. (2004) suggested that it is important for the individual with an intellectual disability to become accustomed to one style of supervision across staff members. Although staff turnover, change in caseload, and changes in staff approach should be avoided as much as possible, a consistent approach to which all staff members have been trained, and the consistency of their implementation has been monitored, will reduce disruption.

Consistency in routine is also critically important. It allows the staff to be able to observe the individual in a consistent manner so that they can be aware of any changes in the behaviors. As well unplanned changes or routines without structure can also set conditions for behavior problems. Change in routine and staffing is sometimes inevitable; however it is important to recognize that seemingly minimal changes in scheduling can greatly increase risk. Similarly, a drastic change in routine and structure, such as a re-location, can affect all aspects of the individual's environment. As Boer and colleagues (2004) pointed out, not all individuals with intellectual disability "cope well with change and the external structure that a familiar place or daily routine brings to such offenders is an important aspect of their sense of self-control and well-being" (p. 280). Although unfamiliar, new staff cannot always be avoided, it is important to recognize that when a new staff member begins working, risk increases as the individual who offended may begin to test boundaries or act out. To prevent this as much as possible, Boer et al. (2004) suggested that new staff begin with limited caseloads, be given sufficient training prior to working with people who have offended, and that the transition to the new staff be gradual and monitored. This period of orientation to new staff may evoke some acting out or testing of boundaries by some individuals who have offended (Boer et al., 2004).

Staff complacency, as noted by Lindsay and Beail (2004) is a significant predictor of recidivism in individuals with intellectual disabilities and offense histories that has been consistently noted in the research (Boer et al., 2004; Craig, Browne, & Stringer, 2003; Lindsay & Beail, 2004). Lindsay and Beail (2004) explored the influence of risk assessment variables as predictive of re-offense in 52 persons with intellectual disabilities and offense histories (18 who re-offended past treatment; 34 who did not). Some of the variables related to consistency including deteriorating treatment compliance and staff complacency. One of the most significant predictors of re-offending was the dynamic risk variable associated with allowances made by staff and deteriorating compliance, with allowances being made by staff as one of the strongest predictive factors (Lindsay & Beail, 2004). This is an important consideration for ongoing training and staff performance evaluation and monitoring.

Level of Supervision

Supervision is a dynamic risk factor that is credited with having some of the largest effects on re-offending. For example, McGrath, Livingstone, and Falk (2007) reported positive recidivism rates which they attributed largely to the provision of 24-hour supervision. Similarly, Hanson and Harris (2000) conducted a comprehensive study comparing 208 persons who sexually re-offended to 201 persons who did not sexually re-offend on many variables through interviews and file reviews. They suggested that the amount of and compliance with supervision were directly related to recidivism in sexual offending and inversely related to an increased risk of re-offense (Hanson & Harris, 2000).

Attention is typically given to the ratios and intensity of staff supervision. The amount of staffing needed to properly supervise and support an individual must be determined by the overall habilitative needs of the individual, the type of supervision needed to ensure safety, the relative risk posed by the person based on the history of behaviors, the person's demonstrated motivation to control or re-offend, as well as the degree of self-regulation that has been exhibited. The intensity of the supervision, whether in 'close-proximity' or merely 'eyes on,' is also dependent on the individual's needs and skill level.

In keeping with the risk principle of the RNR model (Bonta & Andrews, 2017), the amount of supervision is dependent on the level of risk. Consistent supervision must be provided through unique monitoring strategies for every individual who offended (Boer et al., 2004). Ioannou (2013) suggested that supervision varies depending on risk but can involve direct observation of the client at all times by one or more staff members. This level of supervision allows for any change in the client's behavior to be recognized, including changes in emotional state, behavioral stability, or mental health indicators that can inform appropriate intervention. Additionally, consistent supervision can allow for staff to notice any changes in risk factors because of changes in life situations, which will alert the need for additional monitoring. For example, a change in the client's routine (e.g., watching a park from afar) can be extremely significant and may reveal new potential to offend; these changes can only be identified through proper and knowledgeable staff supervision. Boer and colleagues (2004) provided the following scenario to illustrate this point: "The presence of a new family in an apartment block may result in delays in catching public transit by the offender who has taken an extra 5 min[utes] to watch the new children get on the school bus" (p. 280). This is a suitable example of when people at risk to re-offend try to increase their access to potentially vulnerable persons, which is another variable that can be alleviated through adequate supervision. While some people at risk will attempt to actively gain access to vulnerable persons, sometimes these encounters occur accidentally (e.g., when a child or woman might come to visit another individual in the home or building, or when out in community). Staff knowledge of the sort of persons potentially at risk (and staff alertness to respond to those critical situations) is an important element of targeted and effective supervision (Boer et al., 2004).

Although supervision must be carefully and consistently applied according to the established program, the degree of supervision must be fluid so that it can change *systematically* if conditions change. If the conditions shift the potential of risk then supervision levels should be shifted programmatically to respond to the dynamic change. Enhanced supervision may be required to respond to certain periods of time, certain events or occasions, or because of some apparent unrelated life experience (e.g., loss of job or an important relationship) that might make the individual more likely to offend. At these times staff must alert the supervisors of the potential elevation of risk caused by the presence of specific triggers or conditions where the person is less likely to use the self-management strategies because of a change in motivation, so that a change in protocol can be instituted.

3. Planned Opportunities for Learning and Engagement

Griffiths and Fedoroff (2008) suggested that habilitation is based on "two primary and interacting intervention elements: development of habilitative strengths within the individual and exposure to the habilitatively appropriate environment by which the acquired habilitative strengths can become appropriated by the individual" (p. 367). Building a strong prosocial life that has meaningful engaged relationships and activities leaves the individual little time or opportunity in which to commit an offense (Ward, Mann, & Gannon, 2007). Moreover, by instilling a means to gain a reinforcing quality of life, the individual can establish a life worth losing (Ioannou, Griffiths, Owen, Condillac, & Wilson, 2014). The phrase a life worth losing may appear strange to some readers, but it implies that many offenders, particularly those with intellectual disabilities have not been afforded lives that are inherently valued by the offender. Often their lives have been stripped of the privileges, rights, and opportunities that are typically afforded individuals in our society to provide a quality life. Thus, part of appropriate habilitation is to give the person who has offended a life that has value and that is important to the individual, such that the person will behave in a manner to protect it, to not lose it. So whether you wish to call this a life worth losing or a life worth keeping, the assumption is that as psychological well-being increases, risk decreases; as psychological well-being decreases, risk increases. For the rest of this chapter we have chosen to call it a life worth keeping.

Dewhurst and Nielsen (1999) suggested a resiliency-based approach to working with persons who have sexually offended that provides a means for individuals to change and, as such, to bounce back from adversity. Six core resiliencies have been suggested by Wolin and Wolin (1993): initiative, ability to develop relationships, morality, creativity and humour, independence, and insight. In addition, Dewhurst and Nielsen (1999) added empathy as a seventh resiliency factor. They suggested that rather than use these resiliency factors to point out the deficiencies of the individual, effective resiliency strategies should focus on enhancing the core resiliencies by fostering, recognizing, and reinforcing examples of these when demonstrated by the individual. The concepts involved in resiliency closely align with several current approaches in both the treatment of persons who have sexually offended (the Good Lives Model; see Peel Behavioral Services [PBS] & Wilson, 2017; Ward & Stewart, 2003; Yates et al., 2010) and two approaches employed in work with persons with intellectual disabilities: Person Centred Planning (i.e., Kincaid, 1996) and Quality of Life (i.e., Renwick, Brown & Raphael, 1994).

The elements of Quality of Life, the Good Lives Model, and Person-Centered Planning all interact in service planning to provide a framework for resiliency as shown in Figure 8.3.

Figure 8.3: **Resiliency Factors**

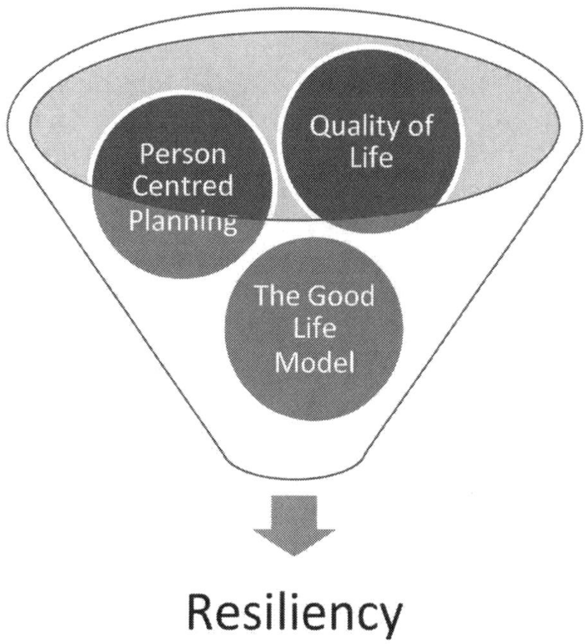

Each of these will be elaborated below.

The Good Lives Model, described earlier in this book (GLM; PBS & Wilson, 2017; Ward & Stewart, 2003), suggested that clients in treatment must be given the means to acquire 'primary human goods' (i.e., experiences and states of mind that all human beings seek to attain) in prosocial ways so that the need to offend (i.e., antisocial behavior) to secure them is no longer necessary (Ward et al., 2007). This way of looking at effective human existence harkens back to the earlier "life skills" constructs of balance and self-determinism identified by Curtiss and Warren (1973). By way of example, Boer and colleagues (2004) identified that one issue that related to manageability of individuals with intellectual disabilities who offend was boredom. They found that routines in activities and a structured and full day can reduce boredom and prevent the occurrence of high-risk behaviors (Boer et al., 2004). Thus, effective treatment ensures that the environment provides external conditions (e.g., activities, resources, social supports, opportunities) to set the occasion for prosocial behaviors to flourish. Early remnants of this approach have been evident in treatment programs for individuals with intellectual disabilities for over 25 years (i.e., Griffiths et al., 1989; Haaven et al., 1990). In their later work, Haaven and Coleman (2000) discussed building a good life with their distinction between the 'old me' and 'new me' in treatment of persons with intellectual disabilities who had sexually offended. The 'old me' was the individual who committed sexual offenses, and his beliefs, values, and goals associated with offending behavior. The construction of a 'new me' involved establishing a new set of goals, values, beliefs, and ways of living that reflected a good life for the individual in which primary goods could be achieved and sustained through socially acceptable ways. In the conceptualization of a 'new me', friends, family, activities, events, and material possessions are highlighted (Haaven & Coleman, 2000). A recent publication (PBS & Wilson, 2017) provides a compendium of exercises aimed at assisting individuals in treatment with opportunities to explore the primary goods suggested by the Good Lives model.

These approaches provide a rebalancing of reinforcement history for an individual with an intellectual disability and can aid in relapse prevention. Many persons with intellectual disabilities had nothing much to lose by re-offending, because the reinforcement density in their lives was typically bereft. The establishment of strong non-contingent reinforcement for a variety of life enriching interactions and activities, contingent reinforcement for appropriate behaviors, and building a better life create conditions under which a re-offense would be costly for the individual in terms of loss of a range of reinforcing opportunities that are afforded for non-occurrence (i.e., a life worth keeping). This perspective has received some correlational support in the literature. For example, Hanson and Harris (2000; see also Hanson et al., 2007) found that that the social environment of those individuals who did not re-offend had more positive influences than negative, whereas the social environment of those who re-offended had more negative influences than positive. What constitutes a good life must be based on identifying the elements of what a good life would look like for each individual; or, what a quality life would be for that person. This idea of a good life can be highly individualized although many constructs will be similarly applicable to a majority of persons. It is also important to remember that many persons with intellectual disabilities will have had difficult experiences in early life meaning that their conception of a "good life" may not be the same as what staff, treatment providers, or other people might think of. Sometimes, it may be better to ask clients to strive for a "better life" rather than get too bogged down in trying to define what a "good life" might actually be.

Quality of Life

The concept of quality of life has been evident in many areas of study dating back to Maslow's early concepts of hierarchy of needs (Maslow, 1943) but has been particularly important in recent years in the evaluation of the lives of persons with intellectual disabilities. There have been numerous papers that have defined and operationalized the concept of quality of life for persons with intellectual disabilities (e.g., Felce & Perry, 1995; Renwick et al., 1994). Renwick and associates (1994) described quality of life in terms of three elements: (i) physical/psychological health and wellbeing, (ii) belonging in the community and with important others, and (iii) engagement and growth in everyday life and of a future. Felce and Perry (1995) proposed a quality of life model that encompassed the dimensions of physical (health and well-being), material (income, possessions, housing quality, and privacy), social (family, friends, and community involvement through activities, events, acceptance, and support), emotional well-being (positive affect, fulfillment, self-esteem, and faith/belief), along with development and activity (employment, housework, leisure/hobbies, education, and independence). All the components that make up quality of life are important enhancements to apply in a systematic approach to assessment and treatment leading to the prevention of relapse(s). For example, in addition to focusing on sex offense risk factors, it is important to provide individuals at risk with opportunities that incorporate the various dimensions of quality of life.

The emphasis on improving quality of life for individuals who have offended is a shift of focus from hopelessness and a lack of control to one of hope and resiliency. Factors such as trusting relationships, encouragement, personal strength and self-esteem, social and interpersonal skills, and communication skills have been identified as pivotal factors in building resilience (Masten, 2001). Additionally, certain qualities of the environment or the individual can compensate for or protect the individual in the face of risk. Applying a resiliency model of intervention to persons with intellectual disabilities who have sexually offended would suggest that recidivism could be decreased by building a supportive, positive, and reinforcing environment, along with helping clients to establish the competencies necessary to respond to risk factors in realistic ways.

Despite the strong emphasis placed on the importance of quality of life and resiliency in the literature, these concepts are not commonly applied as a measure to prevent sexual re-offending to persons with intellectual disabilities. This is ironic because the cornerstone of services for persons with intellectual disabilities is based on providing individualized support directed at enhancing quality of life through person-centered planning. However, when the person with an intellectual disability sexually offends, the principles on which service is provided often neglect to include these fundamental elements.

As noted above, quality of life is an individually determined concept. Although the components in the two quality of life conceptualizations described above have many similarities, the included components may not share the same value for every individual. As Reiss (2001) wrote, it is important to determine the relative motivational influence of various factors, such as social contact, on a case-by-case basis to ascertain the relative reinforcing value of these basic human needs for a particular individual.

Through person-centred planning the relative value of the various components can be analyzed as they relate to the individual, thereby setting the stage for a good quality of life for that person.

To summarize, resiliency is founded on the idea that the individual in question has the skills necessary to cope with future situations similar to those that produced the offending behavior, but also that the individual has been afforded the essential features of a good quality of life, or a 'good life.' However, Ward et al. (2007) caution that providing a quality of life is not entirely sufficient when dealing with people who have offended: "Simply seeking to increase the well-being of an offender without regard for his level of risk may result in a happy but dangerous individual" (Ward et al., 2007, pp. 92-93). They suggested that there should, therefore, be a functional balance between a fulfilling life and risk management. Thus, level of rights must be balanced with community protection; this balance is determined by the level of risk.

Person-Centered Planning

Considered as a best-practice strategy in serving persons with intellectual disabilities (Schalock et al., 2002), person-centered planning is often mandated by funding bodies: "Life plans, lifestyle planning, essential life plans, personal futures planning and functional life planning are all examples of approaches to person-centred planning" (Gahan, Dykstra, & Summers, 2002, p. 194). It is both a philosophy and an approach (Ritchie, 2002) that guides planning for an individual in terms of evaluation and goal setting (Mansell & Beadle-Brown, 2004). The key elements are: (i) that planning is focused on strengths, abilities, and wishes of the individual and not their deficits or challenges; (ii) that the person is not only included, but at the center of the planning process with the support of those closest to him/her; and (iii) that the level and type of support is based in individualized goals, not on pre-existing services (Mansell & Beadle-Brown, 2004). The objective of this type of planning is to enhance individualization of supports to both achieve objectives and improve quality of life. Although literature is lacking on the outcomes for this intuitive approach, a recent study has shown that planning based on these principles demonstrates enhanced personal outcomes and supports when compared to traditional planning approaches (Gosse, Griffiths, Owen, & Feldman, 2017).

This type of planning approach complements and is consistent with the idea of building a quality life. It further ensures that the individual is invested in the chosen outcomes and that others in the individual's social network have identified roles and responsibilities in supporting those outcomes, which is very much in keeping with the responsivity principle of the RNR model (Bonta & Andrews, 2017). For people who have offended, a goal may be to keep them safe (as well as others), but, in addition, it involves choosing future outcomes that they can work towards to gain greater independence, skills, and opportunities. This provides a medium through which the objectives of a quality of life can be framed in terms of an improved life, rather than a model of deficit reduction.

One of the key areas fundamental to person-centered planning is inclusion in the community. Community integration has been a difficult and imperfect process for individuals with intellectual disabilities (Chowdhury & Benson, 2011). However, Lindsay (2005) suggested that community involvement is necessary for persons with intellectual disabilities who have offended to achieve a good life. Otherwise, a lack of engagement in society can lead to two important consequences: "First, if the individual is not engaged in occupational, leisure, and social activities, they have more time to engage in antisocial or deviant activities. Second, their number of prosocial influences is correspondingly reduced" (Lindsay, 2005, p. 435).

While many individuals with intellectual disabilities evade criminal charges, some do incur sanctions from the justice system. Even though court diversion is a common path, probation may still be a requirement, and with it several sanctions for risk management may be applied, such as limits on the locations the individual may go to and the people with whom they are allowed to associate. These sanctions or limitations can be invaluable for individuals in whom motivation to change is a challenge or who lack the skills to manage risk themselves. However, when the concern for community safety and minimizing risk are at odds with the opposing needs for rehabilitation, such measures can also serve to create barriers to community engagement or reintegration. Although the clinical and judicial spheres do not always intersect, working in collaboration with probation officers or other behavioral supervisors can be helpful in working out a coordinated plan that satisfies both risk management and the rehabilitative goals, such as fostering other employment, interests, or hobbies but under set conditions (e.g., times of day, type of required staffing).

Persons with intellectual disabilities who have offended come from a variety of environments and histories and have individual skill sets and abilities. Although inclusion in the community is an important step, it is imperative to consider the skills necessary for successful (re)integration. Individuals with intellectual disabilities who have engaged in offensive conduct need to be educated *prior* to reintegration and provided with training on acceptable social behavior and cultural norms – leading to opportunities for success. These individuals *may* have grown up with a different set of rules, which ultimately renders difficult any situation in which they are expected to instantly adapt to a new set of rules (Hingsburger & Harber, 1998). Indeed, this would be difficult for anyone, not just persons with intellectual disabilities. Individuals need specific skills and knowledge to adapt, and many will require support from staff to facilitatte the learning opportunities required to acclimatize to a non-offending lifestyle.

Griffiths and associates (1989) noted the importance of addressing gaps in the learning components needed for a person to be successfully supported in the community. Determination of the skills needed is individually assessed and training is provided as needed in education, relationships, social competency (social skills), coping skills, and responsibility. These skills will be addressed in Chapter 9, Teaching Alternative and Coping Skills.

4. Social Relationships that Promote Appropriate Behaviors

> *Lack of interpersonal skills throughout adolescence and young adulthood may result in some men avoiding social situations and increasing their personal isolation. Lengthy periods of time alone may allow the individuals to foster deviant sexual fantasies and maladaptive sexual schemata which increase the possibility of a sexual offense. With repeated, ordinary social contact, any propensity to develop these maladaptive sexual schemata will be hampered by constant prosocial influences which constitute repeated 'reality checks'. These are not major significant events, but rather constitute mundane and ordinary social contact. (Lindsay, 2009, p. 103)*

Griffiths and Fedoroff (2008) suggested that "a key factor in the long-term success and generalization of intervention may be the development of habilitatively appropriate *social* environments" (p. 368). They suggested that the role of the social environment is to ensure that opportunities are provided for the individual to develop, perhaps for the first time, the value of positive relationships with a variety of people who are part of a person's life by mutual choice and to learn to maintain these relationships because of mutual enjoyment. An essential element related to creating an habilitatively appropriate social environment is to develop a range of sustaining or stable relationships that can provide the opportunity for personal or, where appropriate, intimate relationships to be reinforced. An habilitatively appropriate social environment will allow the individual to experience success in social interactions and daily life, so that the person emerges with enhanced self-esteem awareness and personal control. The new identity, or "new me" as Haaven et al. (1990) have described it, emerges as a result of these positive social experiences and the development of new and reinforcing social interactions that are based on clear expectations for a new and improved quality of life and knowledge of the consequences of the potential loss of that quality of life if inappropriate sexual expression reoccurs.

Social Relationships

Without social opportunities and social skills, individuals may find it more difficult to establish meaningful relationships later in life. Social relationships can provide motivation to avoid re-offense and provide supervision and support when thoughts of offense emerge. Indeed, supports and community connections can be invaluable in providing motivation and assistance to remain offense free. It is important to include and foster supportive and involved family and community connections. However, in some cases these pre-existing relationships might become strained due to the offending (which may have happened within the same social or support circle) and subsequent sanctions. Offending often ostracizes individuals from their natural support network, and this is especially concerning because many individuals with intellectual disabilities may have had only a small network of social support prior to the offense. Families and friends may be scarce and those relationships become strained with offending, and if these supports leave risk may increase. Although researchers such as Lindsay (2009) have found that having ties to the community and friendships can reduce risk, often persons with intellectual disabilities and, perhaps, more so those who have offended, have significantly fewer connections than the typical population.

For some persons with intellectual disabilities who have sexually offended, staff members may become their primary, if not only, social network. It is, therefore, vital that these interactions form the foundation on which future social relationships can eventually be built. However, staff relationships are not designed to be long term friendships, nor should they. The social relationship with staff should be respectful and supportive, but the fiduciary responsibilities of this role make it imperative that ethical boundaries are established.

When and if appropriate to risk and resiliency, efforts should be made to expand a network of social interactions and supports. However, all too often the only opportunities individuals with an intellectual disability have are at segregated dances and bowling outings, and these occasions are set up by staff and provide little chance for organic friendships. Unpaid relationships for individuals with intellectual disabilities are very rare and difficult to obtain. Friendships and social interaction have benefits in development, providing skill building in reading and responding to social cues, reciprocal conversation, and means of starting and maintaining friendships.

Research has shown that concepts such as Circles of Support and Accountability (Wilson, McWhinnie, Picheca, Prinzo, & Cortoni, 2007; Wilson & McWhinnie, 2017), in which volunteers and professionals provide community support and advocacy, can be of benefit in improving both quality of life and risk management. The program was developed in Canada in 1994 but has proliferated internationally. Several studies have demonstrated that individuals released from secure settings or other care facilities can successfully re-enter society after offenses or legal sanctions and engage in less violent and sexual re-offending behavior than comparison groups (Bates, Williams, Wilson, & Wilson, 2013; Duwe, 2013, 2018; Wilson, Cortoni, & McWhinnie, 2009; Wilson, Picheca, & Prinzo, 2007).

Family and Supports

There are times when the individual who offended can remain living with family or when the individual spends time in the family home even if they reside elsewhere. In these cases, the family needs intensive training and support to be able to follow through on the elements of any treatment program and risk management strategies. If the offense occurred within the family (i.e., against a family member), then significant environmental controls would need to be put into place to ensure that the individual who offended is never left alone with potentially vulnerable persons.

Families may need to be prepared and supported in re-establishing relationships with individuals who offended. Because many offenses occur within family, reunification between the person victimized and the person who did the victimizing may be a concern. Victimized persons may feel a sense of betrayal from the person who offended against them. Depending on the nature of the relationship and level of trust prior to the offense, the trauma can be significant. If force or coercion were used as well, this can further exacerbate the effects. Some families may need to see that the person has benefited from treatment before they are willing open the door to a relationship. This may take time as some families are not ready to reunify.

In all cases, the victimized person should guide the reunification process, taking only the steps that they are willing to take when ready. Typically, when his/her psychologist or therapist and the client who offended feel they are ready to open communication, the person who offended will be allowed to write a letter. The process continues with various forms of communication, but always guided by the person who was victimized. However, despite barriers research has identified factors that increase the likelihood of successful reunification following abuse (Miller, Fisher, Fetrow, & Jordan, 2006), and it can be beneficial in certain cases.

Meetings with mediation may be necessary, and the process may begin slowly and build in both contact and intimacy. It is the family and supports that must drive the process and their consent and guidance are invaluable. Rushing the process with a family can be extremely counterproductive and can prevent opportunities for re-establishing relationships. The family itself may need counselling to deal with issues and reach a decision whether they want the individual back in their lives. Despite the family being an invaluable resource, they must do so willingly and many choose to separate from the person who offended. If they do decide to be part of the offending person's life again, it may be a long process before all parties are prepared.

If all voices and all opinions are not respected when mediating between persons who have been victimized and those who victimized them, the foundation of the process will be tenuous and subject to failure. It goes without saying that a full understanding of the risks involved must be of critical importance during this process. No matter how eager, the degree to which all individuals involved feel secure must always be appropriately managed. Given their prior histories and the presumed lack of recent contact, this process can be very unpredictable, and a conservative approach may be best.

Intimate Relationships

Sexual behaviors are often motivated by functions that are not necessarily inappropriate (paraphilic) in nature. As described in Chapter 6, attention, escape, or other means of non-sexual pleasure could reinforce and maintain the behavior, but the offense can also be motivated by biological needs for sexual gratification or intimacy with another. Hanson and Harris (2000) found that individuals who re-offended experienced more intimacy problems, such as relationship conflicts and lack of intimate partners, whereas the opposite was true for persons without offending histories. Thus, a lack of positive relationships is an important piece of the risk assessment puzzle that has been shown to increase the likelihood of a sexual re-offense. This knowledge can be advantageous, as the function of relationships is relatively clear and readily understood. The disadvantage is that relationship-based intimacy with another cannot simply be sought and procured. Persons with intellectual disabilities rarely have the same opportunities as those in the typical population to engage in sexual relationships. In fact, any sexual behavior, including masturbation, has historically been discouraged, as individuals with intellectual disabilities were often perceived as non-sexual entities (Griffiths, 2003). Griffiths noted that the socioenvironmental contexts in which most persons with intellectual disabilities live have been typically repressive and punitive for all sexual behavior, even that which is appropriate (age-appropriate, consenting, private, and within the limits of social law and mores). Such restrictions can set occasion for a behavior motivated primarily by the goal of achieving sexual satisfaction to be further influenced by the desire to avoid punishment and ridicule rather than the engagement in a consenting, appropriate relationship. As Griffiths and Fedoroff (2008) noted, "the systems in which people with intellectual disabilities live can promote a 'Catch 22' regarding the development of sexually appropriate behavior" (p. 363). The conditions of the environment can promote a higher incidence of sexually inappropriate behavior.

Sexual offending behavior may be rooted, in some cases, in a lack of appropriate education regarding sexuality and interpersonal relations (Griffiths, Hingsburger, Hoath, & Ioannou, 2013). A key component of appropriate and healthy sexuality is also one of the least understood: consent. Consent is a difficult and abstract concept to many in this population and has often been poorly modeled. Research suggests that the ability to provide consent in areas such as making medical decisions can be improved with structured training and teaching (Ferguson & Murphy, 2014). Teaching consent should be targeted as early as possible for two reasons. One, it provides a degree of abuse prevention and ensures that the individual knows how to give (and receive) consent. As well, it decreases the likelihood of future inappropriate behavior that could be the result of inappropriately learned boundaries or counterfeit deviance. This is both a protective and risk management strategy to set the stage for success; one that can be reliably done with some individualized trainings and education.

Although persons who have learned appropriate socio-sexual knowledge would ideally have the opportunity to demonstrate a mastery of this knowledge, this raises a serious ethical dilemma: Is it ever safe to allow individuals who have historically engaged in offending behavior to engage in intimate relationships? There are obvious clinical benefits to individuals with offending behaviors having consensual and age appropriate intimate relationships. As stated previously, the function of inappropriate behavior may be based in the desire for sex and intimacy. However, just teaching socio-sexual skills does not always ensure their application in the real world where interactions cannot be predicted. Griffiths and Fedoroff (2008) noted that although a person may have learned that sexual contact with another must be age-appropriate and consenting, they may still be rejected for unknown reasons. As a result, sexual education must also include learning that sexual attraction is unpredictable and that rejection is a real possibility. They noted, "too often, persons with intellectual disabilities are taught the 'appropriate behaviors' without being taught that the partner may or may not respond as scripted. Thus, it is critical to review the contingencies and prepare alternative responses." (Griffiths & Fedoroff, 2008, p. 368).

There are other risks that must also be managed. Individuals who have engaged in sexually inappropriate behaviors may do so again, and careful planning is required to ensure there is no risk to anyone in the community. Enabling opportunities for intimate relationships to potentially develop should be only fostered under conditions in which the individual has developed and demonstrated non-offending competencies; for some individuals who offended (i.e., those who demonstrate an approach pathway), that may never be possible.

SUMMARY

This chapter highlights many of the important variables that must be considered to set individuals up for treatment success. The foundation for setting the stage for success involves establishing an environment in which it is less likely for offending behavior to reoccur, and where prosocial behaviors are encouraged; where staff are carefully selected, trained and supervised in providing consistent and respectful treatment; where there are planned opportunities for engagement in meaningful activities; and social relationships and community inclusion are encouraged to whatever degree possible. Fundamental to achievement of treatment goals is a focus on teaching alternative and coping skills (which will be the focus of the next chapter), and the establishment of remedial and corrective consequences, as elaborated in Chapter 10.

REFERENCES

Bates, A., Williams, D., Wilson, C., & Wilson, R. J. (2013). Circles South-East: The first ten years 2002-2012. *International Journal of Offender Therapy and Comparative Criminology, 58,* 861-885.

Belva, B. C., & Matson, J. L. (2013). An examination of specific daily living skills deficits in adults with profound intellectual disabilities. *Research in Developmental Disabilities, 34,* 596-604.

Blacker, J., Beech, A. R., Wilcox, D. T., Boer, D. P. (2011). The assessment of dynamic risk and recidivism in a sample of special needs sexual offenders. *Psychology, Crime & Law, 17,* 75-92.

Boer, D. P., Haaven, J. L., Lambrick, F., Lindsay, W. R., McVilly, K. R., Sakdalan, F., & Frize, M. (2013). *The Assessment of Risk and Manageability of Individuals with Developmental and Intellectual Limitations Who Offend – Sexually (ARMIDILO-S).* Retrieved from www.armidilo.net.

Boer, D. P., McVilly, K. R., & Lambrick, F. (2007). Contextualizing risk in the assessment of intellectually disabled individuals. *Sexual Offender Treatment, 2,* 1-5.

Boer, D. P., Tough, S., & Haaven, J. (2004). Assessment of risk manageability of intellectually disabled sex offenders. *Journal of Applied Research in Intellectual Disabilities, 17,* 275-283.

Bonta, J. & Andrews, D.A. (2017). *The psychology of criminal conduct* (6th ed.). Cincinnati, OH: Anderson.

Bratlinger, E. (1983). Measuring variation and change in attitudes of residential care staff toward the sexuality of mentally retarded persons. *Mental Retardation, 21,* 17-22.

Chowdhury, M. & Benson, B. A. (2011). Deinstitutionalization and quality of life of individuals with intellectual disability: A review of the literature. *Journal of Policy and Practice in Intellectual Disabilities, 8,* 256-265.

Craig, L. A., Browne, K., & Stringer, I. (2003). Risk scales and factors predictive of sexual offense recidivism. *Trauma, Violence, & Abuse, 4,* 45-69.

Curtiss, P. R., & Warren, P. W. (1973). *The dynamics of life skills coaching.* Prince Albert, SK, Canada: Saskatchewan NewStart Inc. for the Training Research and Development Station, Department of Manpower and Immigration.

Dewhurst, A. M., & Nielsen, K. M. (1999). A resiliency-based approach to working with sexual offenders. *Sexual Addiction and Compulsivity, 6,* 271-279.

Duwe, G. (2013). Can circles of support and accountability work in the United States? Preliminary results from a randomized experiment in Minnesota. *Sexual Abuse, 25,* 143-165.

Duwe, G. (2018). Can circles of support and accountability (CoSA) significantly reduce sexual recidivism? Results from a randomized controlled trial in Minnesota. *Journal of Experimental Criminology.* Published online first.

Fedoroff, J. P. & Richards, D. A. (2010). Sexual disorders and intellectual disabilities. In S. Levine, C. B. Risen & S. E. Althoff (Eds.), *Handbook of Clinical Sexuality for Mental Health Professionals, 2nd edition* (pp. 451 468). New York: Routledge Publishing.

Felce, D., & Perry, J. (1995). Quality of life: Its definition and measurement. *Research in Developmental Disabilities, 16,* 51-74.

Ferguson, L., & Murphy, G. H. (2014). The effects of training on the ability of adults with an intellectual disability to give informed consent to medication. *Journal of Intellectual Disability Research, 58*, 864-873.

Gahan, S., Dykstra, L, & Summers, J. (2004). Person-centred approaches to services and supports. In D. M. Griffiths, C. Stavrakaki, & J. Summers, *Dual diagnosis: An introduction to mental health needs of persons with intellectual disabilities* (pp191-206). Sudbury, ON: Habilitative Mental Health Resource Network.

Gardner, W. I., Graeber, J. L. & Cole, C. L. (1996). Behavior therapies: A multimodal diagnostic intervention model. In J. Jacobson & J. Mulick (Eds,), *Manual of diagnosis and professional practice in mental retardation* (pp. 355-369). Washington DC: American Psychiatric Press.

Gosse, L., Griffiths, D., Owen, F., & Feldman, M. (2017). Impact of individualized planning approach on personal outcomes and supports for persons with intellectual disabilities. *Journal of Policy and Practice in Intellectual Disabilities, 14*, 198-204.

Griffiths, D. (2003). Sexuality and people with developmental disabilities: From myth to emerging practices. In I. Brown & M. Percy (Eds.), *Developmental disabilities in Ontario* (2nd ed.) (pp. 677–690). Toronto, ON: Ontario Association on Developmental Disabilities.

Griffiths, D., & Fedoroff, P. (2008) Persons with intellectual disabilities who sexually offend. In F. M. Saleh, A. J. Grudzinskas, J. M., Bradford, & D. J. Brodsky (Eds.), *Sex offenders: Identification, risk, assessment, treatment, and legal issues* (pp. 352-374). New York: Oxford University Press.

Griffiths, D., Gardner, W. I., & Nugent, J. (1998). *Behavioral supports: Individual centered behavioral interventions – A multimodal functional approach.* Kingston, NY: NADD Press.

Griffiths, D., Hingsburger, D., Hoath, J., & Ioannou, S. (2013). 'Counterfiet deviance' revisited. *Journal of Applied Research in Intellectual Disabilities, 26*, 471-480.

Griffiths, D. M., Quinsey, V.L., & Hingsburger, D. (1989). *Changing inappropriate sexual behavior: A community-based approach for persons with developmental disabilities.* Baltimore: MD: Paul H. Brookes Publishing Co

Haaven, J. L., & Coleman, E. M. (2000). Treatment of the developmentally disabled sex offender. In D.R. Laws, S.M. Hudson, & T. Ward (Eds.), *Remaking relapse prevention with sex offenders: A sourcebook* (pp. 369-388). Thousand Oaks, CA: Sage Publications Inc.

Haaven, J., Little, R., & Petre-Miller, D. (1990). *Treating intellectually disabled sex offenders: A model residential program.* Orwell, VT: Safer Society Press.

Hanson, R.K., & Harris, A.J.R. (2000). Where should we intervene? Dynamic predictors of sexual offense recidivism. *Criminal Justice and Behavior, 27*, 6-35.

Hanson, R. K., Harris, A. J., Scott, T. L., & Helmus, L. (2007). *Assessing the risk of sexual offenders on community supervision: The Dynamic Supervision Project.* Ottawa, ON: Public Safety Canada.

Hingsburger, D., & Harber, M. (1998). *The ethics of touch: establishing and maintaining boundaries in service to people with developmental disabilities.* Eastman, QC: Diverse City Press.

Ioannou, S. (2013). *Managing risk in a culture of rights: providing support and treatment for sex offenders with intellectual disability in community-based settings.* Unpublished Master of Arts Thesis. St. Catharines, ON: Brock University.

Ioannou, S., Griffiths, D., Owen, F., Condillac, R., & Wilson, R. J. (2014). Managing risk in a culture of rights: Providing support and treatment in community-based settings for persons with intellectual disabilities who sexually offend. *ATSA Forum, 26,* 1-11. Retrieved from http://newsmanager.commpartners.com/atsa/issues/2014-01-11/4.html.

Kincaid, D. (1996). Person-centered planning. In L. K. Koegal, R. L. Koegal, & G. Dunlap (Eds.), *Community, school, family, and social inclusion through positive behavioral support* (pp. 439-465). Baltimore MD: Paul H.Brookes.

Kruttschnitt, C., Uggen, C., & Shelton, K. (2000). Predictors of desistance among sex offenders: The interaction of formal and informal social controls. *Justice Quarterly, 17,* 61-87.

Lindsay, W. R. (2005). Model underpinning treatment for sex offenders with mild intellectual disability: Current theories of sex offending. *Mental Retardation, 43,* 428-441.

Lindsay, W. R. (2009). *The treatment of sex offenders with developmental disabilities.* West Sussex, UK: Wiley-Blackwell.

Lindsay, W. R. & Beail, N. (2004). Risk assessment: Actuarial prediction and clinical judgement of offending incidents and behavior for intellectual disability services. *Journal of Applied Research in Intellectual Disabilities, 17,* 229–234.

Mansell, J., & Beadle-Brown, J. (2004). Person-centred planning or person-centred action? Policy and practice in intellectual disability services. *Journal of Applied Research in Intellectual Disabilities, 17,* 1-9.

Martens, B. K., & Witt, J. C. (1988). Expanding the scope of behavioral consultation: A systems approach to classroom behavior change. Professional *School Psychology, 3,* 271–281.

Maslow, A.H. (1943). A theory of human motivation. *Psychological Review, 50,* 370-396.

Masten, A. S. (2001). Ordinary magic: Resilience processes in development. *American Psychologist, 56,* 227–238

McGrath, R. J., Livingston, J. A., & Falk, G. (2007). Community management of sex offenders with intellectual disabilities: Characteristics, services, and outcome of a statewide program. *Intellectual and Developmental Disabilities, 45,* 391-398.

Miller, K. A., Fisher, P. A., Fetrow, B., & Jordan, K. (2006). Trouble on the journey home: Reunification failures in foster care. *Children and Youth Services Review, 28,* 260-274.

Miltenberger, R. (2004). ***Behavior modification: Principals and procedure*** (3rd ed.). Belmont, CA: Wadsworth Publishing.

Nosik, M. R., Williams, W. L., Garrido, N., & Lee, S. (2013). Comparison of computer based instruction to behavior skills training for teaching staff implementation of discrete-trial instruction with an adult with autism. *Research in developmental disabilities, 34,* 461-468.

Peel Behavioral Service & Wilson, R.J. (2017). *Passport to independence.* Holyoke, MA: NEARI Press.

Proulx J., Perreault, C., & Ouimet, M. (1999). Pathways in the offending process of extra familial sexual child molesters. *Sexual Abuse, 11,* 117-129.

Quinsey, V. L., Book, A., & Skilling, T. A. (2004). A follow-up of deinstitutionalized men with intellectual disabilities and histories of antisocial behavior. *Journal of Applied Research in Intellectual Disabilities, 17,* 243-253.

Reid D. H., Parsons M. B., & Green C. W. (2012). *The supervisor's guidebook: Evidence-based strategies for promoting work quality and enjoyment among human service staff.* Morganton, NC: Habilitative Management Consultants.

Reiss, S. (2001). *Who am I? The 16 basic desires that motivate our actions and define our personalities: Beyond pleasure and pain.* New York: Putnam.

Renwick, R., Brown, I., & Raphael, D. (1994). Quality of life: Linking a conceptual approach to service provision. *Journal on Developmental disabilities, 3,* 32–44.

Ritchie, P. (2002). A turn for the better in implementing person-centered planning: Voices of experience. In J. O'Brien & C. L. O'Brien (Eds.), *Implementing person-centered planning: Voices of experience.* Vol. II (pp., 11-24). Toronto: Inclusion Press.

Schalock, R., Brown, I., Brown, R., Cummins, R., Felce, D., Matikka, L., Keith, K., & Parmenter, T. (2002). Conceptualization, measurement, and application of quality of life for persons with intellectual disabilities: Report of an international panel of experts. *Mental Retardation, 40,* 457-470.

Sobsey, R. & Doe, T. (1991). Patterns of sexual abuse and assault. *Sexuality and Disability, 9,* 243-259.

Touchette, P. E., MacDonald, R. F., & Langer, S. N. (1985). A scatterplot for identifying stimulus control of problem behavior. *Journal of Applied Behavior Analysis, 18,* 343-351.

Ward, T., & Gannon, T. A. (2006). Rehabilitation, etiology, and self-regulation: The comprehensive good lives model of treatment for sexual offenders. *Aggression and Violent Behavior, 11*(1), 77-94.

Ward, T., Mann, R. E., & Gannon, T.A. (2007). The good lives model of offender rehabilitation: Clinical implications. *Aggression and Violent Behavior, 12,* 87-107.

Ward, T., & Stewart, C. A. (2003). The treatment of sex offenders: Risk management and good lives. *Professional Psychology: Research and Practice, 34,* 353–360.

Ward-Horner J. & Sturmey P. (2012). Component analysis of behavior skills training in functional analysis. *Behavioral Interventions, 27,* 75–92.

Wilson, R. J., Cortoni, F., & McWhinnie, A. J. (2009). Circles of support & accountability: A Canadian national replication of outcome findings. *Sexual Abuse, 21,* 412-430.

Wilson, R. J. & McWhinnie, A. J. (2017). *Circles of support & accountability: A "how to" guide for establishing CoSA in your location.* Report compiled under contract to Counseling and Psychotherapy Center, Inc. for the United States Department of Justice, Office of Justice Programs, Office of Sex Offender Sentencing, Monitoring, Apprehending, Registration, and Tracking.

Wilson, R. J., McWhinnie, A., Picheca, J. E., Prinzo, M., & Cortoni, F. (2007). Circles of support and accountability: Engaging community volunteers in the management of high risk sexual offenders. *The Howard Journal of Criminal Justice, 46,* 1-15.

Wilson, R. J., Picheca, J. E., & Prinzo, M. (2007). Evaluating the effectiveness of professionally facilitated volunteerism in the community-based management of high risk sexual offenders: Part two—A comparison of recidivism rates. *Howard Journal of Criminal Justice, 46,* 327-337.

Wolin, S.J., & Wolin, S. (1993). *The resilient self.* New York: Villard Books.

Yates, P. M., Prescott, D. S., & Ward, T. (2010). *Applying the good lives and self-regulation models to sex offender treatment: A practical guide for clinicians.* Brandon, VT: Safer Society Press.

Chapter Nine

Teaching Alternative or Coping Skills for Sex Offending Behavior

We have known since the 1960s that the best way to decrease a challenging behavior is the use of differential reinforcement. Ayllon and Azrin (1968) and Azrin and Holz (1966) demonstrated reductions in inappropriate behavior by providing access to alternative appropriate behaviors that serve the same function, or that bring about the same reward. The application of these principles is critically important when applied to sexual offending behavior, as McGuire (2001) described in the following:

> *The aim of the functional analysis of sexual-offending behavior is two-fold. One is to eliminate the undesirable behavior, in this case sexual-offending behavior, but also to provide alternative, positive behavior to engage in.... if the offender is not taught appropriate behavior to engage in for reinforcement, there will be an eventual return to the previous behavior (p.142).*

EMPLOYING A DECISION MODEL TO DETERMINE INDIVIDUAL HABILITATIVE COMPONENTS OF TREATMENT

Determining alternative functional skills or coping skills is based on the analysis of the antecedents, motivating operations, and maintaining consequences/function. Treatment for persons with intellectual disabilities who have sexually offended is not a one-size-fits-all model. The effectiveness of interventions will depend on identifying the areas of remediation that are relevant to the particular individual and designing individualized programs to meet those targeted needs.

THE ROLE OF FUNCTIONAL REPLACEMENT SKILLS

After a full assessment has been completed and both the function of the problematic behavior and skill deficits have been identified, work must begin on replacing those behaviors and teaching the necessary skills to manage situations that could present with high risk. Often programs for persons who have sexually offended include a range of components that serve to provide alternative means of achieving a function (such as teaching social skills to those seeking attention, providing sex education for those who are seeking out a relationship but lack appropriate knowledge or skills, or emotion management for those who offend when under duress or frustration).

Although it is assumed that deficits in these areas may be related to the likelihood of a re-offense, it should not be assumed that all individuals who offended require the same type of intervention. Behavioral skills training, involves a combination of effective learning principles to maximize treatment effects, including instruction, modeling, rehearsal, and feedback (Miltenberger, 2008). There should be no "one size fits all" approach to treatment of persons who have sexually offended, and behavioral skills training can be used to teach the identified deficits which may mitigate conditions that influence re-offending.

A functional replacement behavior is a new behavior that serves the same function and has the same reinforcing properties as the problematic behavior. The replacement behavior is most effective when it requires less effort and is more reinforcing than the problem behavior (Cooper, Heron, & Heward, 2007). An example would be an individual who steals women's underwear from the store because he enjoys the way it feels but is too embarrassed to purchase it. An intervention can consist of reducing the stigma associated with the clothing, as well as providing easy access to stores without aversive consequences. These conditions will carry none of the negative outcomes that the problematic behavior carries. These strategies can be taught relatively easily based on the individual's skill level and should be reinforced immediately and consistently to shape these responses to oppose the problematic behavior. These replacements are designed to lead to immediate reinforcement with no negative side effects such as guilt or shame, as well as charges, jail, or community restrictions. As such, they should become more reinforcing in a shorter period of time.

In addition to what functionally replacement behaviors *are*, it is important to also consider what they are *not*. Often in clinical practice no consideration is given to replacing sexualized behavior. Rather, there is the expectation that those who have committed a sexually inappropriate or offensive behavior should just 'stop it' or 'make it go away' through responses that bear no relationship to the function, or *why* the person is acting that way. Consider public masturbation as an example. It is not the act itself of masturbation that is inappropriate, but the selection of time or place for engaging in the behavior that is inappropriate or illegal. Let's examine the following example:

> *Through assessment it was determined that an individual has been engaging in masturbation in public places, such as the group home living room, because it feels good to do so; the reinforcement is automatic. The behavior is not mitigated for any biomedical reason or for social reinforcement. In response to this finding the staff members have decided to try to reduce the behavior by keeping the individual's hands busy by doing the dishes when at home or playing with hand held games on the bus. While there may be some merit in distraction under some circumstances, such as if travelling on the bus, this is not an effective or appropriate functional replacement behavior as it will likely not serve the same function nor does it provide opportunity for the individual to learn where it is appropriate to engage in the behavior and where it is not.*

It is important to note that introducing functional replacement behaviors is not as straightforward as it may seem. Rather, to ensure success, it often requires extensive teaching of skills environmental modifications, and the support and consistency of mediators (e.g., family, staff). It may also be helpful to differentiate between inappropriate sexual behavior that has no underlying "deviance" versus inappropriate sexual behavior that has a sexually "deviant" component. However, both must consist of teaching functionally equivalent replacement behaviors.

AN ABSENCE OF SEXUAL DEVIANCE

A functional assessment is likely to reveal the function the behavior serves, which could include sexual touching that serves to provide attention from peers or staff, public exposure to escape from situations of discomfort, or sexual aggression that may serve to reduce anger or frustration. When it is identified that the sexualized behavior provides an attention or escape-based function (e.g., Wright, Herzog, & Seymour, 1992), the person can be taught more prosocial means of escaping a situation or accessing attention (Durand, 1999) such as verbal request, use of a visual cue, or having consistent, frequent breaks scheduled throughout the day. Persons with intellectual disabilities may engage in inappropriate sexual behavior to escape unpleasant or undesired situations, as this type of behavior would typically provide immediate reinforcement, in the form of redirection or removal from the situation as soon as possible. The immediacy of negative reinforcement for the behavior can quickly increase the frequency of this behavior to escape the situation. The same can be said of attention: sexual behaviors are taken seriously and intervention is typically immediate – even if meant to be aversive in nature, staff, peer, or stranger attention is almost guaranteed and will provide reinforcement on every occasion.

A PRESENCE OF SEXUAL DEVIANCE

Teaching functional replacement behaviors for sexual offending behaviors is much more inherently difficult as, by their nature, the majority of sexually inappropriate behaviors serve a sensory function. This means that a replacement behavior must also be as inherently rewarding (and easier to access) to be behaviorally effective. With a sensory-based function, the behavior itself is reinforcing, and any additional steps or behaviors are likely to be even more difficult to obtain reinforcement, which makes them less efficacious. This presents a particularly difficult challenge for a clinician. For a purely physiological self-stimulatory replacement, in certain cases masturbation can be used as a functional replacement. The majority of sexually inappropriate behaviors are motivated by the act itself: the offense and sensations associated with it are the reinforcement. In these cases, the physiological feelings associated with the behavior include sexual arousal and ejaculation, which can largely be replicated with masturbation. Consenting sexual activity with an appropriate partner can be even more reinforcing than inappropriate behaviors but may be more difficult to obtain. Given the living situations of most individuals with intellectual disabilities, relationships may be difficult or impossible, and it is critical that agencies be prepared to support their clients in these pursuits where appropriate. Further, this population traditionally has deficits in social skills (Smith & Matson, 2010) that may make establishing intimate relationships difficult. Treatment programs should aim to fill these gaps and provide appropriate training and opportunities to meet an intimate partner.

There are of course challenges with this method. Masturbation as a replacement behavior is not generalizable in all situations. If the individual is in the community and feeling aroused, masturbation in that moment is not typically a safe or appropriate option. Additionally, there may be inappropriate features of the offending that make it reinforcing, such as the involvement of another individual. If force, degradation, or exhibitionism represents reinforcing aspects of the offenses, they may not be replaceable in an appropriate manner. In these cases, the focus may be multi-faceted. Importance should be placed on the benefits of an appropriate consenting relationship and the negative consequences to the offending behavior, including harm to the individual who was victimized, charges, jail, and other losses the individual may experience. As well, the inappropriate reinforcing properties of the offending, such as deviance or force, should be reduced as much as possible. Although there has been little success in changing male sexual preference (Seto, 2012), work can be done to increase the reinforcing properties of alternate, more appropriate behaviors and teach self-management skills to reduce arousal in the presence of inappropriate stimuli. Consider the following example:

> *A male adult has sexual interests in children and has offended against children in the past. Through phallometric testing or self-report the individual also shows some attraction to male adults. The Good Lives Model (Ward, 2002) would state it may not be the end goal (i.e., function) that is the problem; rather it is the behavior, or how he goes about attaining that goal. An assessment shows attraction to children is due in part to seeking intimacy (social reinforcement through gaining access to something). So, a suggested approach would be to: i) replace the behavior with appropriate ways to attain intimacy, and ii) replace the target group with an appropriate age group in which he has also shown interest.*

TEACHING ALTERNATIVE AND COPING SKILLS

For individuals who engage in sex offending, it is important to teach alternative skills that are appropriate and safe. This requires the assessment of the type of skills that may benefit the person in coping or serve as alternatives to some of the precursor behaviors that lead up to an offense. It may also include identifying various knowledge gaps that may be present that contribute to the behavior, such as knowledge of the law and its consequences. Although teaching appropriate skills that the individual may use to prevent a future offense is important for offenders in general, this element may provide important replacement skills especially for those whose offense, was not mitigated by a desire for inappropriate sexual interaction, but was one of convenience, lack of skill, or a result of emotional dysregulation or a mental health issue. However, even in individuals for whom the offense was influenced by paraphilic factors, such as a preference for children or violence, there are often benefits to skills that would enable them to receive a range of reinforcement that may be social, vocational, or recreational that would serve to provide alternative sources of reinforcement, albeit maybe not a replacement for the offending behavior, *per se*.

Deciding what to teach is based on assessments that determine underlying functions of the sex offending behavior, including any skill and knowledge deficits. Not all individuals who offended will require the same degree of skill development in all areas; however, availability of the various components is important should the assessment determine that these are areas that are lacking or needing improvement. The key is to create a decision model to individualize the treatment of each person. Table 9.1 illustrates examples of alternative skills for the possible functions of inappropriate behavior.

Table 9.1 ***Examples of Alternative Habilitative Skills***

Function	Possible Deficits	Possible Alternative Skills
Social Positive Reinforcement (attention, access to tangible)	Limited communication, social skills, and/or ability to develop or sustain relationships (socio-sexual skills)	Functional communication training, social skills training- relationship training, and/or sex education as appropriate.
Social Negative Reinforcement (avoid, escape an aversive situation)	Limited communication, or lack of skills related to a particular activity or task or alternative social skill to achieve goal, and/or lack of problem-solving skills.	Functional communication training, altering activity or difficulty with which activity is presented (i.e., task analysis to break the task down into smaller steps), teaching alternative means to avoid or stop unwanted event, and/or teach problem solving skills and cost/benefit analysis
Automatic Reinforcement (sensory, feels good)	Lack of impulse control, coping skills, or self-regulation skills, lack of understanding of the risks or triggers of personal arousal, cognitive distortions, limited or no knowledge of appropriate vs. inappropriate behavior, or consent laws, lack of ability to age discriminate, inability to understand the emotions of others or a lack of empathy for victimized persons; influence of addictive substances.	Mindfulness skills (to strengthen executive functioning and reduce impulsivity), emotional regulation skills, increasing awareness of offense progression (steps to offending, risks/triggers that increase arousal and likelihood of offense), socio-sexual education including responsibility training related to the law, social mores and age of consent, increasing understanding of the impact of offending on persons who were victimized; rehabilitation for addiction issues.

Lindsay (2009) noted that the work of Griffiths, Quinsey and Hingsburger (1989) developed a "comprehensive example of behavioral management approaches," further suggesting that "the first significant and influential development in the field was a comprehensive treatment program aimed at improving social functioning, improving sexual awareness and knowledge, extending relationships, improving coping skills, and reducing inappropriate sexuality" (Lindsay, 2009, p. 59). Griffiths et al. (1989) suggested that "standards for the use of behavior modification, whether procedural or legislated, emphasize the efficacy and ethics of replacing inappropriate behaviors with appropriate ones as a first step in treating the client. However, for sexually inappropriate behavior, particularly when exhibited by individuals with developmental disabilities, this standard of practice is not routinely observed" (p. 11). They suggested that the development of appropriate socio-sexual expression should be a standard component of rehabilitative training for all persons with intellectual disabilities who sexually offend. In their integrated model for sexual behavior for the treatment of persons with intellectual disabilities, they highlighted five key areas of skill development: sex education, relationship training, responsibility training, coping skills, and social competency training, in addition to teaching awareness and skills to minimize risks, which should be assessed and incorporated into treatment, as the assessment deems appropriate. See Figure 9.1, below.

***Figure 9.1* Components of Comprehensive Treatment Options**

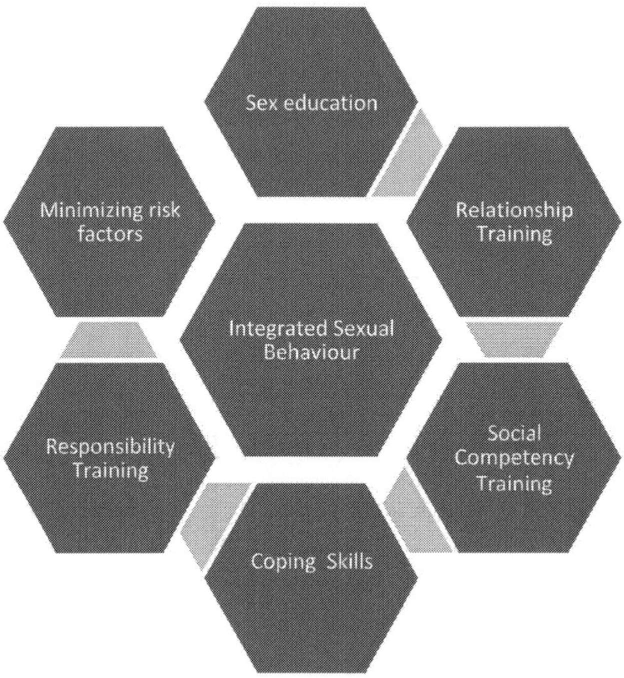

Griffiths and colleagues (1989) further suggested that following assessment, teaching decisions would be made based upon the educational components that were assessed to be associated with the offenses. Thus, if a lack of skill and knowledge were identified then sex education involving responsibility training and relationship training would be provided and/or if social competency was deemed as a variable then relationship training with appropriate coping skills would be introduced into treatment. Lastly, if the individual demonstrated inappropriate sexual arousal (say to children), then coping skills and responsibility training would be introduced, in addition to treatment for the inappropriate arousal.

In the early days of treatment for persons with intellectual disabilities who sexually offended, Haaven, Little, and Petre-Miller (1990) also proposed a comprehensive treatment package emphasizing habilitative elements. As noted in Chapter 8, they suggested that treatment should include components aimed at enhancing sexual knowledge, social skills, and self-control for their individuals who offended within a residential treatment facility. Their model was based on providing individuals who offended the skills to move from an "Old Me" that included the behaviors of concern to a "New Me" that was based on the newly acquired appropriate skills.

The message of alternative and coping skills still has validity as evidenced in the Plaud, Plaud, Kolstoe, and Orvedal (2000) review of behavioral treatment of sexual offending behavior in persons with developmental disabilities. They noted that a therapeutic behavioral change approach should be "tailored to the needs of the individual in all sexual and curriculum areas" with an emphasis on "building new and appropriate sexual behaviors as well as general behavioral skills" (p. 54). Moreover, Lindsay (2009) noted that since the 1980s the treatment of persons with intellectual disabilities who have offended has not only "focused on the criminogenic aspects of the individual's difficulties but also on their general lifestyle" (p. 59). This aspect was not initially evident in the work with persons without intellectual disabilities who have offended; however, this became more apparent for that population with the introduction of the *Good Lives Model* (GLM; Ward & Stewart, 2003). Furthermore, persons with intellectual disabilities and sex offending behavior often present with a range of interpersonal problems that stem from maladaptive learning histories and lived experiences. According to Levenson (2014), "Inadequate skills can cause and reinforce a vicious cycle in which problematic distress-relieving coping strategies contribute to dysfunctional patterns of relating to others" (p. 17). Thus, it is critical to determine all skill deficits through comprehensive assessment, and then provide teaching in these areas.

TEACHING FUNDAMENTAL SOCIO-SEXUAL SKILLS

Sex Education

Sex education encompasses a broad definition of social and sexual knowledge, not only limiting it to anatomy and knowledge of sexual activity but to the social context in which sexual behavior is deemed appropriate in the current culture. Research has shown that persons with intellectual disabilities are generally lacking in sexual knowledge prior to training (Lindsay, Bellshaw, Culross, Staines, & Michie, 1992). Although considerable anecdotal evidence exists, the empirical evidence on the effectiveness of sex education with persons with intellectual disabilities is often lacking (Lindsay et al., 1992; Whithouse & McCabe, 1997). Much of the research in this area fails to provide adequate measurement and control comparisons or typically fails to evaluate generalization (Whitehouse & McCabe, 1997). However, a control group study by Lindsay and colleagues (1992) involving 46 individuals participating in a sex education program demonstrated that after nine months of training regarding topics such as body parts, masturbation, male and female puberty, intercourse, pregnancy and childbirth, birth control, and venereal disease, significant and substantial knowledge increases were apparent in the training group compared to the control group which did not receive training. Follow-up evaluation demonstrated that the effects also maintained. They concluded that individuals with intellectual disabilities could learn through sex education training and that such training is a useful addition to a comprehensive treatment regime.

In recent years, there has been a shift towards providing sex education for persons with intellectual disabilities pre-emptive to a problem, making it more normalized and accepted in this group, as it has been with the nondisabled population. However, in the past, education was denied or only offered following an occurrence of inappropriate behavior. In addition, people with intellectual disabilities have often been taught that even healthy sexual behavior is inappropriate and something to be ashamed of, which may lead to inappropriate expression of sexuality. Some reasons why individuals with intellectual disabilities have not been provided with sex education include fear of abuse or pregnancy. Often the parents of individuals with intellectual disabilities would not allow their child to receive sex education because they feared it would sexualize their child's behavior, despite research showing the contrary (Tarnai, 2006).

If an individual has engaged in inappropriate or offensive sexual behavior, it is vital, as noted in the assessment section, that socio-sexual knowledge be evaluated. If the assessment shows that the sexually offensive behavior was due in part, or in rare cases fully, to a lack of sexual education, then the gaps in knowledge should be targeted as a pivotal part of any intervention. The most common sexual areas requiring intervention that these authors have seen in practice, are: lack of understanding sexual consent and consent laws, sexual acts that are against the law, private versus public including the grey areas (e.g., private bathroom in your home, but not a public bathroom), appropriate ways to ask someone on a date, verbal sexual harassment, and age discrimination.

Most importantly, there is a significant gap in not only teaching these concepts and what they mean, but also the need to practice applying each one across situations. People with intellectual disabilities often 'parrot' the rule or concept, but they do not understand why that rule is in place or have the skills to practice it. For example, an individual may be able to name public and private places or that their room is an appropriate place to masturbate but may not have the skills to act on this knowledge regarding where to go and what to do if they are aroused in public. This learning can be achieved through repetitive teaching and role playing so that the individual learns the skill and not just the concepts and through providing multiple exemplars that include a variety of different situations in which the person might find themselves aroused.

When providing sex education, it is important to evaluate knowledge and attitudes prior to (Edmonson, McCombs, & Wish, 1979), during, and after training (Lumley & Miltenberger, 1997). Griffiths (1999) advocated for the use of evaluating pre- and post-training at a minimum. Without empirical evidence from pre- to post-training and evidence of generalization, assumptions can be made about socio-sexual knowledge that may be both erroneous and dangerous (Griffiths & Lunksy, 2003).

Griffiths and Lunsky (2003) produced a revised *Sociosexual Knowledge and Attitude Assessment Tool* (SSKAAT-R) that evaluates anatomy, women's and men's bodies, intimacy, pregnancy, childbirth, birth control/STDs, and healthy boundaries. This latter area of assessment is unique among socio-sexual evaluation tools because it examines issues such as appropriate and inappropriate sexual behavior, including incest, sex involving children, and forced sexual behavior. As a result, it has particular relevance to assessment for individuals who are engaging in inappropriate sexual behavior. Both knowledge and attitudes are evaluated. The SSKAAT-R was described in Chapter 4.

There are very few standardized, published, and validated teaching curricula for socio-sexual education for people with intellectual disabilities, let alone those who have offended. Typically, structured sex education curricula encompass a vast array of topics that may take a long time to complete. Socio-sexual skills training curricula such as *Life Facts* (Cowardin & Stanfield, 1989) and *Life Horizons I and II* (Kempton, 1988) can provide comprehensive tools to provide this training. The *Life Facts* series (Cowardin & Stanfield, 1989) covers topic areas like sexuality, sexual abuse prevention, emotions management, and health education. The *Life Horizons* series covers topics related to anatomy and sexual health, self-esteem and relationship building, dating skills, and moral, legal, and social aspects of sexual behavior (Kempton, 1988).

It must be emphasized that not every individual who has offended will need sex education or every aspect of a curriculum. The authors have found that most persons with intellectual disabilities who have offended will benefit from education on some aspects of sexuality, if nothing more than issues of consent. The specific individualized curriculum required will depend on the outcome of the SSKAAT-R assessment to ensure that it targets specifically the areas the person needs to learn. An individualized education program can be developed using educational materials such as those noted above to create an individualized and targeted curriculum.

Social Skills Training

Social skills can encompass a variety of areas, including assertiveness skills, conversational skills, and communication skills. Social skills training provided to persons with intellectual disabilities who have offended can either be specific to the offense or focus on general social skills that are not directly related to an offense. Social problem-solving attempts to improve cognitive skills, such as beliefs and attitudes that were related to the offending behavior (Lindsay et al., 2011). This area of teaching "equip[s] offenders with thinking skills which will promote alternative, pro-social means of approaching social situations including high-risk situations in which the person is at risk of offending" (Lindsay et al., 2011, p. 183). One of the most widely used evidence-based, cognitive skills programs is the *Reasoning and Rehabilitation Program* (R&R; Ross, Fabiano, & Ewles, 1988), which focused on developing cognitive, reasoning and social problem-solving skills in individuals who offended in the typically developing population (Ross & Fabiano, 1985). Another important treatment component involves teaching social skills to individuals who offended who have interpersonal skill deficits. Research focusing on generalizing skills learned in a group setting concentrated on targeting social skills related to relationships, problem solving, interactions, and feelings (Griffiths, Feldman, & Tough, 1997). If assessment determines that social skills are lacking, these need to be addressed to complete a comprehensive and wide-ranging treatment package.

Similar to the paucity of empirically based sex education materials, the availability of validated teaching tools for social skills are limited. The *Social Life* is one program that has both validated effects and generalization outcomes (Griffiths, 1990 a, b; Griffiths et al., 1989). The curricula were designed in the form of a board game that could be adapted to match topic areas that had been deemed problematic for the individual (Griffiths et al., 1997). Behavioral generalization strategies have been embedded within the game format to ensure social validity (e.g., see Stokes & Baer list in Table 9.2, below) (Griffiths, 1995). The value of experiential learning through modelling of pro-social peers, caregivers, or support staff should not be dismissed. Providing the individual with opportunities to practice social skills can also be a valuable way to teach in-the-moment while providing immediate feedback. It utilizes role play and concrete scenarios to teach appropriate social-sexual skills in a variety of situations. The content of the game was individualized to avoid provision of a cookie-cutter intervention. Research on the *Social Life* game demonstrated that skills learned were generalized beyond the game to real life settings and situations (Griffiths et al., 1997).

Although the stage of achieving generalization into the community and outside of the therapeutic setting will be discussed again in Chapter 11, generalization is also dependent on how the skills were taught in the teaching setting. Bridging the gap between treatment and generalization is founded on the principles that are applied in all behavioral treatment strategies. Due to the risk posed by the behaviors of individuals who have offended, it would be unethical to just 'train and hope' as Stokes and Baer (1977) cautioned decades ago in their seminal work. Because training and treatment are often conducted in specialized treatment settings, whether inpatient or outpatient, automatic transfer of skills is highly unlikely and can never be assumed. The social validity of the generalization of treatment lies in demonstration of the application of treatment effects in the natural environment and the ethics of practice requires evidence. Thus, skill development programs should include comprehensive elements of the principles of generalization outlined by Stokes and Baer (1977). Applications of those principles are elaborated in Table 9.2: Explicit Strategies to Enhance Generalization. To summarize, within teaching sessions it is important to select behaviors that are contextually relevant and that can be hooked into the natural contingencies of reinforcement following treatment. The training should be loose so as not to confine the learner to only specific stimuli and involve stimuli that are commonly found in the natural settings. Teaching new skills should involve the use of multiple and diverse exemplars that cover a multitude of potential experiences and variations to which the person must respond with differential responses. Embedded within the teaching should be opportunities for the individual to use problem- solving skills to learn to identify and respond to the various situations. The individual should be provided with the opportunity to receive reinforcement for appropriate responses on a changing and indiscriminate schedule and have reinforcement provided when new skills are demonstrated both in the teaching sessions and naturally occurring during the day. Lastly, it is important to ensure that while teaching is occurring, the individual is provided with ample opportunities to use the new skill in their everyday life to receive reinforcement, while at the same time ensuring that the environment does not provide reinforcement for the inappropriate behaviors that had previously been used to attain goals. Ideally, the individual now knows how to achieve the reinforcement appropriately.

Table 9.2: *Explicit Strategies to Enhance Generalization (based on Stokes & Baer, 1977)*

Strategy	Applications
Select contextually relevant behaviors to teach the individual for potential situations and environments in which generalization is required.	Behaviors taught as simple "if/then" responses will be inappropriate if used out of context. The immediate utility and desirability of the behavior and its appropriateness to the physical and social context determine contextual relevance. Individuals who offend must be taught specific and contextually relevant strategies to use in situations where there is an increased risk for re-offense, such as presence of a child. Rather than teach just what not to do, it is important to teach the individual strategies that will keep the person safe and reduce the potential for re-offense. Strategies such as teaching the individual which situations are high risk and how to avoid those (i.e., walking a path to work that does not go past the park) or teaching the person the skills for non-offense if faced with high risk situations (e.g., ensuring that the individual is accompanied to a family gathering by a cohort who will ensure the person acts appropriately) or if faced with an unanticipated situation of risk to have various strategies to escape.
Use common physical and social stimuli to simulate the natural environments.	Generalization is enhanced when there are stimuli common to both training and generalization settings sufficient to gain discriminative value. Training could be conducted *in situ* or in situations that simulate the natural environment. Simulations may include video scenarios, virtual reality, or forward feedback methods.
Train loosely to simulate natural patterns of interaction.	Training that uses simulated social milieu has been shown to achieve enhanced generalization. For instance, utilizing a social game with role play to teach generalization of certain skills.
Provide sufficient stimulus and response examples to encompass a range of possible situations in which the person may need to apply the skills.	Training is not about training an appropriate response but a range of appropriate responses depending upon the stimulus that is presented. The key is to teach not only a skill but a response class that can be applied to other situations in the future. Game approaches or those using video scenarios can introduce a milieu for teaching a range of appropriate responses that serve the same function to various stimuli.
Use self-mediated stimuli, such as social-problem solving, to analyze, select and respond to social situations.	Training should employ strategies to teach the individual responses, as part of their newly learned behavior that can be used as a mediator in new situations. Social problem solving allows the person to learn skills to assess a situation for potential evoking stimuli, select an appropriate response that will abate and is incompatible with the inappropriate response (such as escape or relaxation strategies), then act upon it.

Provide indiscriminate contingencies using schedules of reinforcement.	The use of indiscriminate consequences often involves the use of intermittent or delayed schedules of reinforcement; however, discrimination may also be accomplished by delivery of contingencies in an unpredictable manner, meaning that no clear stimuli are present to signal the delivery of a consequence. An example of the use of this would be vicarious reinforcement, to reinforce the behavior in an individual by attending to the same behavior in others.
Provide reinforcement for unprompted generalization of new skills.	Individuals (staff or non-staff) in the treatment and post- treatment setting need to be trained so that the presentation of unprompted generalization is monitored and reinforced. Treatment effects often fail to maintain because diminished trainer adherence in providing praise. The planned reinforcement for generalized behavior must be systematically designed into the post treatment plan if it is to be maintained and eventually faded to an intermittent schedule.
Introduce into a natural community of reinforcement by ensuring reinforcement is inherently available.	Preparing the post-treatment environment is vital to ensure that there is an abundance of naturally occurring opportunities for the individual to engage in the learned behaviors and ensure that the use of those behaviors is naturally reinforced. Access to non-contingent reinforcement strategies for a variety of appropriate behaviors further decreases the probability of re-offense.
Modify environments that support the maladaptive behavior to provide alternative means to attain goals.	Natural environments present dynamic stimulus control conditions. It is vital that the features of the natural environment support the new therapeutic behaviors. Implementation of a 'Good Life' approach to post-treatment environments ensures that the individual is not subjected to reinforcement trade-down that would create vulnerability for relapse of previous maladaptive behaviors that lead to reinforcement.

Relationship Training

Relationship training may be essential for providing an individual who offended with the opportunities to learn appropriate alternative interpersonal behaviors. This training should include a focused curriculum targeting boundaries, feelings, emotional and physical intimacy, reciprocal conversation, and abuse prevention. Role-playing and social modelling are often key to getting true understanding and application of these abstract concepts. There are curricula already developed (of varying quality and utility); the selection of appropriate resources should be based on the type of training that would best suit the person's goals and learning approach. *Circles* (Walker-Hirsch & Champagne, 1993) is a widely-used curriculum that provides concrete and visual representation of relationships based on levels of intimacy depicted in concentric circles. However, the program may not portray relationships and dynamics that are representative of the person with intellectual disabilities who has sexually offended and may therefore require significant adaptation and modification.

Responsibility Training

Research has suggested that most persons with intellectual disabilities who have offended follow the Approach pathway. Lindsay (2009) concluded that this suggests that "few have significant awareness of the extent to which these acts are socially unacceptable" (p. 98). He suggested that if persons with intellectual disabilities have been led to offend by a combination of sexual preference and adverse experiences in their developmental histories, then by teaching them that these behaviors are considered sexually inappropriate may lead to a reduction in their wish to offend. Lindsay (2009) has, therefore, suggested that one element of teaching is educating the individual that the offending behaviors violate social conventions as a component of self-regulation. Griffiths et al. (1989) proposed a similar concept in their early model. They suggested that responsibility training involves three components: Personal, Interactive, and Moral. Personal Responsibility includes teaching the person about protection of the integrity of oneself sexually (e.g., against abuse or disease); Interactive Responsibility relates to sexual responsibility (personal hygiene, social convention and distance, social coercion, as well as the effects of drugs or alcohol); and Moral Responsibility, which although not legally governed, involves the role of personal choice as a guiding principle in life. Lindsay (2009) emphasized the importance of teaching about the conventions of society and the laws regarding sexual behavior. He noted, "As more and more clients live in the community and a small percentage of them offend, it has been increasingly clear to me that it is extremely important to have a thorough understanding of the conventions and values of society. Where an individual has had a restricted or distorted upbringing, they may have failed to develop a full understanding of these conventions" (p. 72).

The value and efficacy of empathy in understanding victimization with typical persons who sexually offend has been under debate. "A sexual offender is thought to have victim empathy when he has a cognitive and emotional understanding of the experience of the victim of his sexual offense" (Mann & Barnett, 2012, p. 1). There is no consensus in the literature on whether demonstrating empathy for victimized persons is necessary or potentially dangerous (Mann & Barnett, 2012). Furthermore, it has been noted that even if a person who sexually offends is aware of the feelings of persons they victimized, this is not enough to change their behavior and prevent them from offending (Hanson, 2003). There is a lack of evidence that supports empathy work as an effective tool to changing sex offending behavior. However, there may be some utility to use it on an individualized basis, as empathy is an important responsivity issue. Hanson (2003) suggested that persons who offend have different empathy deficits, and these specific deficits should be targeted individually in treatment. For example, a person who sexually offends may know how the people they victimized felt but be too ashamed to admit it. Another person who offends may not understand the harm their actions caused. Otherwise, a person who offended may know the harm they caused, but they show hostility towards the victimized persons (Hanson, 2003). These specific deficits can be targeted in an individualized treatment plan through discussion and role-play.

Empathy for victimized persons can include understanding the severity and long-term implications that the offending individual's actions can have on an individual who was victimized. Lindsay (2009) discussed the importance of perspective-taking in persons with intellectual disabilities who sexually offend. If the individual who offended cannot take the perspective of an individual who was victimized and others who were affected by their offense, it allows them to deflect responsibility for their actions and further reinforces cognitive distortions: "the lack of victim empathy encourages feelings of entitlement and discourages any self-doubt concerning the perpetration of any offenses" (Lindsay, 2009, p. 236). Although empathy for victimized persons focuses largely on the person who was sexually abused, another primary component should include the impact on other individuals who were affected by the offense. Consider the following scenario:

> *A person with an intellectual disability sexually abused his younger cousin over a period of 2 years. The individual who offended was not charged; rather, he was assigned to participate in a treatment program. However, when his cousin's parents discovered the abuse, they wanted nothing to do with him and his parents and cut off all communication. The local community where his family had lived for the past 20 years found out about the offense, forcing his family to move to another city several hours away, leaving their home and jobs.*

The clinician may ask their client in this situation who was affected by the offense, to which the obvious answer is the individual who was victimized. However, with further exploration the individual who offended may come to appreciate the wider scope of harm committed by the offense, such as how the offending individual's family were also affected through harm to family relationships and loss of their home, jobs, and community ties. Victimization often resembles ripples in water after a pebble has been dropped – with ever expanding circles of potential harm. Becoming aware of how their actions affected everyone around them can provide a good starting point for working on empathy for some individuals who offended.

The Bumby MOLEST and RAPE Scales (Bumby, 1996) are often used to assess the cognitive distortions of persons who engaged in child molestation or rape and can be used to determine where empathy for victimized persons may be lacking. The statements on these scales are rated from 1 ("strongly disagree") to 5 ("strongly agree"). Certain items on these scales can identify the presence of attitudes that minimize the impact a sexual offense has on the individual who was victimized and identify where empathy work is needed. The following items on the MOLEST scale can help identify where there is a lack of empathy and understanding the severity of the offense on the individual who was victimized: Item 3 ("Many children who are sexually assaulted do not experience many major problems because of the assaults"), Item 8 ("If a person does not use force to have sexual activity with a child, it will not harm the child"), Item 10 ("Just fondling a child is not as bad as penetrating a child and will probably not affect the child as much"), Item 23 ("Children who have been involved in sexual activity with an adult will eventually get over it and go on with their lives"), and Item 37 ("I think the main thing wrong with sexual activity with children is that it is against the law"). Although these are not empirically validated for measuring empathy for victimized persons, they can provide the clinician some helpful insight into the offending individual's attitudes on how their actions impact the individual who was victimized.

TEACHING COPING SKILLS

The long-term goal of treatment is to ensure that the individual who offended acquires the skills to deal with current problems and to learn how to apply those skills to manage future problems (McKain, 1982; Meichenbaum, 1975). McKain (1982) suggested that there are several benefits to teaching coping skills, which include providing a concrete understanding of the nature of the problem and the strategies to manage or prevent them, demystifying the circumstances that led to the problem to common occurring events so that they can be put within the person's control, demonstrating methods for regaining control (and, as such, to enhance self-worth and confidence), providing new responses to previous situations that provided the problem and, lastly, enhancing generalization of the combined skills to use in other settings outside of treatment.

Coping strategies encompass a broad range of skills that can be used as alternative skills when the person has certain skill deficits that contribute to offending behavior. Some of the key skills that are often taught as part of coping skills for persons with intellectual disabilities include cognitive restructuring, self-regulation, anger management, problem solving, and relaxation skills. These skills are all areas that fall under coping skills and can be targeted in treatment. However, this list of coping skills is not exhaustive of areas that may need to be addressed in a comprehensive treatment plan.

Cognitive Restructuring

Individual attitudes that are false (cognitive distortions) have been the subject of much interest in the field of assessment and treatment for individuals who have offended. The role of attitudes and information processing have been highlighted as critical in the development of sexual offending behavior (Hudson, Ward, & McCormack, 1999). Although this has been more widely researched in the sexual offending literature, little had been done to explore this with persons with intellectual disabilities until the development of the *Questionnaire on Attitudes Consistent with Sex Offenses* (QASCO; Lindsay, Whitefield, & Carson, 2007).

In addressing attitudes and beliefs that influence offending in treatment, the terms cognitive distortions or cognitive schemas may be used, and there is a distinct difference between the two. Cognitive distortions encompass more specific attitudes or judgments about a situation, for example, "the woman smiled at me, which means she wants to have sex." Cognitive schemas are broader attitudes that influence offending, such as "when women smile at men it means they want to have sex." The presence of cognitive distortions and schemas can take years to work through in treatment, especially when these attitudes have been ingrained and reinforced throughout a long learning history. In his practice workbook on the treatment of persons with intellectual disabilities who have sexually offended, Lindsay (2009) discussed doing group work with individuals who had different offenses and targeting their distortions through peer challenging. A peer challenging a person's belief that the child was playful because he wanted to have sex can resonate more with the individual than the same message coming from a clinician who is typically seen as an authority position who hasn't offended and who does not have an intellectual disability. Lindsay (2009) further described the use of problem solving scenarios to work through distortions, both by the individual participating in different role plays and by helping others problem solve through various circumstances related to individual offenses.

Challenging cognitive distortions is a critical first step. Once challenged, these distortions and schemas need to be replaced by something more functional and appropriate. This process should be driven by the individual who offended, as it is important to develop alternative, more accurate explanations of his own actions and those of the person he victimized (Ward, 2000). Take the individual above: the schema "when women smile at men, it means they want to have sex," leads to the distortion that "the woman smiled at me, which means she wants to have sex." Once challenged, this schema needs to be replaced with something more appropriate (e.g., "people smile when they are happy"), which leads to distortions being reassessed (e.g., "that woman smiled because she was happy; it had nothing to do with sex"). These alternative schemas should be established by the individual through the course of treatment. As schemas and distortions are challenged, new private verbal behavior (i.e., rule statements) will be formed and can lead to a re-evaluation not only of the motives of the person who was victimized but the motives of the individual who offended. Schemas that attributed the offenses to external factors may be adjusted, and the individual takes more responsibility for the offenses. Though research is mixed on the overall efficacy and necessity of addressing cognitive distortions (Marshall, Marshall, & Kingston, 2011; Ó Ciardha & Gannon, 2011), for some individuals it can be a valuable treatment option and may lower risk of re-offense.

Self-Regulation

Throughout assessment, the individual's offense progression or pattern should be clearly established. In this progression, there may be the presence of highly emotional states that led to poor decision making and problem solving, which consequently led to an offense. These emotional states could include any feelings of anger, sadness, fear, arousal, or happiness. Part of treatment should then include teaching the individual to regulate the emotions that can lead them to poor decision making. For resources on self-regulation with persons with intellectual disabilities see, *The Skills System Instructor's Guide: An Emotion-Regulation Skills Curriculum for All Learning Abilities* (Brown, 2011), and *Pathways: A Guided Workbook for Youth Beginning Treatment* (Kahn, 2011).

Impulsivity may or may not be a significant contributor to sexual offending for some persons with intellectual disabilities who offended (Parry & Lindsay, 2003); however, delay of reinforcement (especially primary reinforcers, such as sexual gratification) and ability to self-regulate may be difficult for a portion of this population. Hanson and Harris (2000) found that anger and distress before an offense are predictors of future offenses. These challenges can be exacerbated by the presence of arousing stimuli, which may serve as antecedents to behavior patterns that have been reinforced in the past. An individual must have the ability to cope with situations when they are in an environment that has potential to evoke offending behavior. For instance, seeing an attractive woman may lead to feelings of arousal and, consequently, a desire to touch her. Without the appropriate coping and self-regulation skills, the person may engage in an offense. Additionally, in the past, this behavior could have been immediately gratifying with no aversive consequences. As a result, this behavior is more likely to occur again. To combat these situations, strategies are needed to manage arousal and cope with potentially risky environmental circumstances.

Individuals can learn to suppress or otherwise interfere with their arousal (e.g., Laws & Rubin, 1969; Wilson, 1998). Vollmer, Reyes, and Walker (2012) suggested that treatment should include a component to teach the individual to suppress arousal using self-control techniques. They demonstrated, using single-subject reversal design, that individuals with intellectual disabilities acquired the ability to suppress their arousal. If participants were unable to generate a strategy on their own, participants were instructed to count backwards from 100 loudly while arousing stimuli was presented. This can also be a helpful self-regulation technique for the individual to have in their repertoire; however, it is important to note that research has been inconclusive as to whether skills learned in laboratory settings generalize to real-life situations in the community (see Wilson, 2016; Wilson & Miner, 2016). As such, it will be important for individuals with these difficulties to also have other skills available in their risk management repertoires.

Dialectical behavior therapy (DBT), "a manualized treatment that combines treatment strategies from behavioral, cognitive and supportive psychotherapies" (Linehan, Armstrong, Suarez, Allmon, & Heard, 1991 p. 1061), has proven effective in the management and regulation of aggressive behavior (Evershed et al. 2003). It identifies the triggers that led to problematic behaviors and provides a variety of coping skills to increase control over physical reactions, emotions, and thoughts. DBT can also be used to help individuals recognize their own arousal patterns by being aware of environmental triggers and internal cues, which allows individuals the time to utilize an appropriate strategy to either manage or escape from the situation. Evidence also suggests that mindfulness techniques can be successfully utilized with individuals with intellectual disabilities to help manage arousal (Singh, Wahler, Adkins, Myers, & Mindfulness Research Group, 2003). Strategies can be either simple or complex, depending on the individual. Individuals with more significant levels of intellectual disability may have difficulty with abstract concepts and would find more success with concrete strategies. Singh et al. (2011) conducted a study to evaluate effectiveness in teaching skills to enable control of sexual arousal to persons who have an intellectual disability and offending histories. Participants were taught a mindfulness-based meditation technique that taught them to observe their thoughts and take time to stop, think, and plan before immediately reacting. The participants were provided with individualized instruction, a self-practice homework, and engaged in discussions with a therapist to learn mindful observation of thoughts. Their findings indicated that individuals who employed their own self-management strategies failed to maintain self-control. However, when taught a meditation technique, *Mindful Observation of Thoughts*, they reported significantly greater self-control over their own arousal patterns. A takeaway from this study was feedback from participants that the more complicated mindfulness techniques were (e.g., abstract in nature), the more difficult they were to utilize. The meditation, for example, was not efficacious but participants reported success when detaching themselves from their own inappropriate thoughts observing and acknowledging those thoughts rather than reacting to them. It is important to note that all participants in this study had a diagnosis of mild intellectual disability; individuals with more profound cognitive impairments may have less success with these techniques.

Anger Management

Anger and distress before an offense have been found to increase the likelihood of future offenses (Hanson & Harris, 2000; Lindsay & Beail, 2004). For some individuals, the inability to control and regulate these emotions could be a risk factor, and if so it should be targeted in treatment (Landenberger & Lipsey, 2005). In fact, anger may be attached to the individual's offense cycle and could serve as an antecedent or precipitating factor to the offending behaviosr. The anger could be connected specifically to the individual who was victimized and rooted in maladaptive thinking. This type of anger could emerge from a schema or distortion; however, this should also be addressed through challenging the rooted schemas and distortions. The anger could also be external to the individual who was victimized and the sexual assault a means of emotional regulation.

Consider a man who has offended twice in the past, both against female adults and both following problems at work. Work troubles caused stress, which quickly led to anger; he has no appropriate or functional means of dealing with this anger. Instead, he used "sex" or more accurately, sexual assault, to cope with negative emotions. However, with more effective regulation and management of emotions, he could interrupt and prevent escalation of the offense cycle so that alternatives could be considered.

Because persons with intellectual disabilities who have offended will have acquired their disability in different ways (e.g., a syndrome, a birth injury, or head trauma), it is important to recognize that different learning approaches might be required to ensure that teaching style matches the learning style of the learner (this is the essence of the responsivity principle, to which we have referred variously throughout this book). It used to be that we spoke of one, best way to teach persons with intellectual disabilities; however, with emergent genetic research it is now evident that individuals with different genetic syndromes learn in diverse ways and present with strengths and challenges that are unique to their syndrome and often dissimilar to other syndromes. For more information on how this may influence the type of intervention that is selected see: *Genetic Syndromes and Applied Behavior Analysis: A Handbook for ABA Practitioners* (Griffiths, Condillac, & Legree, 2014).

Often, dealing with the individual's anger should be one of the first lines of treatment so that other skills can be taught. When there is excess anger present and a lack of ability to cope with this emotion, the anger overshadows the ability to cope and learn other skills. Anger or emotions management interventions are particularly important for people with intellectual disabilities given their higher rates of aggression (Taylor, 2002) and impulsivity. Teaching appropriate anger management techniques must include skills that are within the person's repertoire and that are practical in nature. For example, teaching anger management skills to persons with intellectual disabilities should include concrete visuals, role-play, practice, and repetition in teaching rather than trying to teach abstract concepts. For example, using an entire binder of visual reminders may not be practical for community participation, but using a key chain of visual reminders that the person can keep with them may be more practical. Remember our ongoing message that the responsivity principle is very important with this population.

In an effort to determine if teaching anger management is an effective evidence-based practice, Hamelin, Travis & Sturmey (2013) conducted a review of the empirical literature on anger management training. Throughout their review, they found that interventions lasted nine weeks to nine months and involved sessions of 30 to 120 minutes. They reported that there were limited studies showing follow-up data or generalization. Overall, the authors cautioned that there is little empirical evidence showing long-term effects of anger management training. As such, although anger may be identified as a variable in the commission of a particular individual's offense, caution must be taken if utilizing a teaching tool that has not been empirically validated.

Problem Solving

Individuals may lack sufficient problem-solving skills, depending on learning history and cognitive level. This is a concern as, even with sufficient motivation to remain offense-free, poor problem-solving skills can lead an individual to risky situations with insufficient means of navigating them. Research has shown that social problem solving could be a valuable component of treatment for persons with sexual behavior problems in this population (Lindsay et al., 2011). As well, there is support that with individualization, persons with disabilities who have offended can demonstrate gains using problem-solving interventions developed for neurotypical persons who have offended (O'Connor, 1996).

A cost-benefit analysis can be a simple method of weighing the pros and cons of offending. The individual who offended has a well-rehearsed inventory of valuable things in his life that he stands to lose (e.g., job, nice home, family and friends) against which he needs to balance what he stands to gain or acquire (e.g., temporary pleasure, negative emotional state). In the moment, the urge to offend may override more rational thoughts about long-term consequences; however, with training, maladaptive thought patterns can be interrupted and allow consideration to be given to the consequences.

With careful planning, situations of potential risk are minimized and individuals can adapt to changing environments to limit exposure to persons at risk for victimization. Strategies may be preventative in nature or reactionary; they may involve changes of route to work or leaving a bus when aroused. All strategies should be individualized, but the more concrete, generalizable, and simple they are, the more likely they are to be efficacious and practical. Within treatment, the clinician can help the client to identify when risky situations are present and to identify a variety of actions they can employ in those circumstances. Some examples of 'what to do' may include deep breaths, walk away, phone a trusted person, talk to a staff member, listen to music, or other skills learned in treatment.

Relaxation Skills

Sometimes individuals with intellectual disabilities are not able to identify the early signs of when to engage their relaxation skills. Behavioral Relaxation Training (Lindsay & Baty, 1986) is one technique that can be used to help an individual recognize what his/her body feels like when it is tense versus relaxed and when they should start relaxation techniques. Relaxation techniques that focus on controlled breathing exercises can be simple and easily transferable across locations and scenarios. Although there are different techniques and strategies available, most involve becoming aware of body cues (e.g., sweaty palms, elevated heartrate), the emotions that caused them (e.g., fear and distress), and the situations that elicit those emotions (e.g., a child knocking on my door). In treatment, breathing techniques are taught to lower the heartrate and return regulation. Those distressing situations are visualized to elicit the emotions, and the techniques are used in controlled settings to increase fluency and ease of use.

Additionally, DBT, as previously described, can also be an effective relaxation and grounding technique for individuals who have sexually offended. Part of understanding an offense progression is an awareness of the associated thoughts and emotions. For persons with intellectual disabilities who have sufficient cognitive skills, DBT can be an effective technique to enhance awareness of thoughts and emotions, and it has been applied to the population of those who have offended. Sakdalan, Shaw, and Collier (2010) demonstrated that DBT was effective in decreasing risk and improving coping skills with a forensic population of persons with intellectual disabilities.

TEACHING STRATEGIES TO MINIMIZE RISK

Risk Management

Risk management strategies typically consist of avoidant strategies that can be used until the individual has mastered the replacement or coping skills to be safe in the community. These strategies can include teaching the individual to avoid situations with numerous triggers that have led to offending behavior in the past. In addition, the focus would also be to remove the individual from the situation or, if that is not possible, to provide simple strategies to manage the situation until removal is feasible. Looking away and walking away are basic avoidant strategies derived from relapse prevention in which the individual redirects himself away from potentially vulnerable persons or uses preferred items to distract himself until leaving is possible (e.g., reading material, hand held games). These avoidant strategies may be used if assessment has determined that the individual does not have the coping skills to keep themselves and others safe when presented with certain situations or people. However, it is important to note that such strategies should be used only if assessment results deem there is a problem with their safety skills in the community that increases risk to themselves or others.

Avoidant strategies may be used as a short-term approach until they learn effective coping skills, principally including approach strategies in which the individual makes critical life changes so as to "approach" a good life, rather than simply trying to avoid a bad one. Individuals often use their staff supervision as a risk management strategy; even without intervention, staff presence can drastically reduce the likelihood of an offense. This can also include calling staff or a caregiver in dangerous situations so that they can provide support and guidance. The individual must be set up for success to use these strategies; for example, by making sure they have the means to call staff when needed and that the staff are available.

Avoiding all potentially risky situations is not always possible and cannot be sustained successfully long term. Therefore, it is critical that additional risk management strategies deemed necessary through assessment become part of a holistic and long-term intervention approach for individuals.

Sometimes, the assessment may indicate that an individual has extremely high levels of inappropriate sexual arousal that cannot be managed adequately through supervision alone. Depending on the arousal levels and inappropriate fantasies that are present, specialised risk management strategies may be necessary until the individual has mastered management of their arousal patterns. At the same time, in such a heightened state of arousal it may be impossible for the individual to utilize any avoidant skills or to even be in a place where they are able to learn new skills. When an individual is in a heightened physiological state, it is less likely that new information will be readily learned. In such circumstances, under the close supervision of specialized psychiatrists, anti-androgen or otherwise antilibidinal medications may be considered for short-term risk management, until replacement coping skills can be taught. The use of these medications requires careful consideration of ethical and human rights aspects (e.g., potentially detrimental side-effects). However, anti-androgens and other such pharmacological agents can be useful in "turning down the volume," so to speak, of the individual's sex drive to a level at which presence in the community is possible and the individual can focus on learning new skills without intrusive sexual thoughts, fantasies, and urges (R. Dickey, personal communication).

IMPORTANT CONSIDERATIONS DURING PROVISION OF TREATMENT

The complex abuse and trauma histories of persons with intellectual disabilities were discussed in the introduction section of this book. A recent study showed that in comparison to males in the general population, persons who have sexually offended have experienced much higher levels of abuse and trauma (Levenson, Willis, & Prescott, 2016; see also Reavis, Looman, Franco, & Rojas, 2013), with populations of persons with intellectual disabilities being even more greatly impacted (Sobsey & Doe, 1991). These early adverse experiences can contribute to emotional, social, and cognitive impairments and lead to harmful coping and interpersonal behaviors. Therefore, the role of early trauma and its development of high-risk behaviors is an important consideration in providing holistic treatment and understanding the clinical needs of this population (Levenson et al., 2016).

Trauma-informed care for persons with sex offending behavior in the neurotypical population has recently become a necessary component of treatment. Trauma-informed care incorporates evidence of early trauma and its impact on behavior across the lifespan (Levenson et al., 2016). Specifically, "By viewing maladaptive and abusive behavior through the lens of early trauma, clinicians can help sex offender clients recognize negative interaction patterns, learn and generalize new skills, enhance their interpersonal relationships and improve their general well-being" (Levenson et al., 2016, p. 9). A traditional approach to treatment for sexual behavior problems may focus only on the current high-risk behaviors as being problematic. Trauma-informed care differs by viewing a history of trauma and abuse as experiences that have shaped and contributed to the individual's behavior. The clinician should create a safe setting with a focus on choice, working together, and empowerment. By understanding that the person's developmental and learning histories have occurred through repeated traumatic experiences, the clinician can provide a more holistic understanding of the individual and their maladaptive behaviors, and thus provide more holistic and tailored treatment (Levenson et al., 2016).

From a trauma-informed care model, three ingredients must be present in treatment: perceived safety, empowerment, and connection (Harvey, 2016). Important components for perceived safety within the context of treatment include having understanding and responsive staff, comfort in the form of food, shelter, and emotional support, preventing physical harm by self or others, and the person having someone they can go to for support (Harvey, 2016). The key to providing empowerment within treatment includes allowing the individual to have real choices where it is safe to do so, real input into their daily life, and being listened to and validated regarding their emotions and things that bother them. Finally, the person in treatment must also have a sense of connection, through opportunities for positive peer relationships, and a sense of feeling heard by caregivers (Harvey, 2016).

In our collective opinion, trauma-informed care is a necessary component in teaching persons with intellectual disabilities who have sexually offended. With a focus on choice and empowerment, the trauma-informed care approach must also be used in conjunction with appropriate risk management techniques so that risk to the individual and the community is not increased.

EVALUATING TREATMENT EFFECTS

Fundamental to the concept of applied behavior analysis is systematic evaluation of the factors that contribute to the behavior as well as the effects of intervention on decreasing the problem behavior and teaching replacement behavior. In teaching alternative and coping skills, it is critical to determine whether training has achieved the desired goals and if the individual has achieved the status of *offense-free*. As Lindsay (2014) noted, this is one behavior for which there should be no tolerance for a degree of success that is not 100%.

Plaud and colleagues (2000) noted that behavioral responses to treatment must be functionally and operationally defined, directly measured, and graphically represented (which goes beyond typical treatment charting). To measure a behavior or skill that is being taught, the skill to increase should be functionally relevant and objectively defined with a clearly identified target goal or mastery criteria. In other words, it should be clearly stated using behavioral indicators of when the skill has been achieved. Measuring the individual's knowledge on a topic area may be necessary; however, it is essential to also measure how well the individual applies the skill in various situations when faced with precursors that have previously led to risky behavior or an offense.

Although ongoing monitoring is the preferred form of data collection, the use of pre/post-tests is also a useful method to measure a skill from pre-intervention to post-intervention. These types of pre/post-tests are best used to determine the person's level of knowledge after teaching about specific concepts such as consent, anatomy, sexual acts against the law, and boundaries. It is important that the person has the knowledge about specific concepts and can practice it in role-play, but they also must show their understanding through their behavior *in situ*. Knowing a concept does not necessarily translate into practice in real life situations. Therefore, various forms of behavioral data collection are critical to determine if skills are being used in real life situations and if intervention is effective. Behavioral data collection of antecedents-behaviors-consequences (ABCs) can be used when the individual is in the *in situ* setting where the opportunity to use the learned skill can be observed to determine what he did well and where adaptations or additional teaching may be required.

Sometimes data collection will show that the person with an intellectual disability is displaying problematic or risky behaviors yet, upon further analysis, it is the environment that requires changes. When a person with an intellectual disability is residing in a group home, family home, or facility with staff support, detailed data collection can often show that simple environmental adaptations are needed to support the person in the use of the new skills. Also, data can show that the caregivers require adaptations in their approach and responses to facilitate opportunities for adaptive skills by the person with an intellectual disability. Modifications to approaches or practices in the individual's environment must be considered alongside their personal skill development.

Self-evaluations are another form of behavioral data collection that can empower the person with an intellectual disability to monitor and evaluate their own progress. For community participation, this can be achieved through post-community outing checks in which the individual documents how their outing went, what they did well, and what they might do better next time. The frequency of self-evaluations depends on the individual, the skills they are trying to learn, and where they are at in treatment. For example, self-evaluations may be completed after a social interaction the individual had with a peer or a caregiver or after the end of each day documenting how their day went and what could be improved for next time.

Sometimes a person's response to not offend or show appropriate behavioral responses may be under the stimulus control of caregiver supervision. In other words, the individual may use their skills and risk management strategies in the presence of staff or caregivers only because they know they are being supervised. Measuring the person's behavior when they do not think they are being supervised is a necessary post-treatment component. This can be done through blind supervisions or community trust programs. Strategies for blind supervision, which entails having someone unknown to the individual provide supervision from a distance and track how they use their skills in various situations that the person may have struggled with pre-treatment, will be discussed fully in Chapter 11. These strategies would be done with the individual's consent, with an understanding that blind supervisions help to determine success and where more work is needed.

Community trust programs have been used in community-based treatment programs for persons with intellectual disabilities and sex offending behavior (Stevenson, Lynn, Miller, & Hingsburger, 2010). Community trust programs provide individuals with "real life opportunities to practice skills and thus transfer what is learned in therapeutic sessions to practical application," (p. 1) while under carefully guided systematic supervision (Stevenson et al., 2010). They are carefully planned, gradual increases in independent community access that are based on the individual showing self-management skills that were learned in treatment (Stevenson et al., 2010). There are specific criteria that should be met prior to community trust programs being considered, all of which must be based on data. Some criteria include the person's consistent participation in treatment, their use of learned skills across people, settings, and situations over a period of at least 6 months, and their ability to identify their environmental risk factors and antecedents to sexual offending (Stevenson et al., 2010). When facilitated and supervised by a clinician with expertise in working with persons with sex offending behavior, community trust programs can be a useful tool to objectively evaluate an individual's progress and treatment effectiveness.

In summary, there are many objective ways to evaluate treatment progress, which require ongoing data collection, monitoring, and analysis, and making any necessary adaptations to the treatment plan on a consistent basis.

SUMMARY

Persons with intellectual disabilities and sex offending behavior often display other behavioral concerns and skill deficits that can result from a complex learning history, unfortunately, also frequently including trauma. The offending and concerning behaviors must be clearly and objectively identified and the areas that require teaching and skill development must be functional replacements of the problem behavior. Identifying whether sexually inappropriate interests or preferences are present will play a crucial role in the teaching component of treatment, including risk management techniques and finding appropriate long-term functional replacement behaviors. There are many socio-sexual and coping skills that may need to be taught depending on assessment results; the areas provided in this chapter were not meant to be an exhaustive list of the issues to be potentially addressed in treatment. When a history of abuse and trauma is present, it is critical that a trauma-informed approach be used alongside an evidence-based treatment plan. Throughout any teaching or intervention, there must also be a way to monitor whether the teaching method is working or if it needs to be adapted – in keeping with the responsivity principle. This can be done through pre/post tests and ongoing behavioral data collection.

REFERENCES

Ayllon, T. & Azrin, N. (1968). *The token economy: A motivation system for therapy and rehabilitation.* New York: Appleton-Century-Crofts.

Azrin, N. & Hotz, W.C. (1966). Punishment. In W. K. Honig (Ed.), *Operant behavior: Areas of research and application* (pp.380-447). New York: Appleton-Century-Crofts.

Brown, J. F. (2011). *The skills system instructor's guide: An emotion-regulation skills curriculum for all learning abilities.* Bloomington, IN: iUniverse.

Bumby, K. M. (1996). Assessing the cognitive distortions of child molesters and rapists: Development and validation of the MOLEST and RAPE Scales. *Sexual Abuse, 8*, 37–54.

Cooper, J. O., Heron, T. E., & Heward, W. L. (2007). *Applied behavior analysis* (2nd ed.). Upper Saddle River, NJ: Pearson Education Inc.

Cowardin, N. & Stanfield, J. (1989). *Lifefacts.* Santa Monica, CA: James Stanfield Publishing.

Durand, V. M. (1999). Functional communication training using assistive devices: Recruiting natural communities of reinforcement. *Journal of Applied Behavior Analysis, 32*(3), 247-267.

Edmonson, B., McCombs, K., & Wish, J. (1979). What retarded adults believe about sex. *American Journal of Mental Deficiency, 84*, 11-18.

Evershed, S., Tennant, A., Boomer, D., Rees, A., Barkham, M., & Watson, A. (2003). Practice-based outcomes of dialectical behavior therapy (DBT) targeting anger and violence, with male forensic patients: A pragmatic and non-contemporaneous comparison. *Criminal Behavior and Mental Health, 13,* 198-213.

Griffiths, D. (1990a, January). Practical considerations for teaching social skills- Part I. *Habilitative Mental Health Care Newsletter, 9,* 1-5.

Griffiths, D. (1990b, February). Practical considerations for teaching social skills- Part II. *Habilitative Mental Health Care, 9,* 9-13.

Griffiths, D. (1995). Teaching for generalization of social skills for persons who have a developmental disability. *Developmental Disabilities Bulletin, 23,* 43-58.

Griffiths, D. (1999). Sexuality and people with developmental disabilities: Mythconceptions and facts. In I. Brown & M. Percy (Eds.), *Developmental Disabilities in Ontario* (pp.443-452). Toronto, ON: Porch.

Griffiths, D., Condillac, R. A., & Legree, M. (2014). *Genetic syndromes and applied behavior analysis: A handbook for ABA practitioners.* London, UK: Jessica King.

Griffiths, D., Feldman, M., & Tough, S. (1997). Programming generalization when teaching social skills to adults with mental retardation: effects on generalization, social validity and self-report. *Behavior Therapy, 28,* 253-269.

Griffiths, D. & Lunsky, Y. (2003). *Socio-sexual knowledge and attitude assessment tool (SS-KAAT-R).* Wood Dale, IL: Stoelting Company

Griffiths, D. M., Quinsey, V. L., & Hingsburger, D. (1989). *Changing inappropriate sexual behavior: A community-based approach for persons with developmental disabilities.* Baltimore, MD: Paul H. Brookes Publishing.

Haaven, J., Little, R., & Petre-Miller, D. (1990). *Training intellectually disabled sex offender: A model residential program.* Orwell, VT: Safer Society Press.

Hamelin, J. Travis, R., & Sturmey, P. (2013). Anger management and intellectual disabilities: A systematic review. *Journal of Mental Health Research in Intellectual Disabilities,* 6, 60-70.

Hanson, R. K. (2003). Empathy deficits of sexual offenders: A conceptual model. *Journal of Sexual Aggression, 9,* 13-23.

Hanson, R. K., & Harris, A. J. R. (2000). Where should we intervene? Dynamic predictors of sexual offense recidivism. *Criminal Justice and Behavior, 27,* 6-35.

Harvey, K. (2016). *Trauma-informed behavioral interventions.* Annual Conference of the American Association of Intellectual and Developmental Disabilities. Glacier Canyon Conference, Wisconsin Dells, WI.

Hudson, S. M., Ward, T., & McCormack, J. C. (1999). Offense pathways in sexual offenders. *Journal of Interpersonal Violence, 14,* 779–798.

Kahn, T. (2011). *Pathways: A guided workbook for youth beginning treatment.* Fourth Edition. Brandon, VT: Safer Society Press._

Kempton, W. (1988). *Life Horizons I and II.* Santa Barbara, CA: James Stanfield Publishing.

Landenberger, N. A., & Lipsey, M. W. (2005). The positive effects of cognitive–behavioral programs for offenders: A meta-analysis of factors associated with effective treatment. *Journal of Experimental Criminology, 1,* 451-476.

Laws, D. R., & Rubin, H. B. (1969). Instructional control of an automatic response. *Journal of Applied Behavior Analysis, 2,* 93-99.

Levenson, J. (2014). Incorporating trauma-informed care into evidence-based sex offender treatment. *Journal of Sexual Aggression, 20*(1), 9-22.

Levenson, J. S., Willis, G. M., & Prescott, D. S. (2016). Adverse childhood experiences in the lives of male sex offenders: Implications for trauma-informed care. *Sexual Abuse, 28* 340-359.

Lindsay, W. R. (2009). *The treatment of sex offenders with developmental disabilities: A practice workbook.* Chichester, UK: Wiley-Blackwell.

Lindsay, W. R. (2014). *Behavioral assessment and treatment of sex offenders with intellectual disabilities and autism.* International Dual Diagnosis Certificate Program, Brock University, St. Catharines, ON, CA.

Lindsay, W. R., & Baty, F. J. (1986). Behavioral relaxation training: Exploration with adults who are mentally handicapped. *Mental Handicap, 14,* 160-162.

Lindsay, W. R., & Beail, N. (2004). Risk assessment: Actuarial prediction and clinical judgment of offending incidents and behavior for intellectual disability services. *Journal of Applied Research in Intellectual Disabilities, 17,* 229-234.

Lindsay, W. R., Bellshaw, E., Culross, G., Staines, E., & Michie, A. (1992). Increases in knowledge following a course of sex education for people with intellectual disabilities. *Journal of Intellectual Disability Research, 36,* 531-539.

Lindsay, W. R., Hamilton, C., Moulton, S., Scott, S., Doyle, M., & McMurran, M. (2011). Assessment and treatment of social problem solving in offenders with intellectual disability. *Psychology, Crime & Law, 17,* 181-197.

Lindsay, W. R., Whitefield, E., & Carson, D. (2007). An assessment for attitudes consistent with sexual offending for use with offenders with intellectual disabilities. *Legal and Criminological Society, 12, 55-68.*

Linehan, M. M., Armstrong, H. E., Suarez, A., Allmon, D., & Heard, H. L. (1991). Cognitive-behavioral treatment of chronically parasuicidal borderline patients. *Archives of General Psychiatry, 48,* 1060-1064.

Lumley, V. A., & Miltenberger, R G. (1997). Sexual abuse prevention for persons with mental retardation. *American Journal of Mental Retardation, 101,* 459-472.

Mann, R. E., & Barnett, G. D. (2012). Victim empathy intervention with sexual offenders: Rehabilitation, punishment, or correctional quackery? *Sexual Abuse, 25,* 1-20.

Marshall, W. L., Marshall, L. E., & Kingston, D. A. (2011). Are the cognitive distortions of child molesters in need of treatment? *Journal of Sexual Aggression, 17,* 118-129.

McGuire, T. (2001). Sex offending: behavioral analysis perspective. *Advances in Psychology Review, 6,* 129-155.

McKain, T. L. (1982). Coping skills training and cognitive behavior therapy. In L. Sank & C. S. Schaffer (Eds.), *A therapist's manual for cognitive behavior therapy in groups* (pp. 9-24). New York: Plenum.

Meichenbaum, D. H. (1975). Self-instructional methods. In F. H. Kanfer & A. P. Goldstein (Eds.), *Helping people change* (pp. 346-380). Elmsford, NY: Pergamon.

Miltenberger, R. G. (2008). *Behavior modification: Principles and procedures* (4th ed.). Belmont, CA: Wadsworth.

Ó Ciardha, C., & Gannon, T. A. (2011). The cognitive distortions of child molesters are in need of treatment. *Journal of Sexual Aggression, 17,* 130-141.

O'Connor, W. (1996). A problem-solving intervention for sex offenders with an intellectual disability. *Journal of Intellectual and Developmental Disability, 21*(3), 219-235.

Parry, C. J. & Lindsay, W. R. (2003). Impulsiveness as a factor in sexual offending by people with mild intellectual disability. *Journal of Intellectual Disability Research, 47, 6,* 483-487.

Plaud, J. J., Plaud, D. M., Kolstoe, P. D. & Orvedal, L., (2000). Behavioral treatment of sexually offending behavior. *Mental Health Aspects of Developmental Disabilities, 3,* 54-61.

Reavis, J., Looman, J., Franco, K., & Rojas, B. (2013). Adverse childhood experiences and adult criminality: How long must we live before we possess our own lives? *The Permanente Journal, 17,* 44-48.

Ross, R. R., & Fabiano, E. A. (1985). *Time to think: A cognitive model on delinquency prevention and offender rehabilitation.* Johnson City, TN: Institute of Social Sciences and Arts.

Ross, R. R., Fabiano, E. A., & Ewles, C. D. (1988). Reasoning and rehabilitation. *International Journal of Offender Therapy and Comparative Criminology, 32,* 29-35.

Sakdalan, J. A., Shaw, J., & Collier, V. (2010). Staying in the here-and-now: A pilot study on the use of dialectical behavior therapy group skills training for forensic clients with intellectual disability. *Journal of Intellectual Disability Research, 54,* 568-572.

Seto, M. C. (2012). Is pedophilia a sexual orientation? *Archives of Sexual Behavior, 41,* 231-236.

Singh, N. N., Lancioni, G. E., Winton, A. S., Singh, A. N., Adkins, A. D., & Singh, J. (2011). Can adult offenders with intellectual disabilities use mindfulness-based procedures to control their deviant sexual arousal? *Psychology, Crime & Law, 17,* 165-179.

Singh, N. N., Wahler, R. G., Adkins, A. D., Myers, R. E., & Mindfulness Research Group. (2003). Soles of the feet: A mindfulness-based self-control intervention for aggression by an individual with mild mental retardation and mental illness. *Research in Developmental Disabilities, 24,* 158-169.

Smith, K. R., & Matson, J. L. (2010). Social skills: Differences among adults with intellectual disabilities, co-morbid autism spectrum disorders and epilepsy. *Research in Developmental Disabilities, 31,* 1366-1372.

Sobsey, R. & Doe, T. (1991). Patterns of sexual abuse and assault. *Sexuality and Disability, 9,* 243-259.

Stevenson, B., Lynn, L., Miller, K., & Hingsburger, D. (2010). The way back: A reasoned and data-based approach to increasing community access for sex offenders during and post treatment. *Journal of Learning Disabilities and Offending Behavior, 2,* 63-71.

Stokes, T. F. & Baer, D. M. (1977). An explicit technology of generalization. *Journal of Applied Behavior Analysis, 10,* 349-367.

Tarnai, B. (2006). Review of effective interventions for socially inappropriate masturbation in persons with cognitive disabilities. *Sex Disability, 24,* 151-168.

Taylor, J. L. (2002). A review of the assessment and treatment of anger and aggression in offenders with intellectual disability. *Journal of Intellectual Disability Research, 46,* 57-73.

Vollmer, T. R., Reyes, J. R., & Walker, S. F. (2012). Behavioral assessment and intervention for sex offenders with intellectual and developmental disabilities. In. J.K. Luiselli (Ed.). *A handbook of high-risk challenging behaviors in people with intellectual and developmental disabilities* (pp. 121-144). Baltimore, MD: Paul H. Brookes.

Walker-Hirsch, L. & Champagne, M. (1993). *Circles*. Santa Barbara, CA: James Stanfield Co.

Ward, T. (2000). Sexual offenders' cognitive distortions as implicit theories. *Aggression and Violent Behavior, 5*, 491-507.

Ward, T. (2002). Good lives and the rehabilitation of offenders: Promises and problems. *Aggression and Violent Behavior, 7*, 513-528.

Ward, T., & Stewart, C. A. (2003). The treatment of sex offenders: risk management and good lives. *Professional Psychology, Research and Practice, 34*, 353-60.

Whitehouse, M. A. & McCabe, M. P. (1997). Sex education programs for people with intellectual disability: How effective are they? *Education and Training in Mental Retardation and Developmental Disabilities, 32*, 229-240.

Wilson, R. J. (1998). Psychophysiological indicators of faking in the phallometric test. *Sexual Abuse, 10*, 113-126.

Wilson, R. J. (2016). The use of phallometric testing in the diagnosis, treatment, and risk management of male adults who have sexually offended. In L. Craig & M. Rettenberger (Eds.), *The Wiley handbook on the theories, assessment & treatment of sexual offending: Volume 2* (pp. 823-849). Chichester, UK: Wiley-Blackwell.

Wilson, R. J. & Miner, M. H. (2016). Measurement of male sexual arousal and interest using penile plethysmography and viewing time. In D.R. Laws & W.T. O'Donohue (Eds.), *Treatment of sex offenders: Strengths and weaknesses in assessment and intervention.* New York: Springer.

Wright, D., Herzog. G., & Seymour, J. (1992). Treatment of a constellation of inappropriate sexual and social behaviors in a 20-year old man with Down syndrome. *Sexuality and Disability, 10*, 57-61.

Chapter Ten

Corrective and Remedial Consequences

Behaviorally, consequences are either reinforcement- or punishment-based. Reinforcement results in an increase in a behavior under similar stimulus conditions in the future by either adding something that the individual finds desirable (positive reinforcement) or eliminating/avoiding something that the person finds aversive (negative reinforcement). Punishment is a basic law of behavior and occurs when the behavior is followed by a consequence that reduces the probability of the behavior occurring under similar conditions in the future. It is accomplished by either presenting a stimulus that the person finds unpleasant following a behavior (positive punishment, or Type I) or by removing a stimulus event that the person finds pleasant following a behavior (negative punishment, or Type II).

Punishers, however, do not always represent consequences that are extremely aversive stimuli, such as electric shock or smelling a noxious odor, both of which have been historically used in treating persons who have sexually offended (see Maletzky & McGovern, 1991). The definition of punishment implies a future decrease of the behavior under similar conditions due to a stimulus change following the behavior (i.e., not necessarily aversive). As in any treatment plan, reinforcement-based strategies should be attempted before punishment procedures (Behavior Analysis Certification Board, 2014).

Punishing events for persons with intellectual disabilities often involve a loss of privileges or the addition of supervision. Miltenberger (1997) noted that there are three functional, non-aversive strategies to decrease problem behavior: extinction, differential reinforcement, and antecedent manipulations. Extinction occurs when the reinforcer that maintained the problem behavior no longer occurs following the behavior. Differential reinforcement (described in more detail later) involves either reinforcing zero or low rates of the inappropriate behavior (differential reinforcement of zero or low rates, DRO), reinforcing any alternative behavior (differential reinforcement of alternative behavior, DRA), or reinforcing incompatible appropriate behavior (differential reinforcement of incompatible behavior, DRI) in an attempt to reduce/replace inappropriate behavior. Antecedent manipulations to the environment reduce the likelihood of the inappropriate behavior, while at the same time increasing the likelihood of desirable behavior. For example, capitalizing on motivating operations (as described in Ch. 5) can be a non-intrusive antecedent strategy to effect behavior change.

PUNITIVE APPROACHES

"Sexual offender recidivism with even low levels of sexual misbehavior has serious consequences for people with developmental disabilities" (Tough, 2001, p. 21, unpublished Master of Arts thesis). The consequences for this population typically fall on each end of the spectrum: minor sexual misbehaviors, ones that would result in no sanctions for a typically developing person, can result in severe restrictions of rights, residential moves, and intensive supervision. On the other end, significant and serious sexual offending by persons with intellectual disability is ignored or dealt with "internally," where the individual never learns normative standards nor that they have a responsibility to do no harm and follow the law. One study showed that 43% of individuals who had serious sexual offenses received no judicial sanctions (Tough, 2001).

For some individuals with an intellectual disability who have displayed sexual offending behavior, treatment has historically been confrontational and restrictive rather than rehabilitative. Consequences applied were typically punitive in nature with the aim of eliminating all sexual behavior. This latter part is of note considering our earlier comments about unfortunately common perceptions of persons with disabilities as being either asexual or disinterested in sex.

Whether punitive strategies serve as punishment of an individual's sexual offending behavior depends on the resultant outcome (i.e., if there is a decrease in future instances of inappropriate sexual behavior, then the punishment procedure was effective). For example, if an individual loses privileges that are less reinforcing than the sexual offending behavior, it may not decrease the inappropriate behavior. Just because something may be deemed "aversive" does not guarantee that it will be effective for decreasing behavior. It depends on what the individual finds aversive and what other schedules of reinforcement and punishment are operating at the same time.

Towards the end of the 20th century, people with disabilities and sexually inappropriate behavior were treated with highly intrusive consequences that were not based on function such as, "facial screening, overcorrection, the use of contingent lemon juice, and time-out"[1] (Griffiths, Quinsey, & Hingsburger, 1989, pp. 9-10). As noted earlier, the treatment of persons who have sexually offended has sometimes applied highly punitive consequences that did not match the seriousness of the act, including aversion therapy (e.g., smelling of noxious stimuli and even faradic stimulation). Aversion therapy techniques were among the behavioral applications to treating persons who have sexually offended (Gaither, Rosenkranz, & Plaud, 1998; Plaud, Plaud, Kolstoe, & Orvedal, 2000). Early aversive approaches to the treatment of sexualized

[1] *Facial screening is the "blocking of an individual's field of vision contingent upon the performance of a behavior." (Singh, Lloyd, & Kendell, 1999, p.5).*

Overcorrection is the "institution of a more appropriate response and repeated practice of it contingent upon the behavior occurring." (Singh et al., 1999, p.5).

Contingent lemon juice is the administration of a squirt of lemon juice in the mouth contingent upon the performance of a behavior.

Time-out is the "imposition of a brief time period when reinforcement is not available." (Singh et al., 1999, p.5).

offending behavior were built on the belief that the individual had experiences in the developing years that led to respondent conditioning of inappropriate sexual interests (Laws & Marshall, 1990).

Following this theory, early behaviorally-based treatment sought to reduce or eliminate the inappropriate sexual preferences through such procedures as covert sensitization, orgasmic reconditioning, satiation therapy, odor aversion therapy (such as olfactory aversion), and faradic or electrical aversion therapy (Marshall, & Laws, 2003; Plaud et al., 2000). Aversion therapies have been applied to decrease arousal to inappropriate stimuli (e.g., children or violence) and to recondition (i.e., through respondent conditioning) the orgasmic response to appropriate stimuli (e.g., consenting adults). Restrictive practices, such as loss of privileges for community access, were routinely employed as both a safety and punitive practice. However, arousal reduction approaches have been found to be largely ineffective over the long term because they fail to account for both the respondent and operant features of behavior. That is, focusing only on respondent conditioning failed to consider other contingencies in the environment that may have been maintaining sexually inappropriate behavior (see Chapter 4). These aversive approaches typically failed to yield the desired results, largely because sex is a natural phenomenon, or unconditioned response, and as with all behaviors maintained through naturally occurring reinforcement they are extremely hard to eliminate. As a result, current models for treatment now involve both arousal reduction methods combined with operant conditioning to provide behavioral skills training (e.g., instructions, modelling, rehearsal and feedback) to teach replacement and compensatory skills.

Behavioral replacement skills were described in Chapter 9 and are determined through a series of approaches including reviewing the records related to the offense, interviewing the individuals who offended and others about the index offense, conducting plethysmography, conducting preference assessments, completing socio-sexual knowledge and attitude measures, and conducting covert probes.

Natural Social Consequences

Just as with the typically developing population, a person with an intellectual disability who commits a sexual offense could face jail or prison time or receive other legal sanctions, such as probation. In treatment, Lindsay (2007) has suggested that it is extremely important to ensure that individuals who offended have a thorough understanding of the mores and conventions of society: "Where an individual has had a restricted or distorted upbringing, they may have failed to develop a full understanding of these conventions" including "society's laws" (p. 72). Knowledge of the offenses may serve as a deterrent. However behavioral therapists have also used the potential of legal punishment to teach individuals who offended about the logical consequences for a convicted person within treatment. For example, if an individual in treatment who is on probation violates a condition of their probation, therapists are required to report the breach to the probation officer. The offending individual in treatment would be informed prior to becoming involved in the intervention that they would be obliged to report a breach of violation; although a duty of ethical practice, this also allows the individual who offended to learn natural and logical consequences of their behavior which may lead to fewer breaches in the future to avoid the punishment.

Contingency Management

> *Behavioral residential services should employ contingency management of daily living skills (through the utilization of behavioral contracts, appropriate staffing, and adequate security precautions), individual education (individualized using precision teaching methods), and specialized behavioral programming for sexual offending (through individual and group behavioral skills training and sexual arousal conditioning approaches). (Plaud et al., 2000, p. 55).*

In the approaches used today, there are both natural and contrived consequences that are typically used with individuals with intellectual disabilities who offend sexually. In addition to the naturally occurring punitive consequences for sexual offending described above, persons with intellectual disabilities are often subject to a range of contrived consequences. The goal of a behavioral treatment program is to achieve behavioral competency by providing opportunities to learn appropriate adaptive and coping skills, which will then be utilized and reinforced in the natural environment. The integration of the educational elements into daily living is an attempt to "trap" the new behaviors so that they eventually fall under the control of natural contingencies in the environment.

Unfortunately, too often contingency systems are used, in residential settings that provide services to individuals who offended, that focus more on management than treatment, and the nature of the consequences are often restrictive and punitive. Griffiths et al. (2003) identified four distinct categories in which rights restrictions occur within residential settings: access and autonomy; relationships and community; safety, security, and privacy; and control and decision-making. Although "restrictions are taken very seriously by those who write behavioral programs and by the governing bodies that oversee the use of behavioral technology," too often "restrictions are used haphazardly and inconsistency within the dynamic of the relationship" between staff and the individual (Ioannou, 2016, p. 2). Ioannou noted that restrictions are employed by individual staff members as a method of controlling behaviors that they have deemed inappropriate. Ioannou refers to these as "random acts of power;" sanctions that are provided in the operation of a residential setting that are not part of a carefully crafted habilitative plan. The nature of restrictions that have been applied to people with intellectual disabilities often has included sanctions that were not directly related to the behavior, such as loss of privileges unrelated to the offense (e.g., taking away television privileges or activity preferences because the person has not showered), nor presented close enough in time to the actual offense to affect the behavior (denying a community activity or access to a family visit for a breach of behavioral contract several days prior).

From a behavioral perspective, the typical management paradigm used can often create conditions in which the individual has been so restricted and punished that they fall into a reinforcement abyss where there is little reinforcement for non-offense behaviors; so the reinforcing value of offending behaviors might increase. Alternatively, because they are deprived of any reinforcement they may be more likely to seek reinforcement of any type, including sexual behaviors. In other words, the potential for recidivism may increase because alternative appropriate behaviors are not receiving reinforcement contingencies potentially; this creates a "nothing to lose" situation, or an establishing operation which increases the potential value of reinforcement through offending. See Figure 10.1, below, to see how the overuse of restrictive consequences can leave the individual in a reinforcement void.

Figure 10.1 **Typical Management Paradigm Following a Sexual Offense**

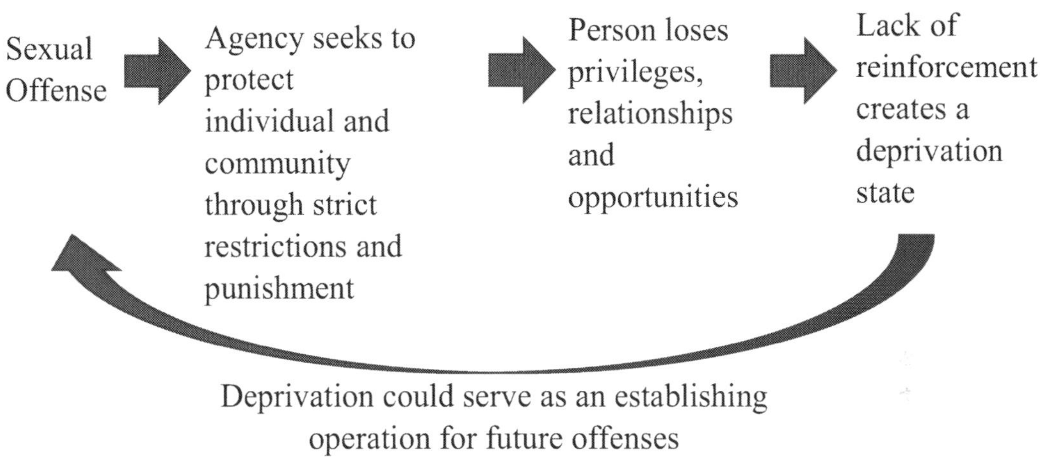

Punitive consequences can be contrasted with remedial consequences that are corrective in nature and designed to teach the individual a more appropriate behavior in place of the inappropriate one. The literature regarding the effects of sanctions versus rehabilitative options has been unanimous in stating that punishment alone will reduce the likelihood of future offensive behavior only temporarily and is not ultimately an ideal long term solution (see Smith, Goggin, & Gendreau, 2002). Although risk management is an important element of intervention as elaborated in the Risk-Need-Responsibility Model (Bonta & Andrews, 2017), approaches that focus primarily on diminishing the risks of re-offense have been criticized in the literature as failing to focus on establishing competing alternative behaviors, strengths, and well-being as a mechanism to reduce recidivism (Ward & Stewart, 2003). An emerging trend regarding treatment efficacy is to not just focus on punishment for the offense, or even suppression, but rather on increasing reinforcement of appropriate or alternative behaviors: "Behavior analysis is at its best when it takes a constructional approach, by concentrating on building repertoires of behavior that people can use to function independently and successfully" (Grant & Evans, 1994, p81).

Ioannou (2016, p.3) cautioned that:

> *[P]utting a restriction in place as a means to reach habilitation should always be at the forefront of implementing restrictions. During the time that the individual has a restrictive measure, they should still be given as much choice, as possible, within the context of the restriction. A restriction should never hinder an individual's habilitation or opportunity for community participation. If the individual requires a staff to supervise them in the community while they are learning community safety skills, then a staff should be available to ensure the individual can go to the community.*

With the population of persons who have offended, some restrictions may be necessary long-term because of imminent risk to the individual who offended, other individuals, or the community at large. However, the use of these restrictions must be based on a written plan that has been properly approved, implemented by trained staff, monitored through data collection and a qualified behavior analyst, and balanced against enhanced quality of life elements including reinforcement and skill development (Ioannou, 2016).

Covert Sensitization

Another way of reinforcing the notion of logical and natural consequences has been introduced into therapy directly using covert sensitization to control sexual arousal, as described by Quinsey and Marshall (1983). Covert sensitization conditioning involves pairing the inappropriate sexual behavior and its antecedents with known aversive stimuli to enhance avoidance of the precipitative events (Plaud et al., 2000, p. 57). Variations of covert sensitization include olfactory and faradic aversion. In olfactory aversion, the aversive stimulus is a noxious odor (e.g., rotten raw hamburger, valeric acid, ammonia). In this process, the individual self-administers the noxious odor (Marshall, Eccles, & Barbaree, 1991). The literature has also described the use of faradic stimulation, in which a mild electric shock is administered (Marshall et al., 1991). This approach (i.e., aversion) has been subject to significant ethical and controversial issues that will be discussed more fully in Chapter 13.

The theoretical base for this type of treatment involves both classical and operant conditioning.

> *Covert conditioning refers to a family of behavioral therapy procedures which combine the use of imagery with the principles of operant conditioning. Covert conditioning is a process through which private events such as thoughts, images and feelings are manipulated in accordance with the principles of learning, usually operant conditioning, to bring about changes in overt behavior, covert psychological behavior (i.e. thoughts, images, feelings), and/or physiological behavior (e.g., glandular secretions). (Cautela & Kearney, 1990, p. 86).*

Covert sensitization is a variation of aversive counter-conditioning (McGrath, Hoke & Vojtisek, 1998), which involves having the individual imagine potential consequences to teach the individual how to stop the imagery associated with inappropriate arousal and stimulation and to replace it with imagery that demonstrates appropriate control and sexuality whenever possible. In other words, the individual imagines performing a behavior chain that has led to sexually inappropriate behavior in the past and, once ensconced in this visualization, is prompted to interrupt the offense behavior chain leading to offense by imagining aversive consequences. "In covert sensitization, the aversive stimulus usually consists of an anxiety-inducing or nausea-inducing images that is presented verbally by the therapist and imagined by the individual" (Plaud et al., 2000, p. 57). The aversive scene is individualized to match the individual's specific triggers. In this procedure, the therapist describes a scene that is known to produce inappropriate arousal for the individual, such as walking through a park with children for a person who experiences sexual arousal to children. The therapist would be aware of the stimuli and setting events that represent a known arousal-producing scenario because of previous interviews with the individual that revealed what inappropriate situations have created arousal in the past. The individual is then asked to imagine themselves in this state and, once the individual can visualize themselves in the described scenes, the therapist would then introduce the image of a realistic but aversive consequence, such as being caught by the child's father, being arrested, or being removed from one's family to a place without favorite items like TV, computer, etc. Again, the circumstances of the punitive consequence would be individualized based upon knowledge of the individual and what was feared or valued by the person. The underlying behavioral process is that of classical conditioning:

> *The therapist works with the individual to develop an aversive image that will be paired with the precipitative events, and with the image of the deviant behavior itself, according to classical conditioning paradigm. The aversive image serves as the unconditioned stimulus (UCS). The images of the precipitative events, being continually paired with the UCS, become the conditioned stimulus (CS). Both the conditioned response (CR) and the unconditioned response (UCR) consists of a negative reaction which may be emotional (e.g. fear), physiological (e.g., nausea), or in some other way repulsive. (Plaud et al., 2000, pp. 57-58).*

The therapeutic result is that the individual should attempt to avoid or evade situations including both the inappropriate sexual behavior and the precipitative events that elicited the behavior in the past due to the negative association that has been conditioned.

In this type of intervention, the individual learns to associate the natural aversive consequences associated with assault, such as jail, removal from the community, and/or rejection and shame that could occur if they acted upon that fantasy. If possible, the aversive consequence is introduced early, in an attempt to interrupt the behavioral chain as soon as possible. If the conditioning is highly effective the person may not be able to engage in the behavior because it may inhibit arousal by introducing fear and anxiety that are incompatible with arousal and, at the very least, may lead to a lower frequency of the behavior (Plaud et al., 2000).

Treatment does not stop with creating an association between the sexual offending behavior, its precipitated events, and an unpleasant event. Although the first part of the scenario ends with the person imagining aversive consequences (which in theory should act as positive punishment of the offending behavior), the scenario is then continued and the person is asked to imagine being in the same scenario but, in this second scenario, the person elects to use coping skills to escape the situation without offending against the child. By adding this second element, the individual can see that by walking away or using some other coping strategy, they are then able to return to their home, see their parents, be free of humiliation and harm, and take advantage of their freedoms and privileges which, in theory, should act as positive reinforcement of the coping behavior.

The second part of the treatment involves a form of negative reinforcement in which an alternative appropriate behavior leads to the removal or avoidance of the punitive consequence. In this process, the therapist is introducing imagery with known punishing qualities to create an association with the inappropriate sexual response behavior. This serves to decrease the behavior, combined with reinforcement following the performance of an appropriate control strategy to increase or strengthen the use of self-control (appropriate responses) in high risk situations. The theory of the strategy is that it will not only teach about social mores and realistic consequence of offending, it reinforces the concept that the use of self-control strategies or appropriate sexuality can lead to maintenance of freedom, access to desired people and conditions, and other positive elements. Of course, in the above example, the effectiveness of the assumed punisher is dependent upon whether the individual experiences the imagery as aversive or not, as well as whether it will serve as a punisher in terms of causing a reduction in the behavior. Even if reduction of the inappropriate behavior occurs it does not guarantee generalization to the natural environment (Rea et al., 2003).

Let's explore how this looks in the Punishment Chart in Table 10.1 below:

Table 10.1 ***Punishment in Covert Sensitization.***

Consequences	Punishment
Positive	The application of an imagined aversive event following an imagined instance of the inappropriate sexual behavior to decrease the probability that the behavior will occur in the future under similar stimulus conditions.
Negative	The imagined removal of positive or rewarding events because of imagined performance of a sexually inappropriate behavior. This might include loss of privileges, opportunities, or even freedoms that will decrease the probability that the behavior will occur in the future under similar stimulus conditions.

The application of covert sensitization also employs the use of reinforcement strategies as seen in Table 10.2 below.

Table 10.2 ***Reinforcement in Covert Sensitization.***

Consequences	Reinforcement
Positive	The application of a pleasant event or stimulus following an imagined instance of an appropriate or alternative behavior (to offending), often one that served the same function, with the goal of increasing the desirable behavior which might serve as a replacement for the inappropriate sexual behavior. The imagined use of an appropriate control or protective strategy is rewarded by ending the scene with the person engaged in an appropriate activity that is known to be reinforcing because the person used their control strategy.
Negative	The removal of an aversive stimulus following the imagined performance of an appropriate response or alternative behavior (to offending). In covert sensitization, the individual is initially faced with the threat of punishment or imprisonment; however, when appropriate non-offending/coping behavior is demonstrated the aversive imagery is terminated and the person is asked to imagine walking away from the situation, leaving the park, and finding a staff or other individual who might trigger non-offense (e.g., parent). This is then followed by imagery of going home or engaging in some desired and valued activity with individuals that the person enjoys.

There are some caveats to the use of covert sensitization with persons with intellectual disabilities. First, although a theoretically logical form of treatment, some individuals with intellectual disabilities will likely have difficulty creating the images necessary to allow this form of therapy to be effective, although social stories and the use of video cameras to make social stories might assist in opportunities for individuals to be directed to use the behaviors as the film is shot.

Second, in the example above, it is important to recognize that if the individual lives in an environment where there is deprivation of reinforcement, or where appropriate behaviors are not positively reinforced, they have not contacted the necessary reinforcement contingencies to maintain the appropriate behavior. There may also be no reason to demonstrate coping or self-control when an opportunity arises when one's life is bereft of positive elements, either in terms of appropriate relationships, activities, or potentialities for positive outcomes. The reinforcement deprivation for appropriate skills may diminish the motivating operation for learning and applying new (appropriate coping) skills thereby creating an evocative effect for inappropriate sexual behaviors if that is what the individual receives the most reinforcement for. It is therefore important to evaluate the schedules of reinforcement that are available in the individual's life prior to, and when providing, treatment strategies so that an enhanced and richer reinforcement milieu is built into the plan in an attempt to build a good life.

Third and vitally important is that these techniques should only be employed by clinicians who have been specifically trained in the use of these techniques.

Shaping Appropriate Masturbation

Historically, Plaud and colleagues (2000) described several techniques that were used to shape appropriate masturbation. The first was *masturbatory satiation,* in which the reduction of arousal to the inappropriate stimuli was designed to be achieved by satiating the individual to the problematic fantasies for a prolonged period, until a prescribed time-period has lapsed. The second was masturbatory extinction, which not only targeted a decrease in the arousal to inappropriate stimuli but also targeted an increase in the arousal to appropriate stimuli. In this approach, the person masturbated to appropriate imagery until completion, then masturbated to nonsexual fantasies until completion, and lastly, masturbated for an extended period of time while engaging in inappropriate fantasy, without ejaculation, thereby decreasing the likelihood that orgasm will occur in association with the inappropriate imagery. Lastly, orgasmic reconditioning, involved creating a strong association with appropriate imagery and arousal while reducing the association between arousal and inappropriate imagery.

The previous examples that involved shaping masturbation have been used in the past with persons with intellectual disabilities but have been questioned due to the cognitive or even physical challenges that these individuals have (Plaud et al., 2000). Others have suggested that these theories did not make a lot of real-world sense regarding male sexuality. What these theories did accomplish was create an unpleasant practice that was devoid of the understanding that, aside from their offending, these are otherwise typical men who do not have the same cognitive profiles as men with intellectual disabilities (R. Wilson, Personal Communication, April 12, 2018). The use of aversive conditioning as used in these procedures may be both socially and ethically challenged. The shaping of appropriate masturbation should, therefore, be contained to the use of antecedent strategies (ensuring that only legal erotic stimuli are available, the person has access to privacy) and teaching strategies that focus on when and where it is okay to masturbate and when and where it is not okay to masturbate.

NON-PUNISHMENT BASED APPROACHES

Research in the 1980s highlighted the importance of paying attention to both what happens and what does not happen (i.e., Kazdin 1982). The most widely used behavioral treatment in the literature in the 1980s was differential reinforcement (Lennox, Miltenberger, Spengler, & Erfanian, 1988). The use of reinforcement techniques is both socially and culturally accepted (Skinner, 1953), preferred within the professional field (Tarnowski, Rasnake, Mulick, & Kelly, 1989), and often not subject to the ethical and practical challenges associated with the use of aversive strategies.

As mentioned earlier, differential reinforcement attempts to decrease the inappropriate behavior and, at times, increase more appropriate and desirable behavior. Differential reinforcement procedures involve providing reinforcement contingent on desirable responses and withholding reinforcement for undesirable responses (i.e., extinction). Positive reinforcement of alternative behaviors holds that the use of differential reinforcement both strengthens the behaviors that are occurring at the moment of the delivery of reinforcement, as well as behaviors that share the same response properties. Differential reinforcement also decreases the likelihood of avoidance and escape behaviors, which are common in punishment and extinction procedures.

Vollmer and Iwata (1992, p. 394) noted that, "it is sometimes difficult to identify and or control the variables responsible for maintaining behavior. Furthermore, the development of effective reinforcement procedures can be highly complex when behavior is multiply controlled." A response to this limitation is differential reinforcement of other behavior (DRO), a reinforcement schedule in which reinforcement is provided for low levels or non-occurrence of a targeted undesirable behavior (time-based). DRO has also been referred to as "omission training" (Uhl & Garcia, 1969) and differential reinforcement of non-responding or zero responding (Poling & Ryan, 1982). DRO is commonly used if it is not possible to identify the specific antecedent events to the offending behavior or if the behavior is occurring at a high rate and no alternative behavior is available. Procedures involving differential reinforcement of other behaviors "have always had a curious place within behavior analysis" (Grant & Evans, 1994, p. 79). A debate has loomed as to whether it represents a reinforcement or punishment procedure, since the ultimate goal is the reduction of behavior, and the occurrence of the behavior results in a delay of reinforcement. Grant and Evans (1994) suggest that DRO can also be viewed as a reinforcement procedure; however, the reinforcing consequence in DRO is immediately dependent on the absence of the target behavior vs. the occurrence of behavior: "When the target behavior occurs under DRO, nothing happens (i.e., no stimulus change occurs)" (Grant & Evans, 1994, p. 79). This presents the possibility for other problem behaviors that may occur during this time being inadvertently reinforced. The use of DRO is often part of a treatment package that additionally specifies some contingency for the occurrence of the target behavior, usually in the form of some sanction or loss of privilege and in combination with differential positive reinforcement.

Positive reinforcement can be either automatic or socially mediated (Iwata, Dorsey, Slifer, Bauman & Richman, 1992). Functionally relevant positive reinforcement is an important element in most contemporary behavioral programming. It employs socially mediated consequences contingent on appropriate behavior, whether it be an alternative to the inappropriate behavior or other appropriate behavior. Two differential reinforcement procedures (described previously) that may assist in establishing competing contingencies for problem behaviors include differential reinforcement of alternative behavior (DRA) and differential reinforcement of incompatible behavior (DRI). Both involve extinction of problem behavior and reinforcing behaviors that are alternative or incompatible with the inappropriate behavior respectively.

Remedial consequences are determined from the analysis of the antecedents/motivating operations and the maintaining consequences (function) of the behavior. Remedial consequences are not meant to be punitive but to provide better replacement behaviors for individuals who may not have those in their repertoire. Take for instance public masturbation: Traditional punishment procedures would target decreasing all masturbation but provide no support in alternative sexual behaviors. A more balanced approach to treatment would be to assess knowledge of public and private behaviors and the precursors to public masturbation, then teach and reinforce private masturbation (DRI). If the inappropriate behavior was the result of lack of knowledge, then the individual could be taught where and when it would be appropriate to engage in this behavior. If the inappropriate behavior is the result of a lack of appropriate imagery, then masturbation can be enhanced by providing age appropriate sexual imagery for use in a private location. However, if the individual engages in public masturbation because of the reaction he receives from others when engaging in the offense, then in addition to the above strategies or providing appropriate opportunities for self-gratification, it is also important to address the function of the offense. That is, if the offense is maintained by attention, withholding attention for the behavior (extinction) and providing attention for more appropriate alternative behaviors is warranted (DRA), as previously discussed.

The concept of DRA in the treatment of persons who have sexually offended relates directly to *the Good Lives Model* (GLM), involving reinforcement for alternative prosocial behaviors. Ward and colleagues (Ward & Gannon, 2006; Ward & Stewart, 2003) proposed the GLM as a broad rehabilitative framework and the integration of a self-regulation approach. The GLM is a strength-based approach that focuses on individuals as goal seeking, attempting to acquire primary human goals (as described in detail in Chapter 6), that, if achieved, can increase overall well-being. Ward, Mann and Gannon (2007) suggested that building a strong prosocial life, that has meaningful engaged relationships and activities, leaves the individual little time or opportunity in which to commit an offense. Moreover, by instilling a means to gain a reinforcing quality of life, the individual can establish a life worth keeping. The assumption is that as psychological well-being and appropriate behaviors increase, risk decreases; as psychological well-being and appropriate behaviors decrease, risk increases.

Non-contingent reinforcement (NCR) is a method whereby the person receives reinforcement that is not contingent on a particular behavior at fixed or variable intervals. It has emerged as part of treatment packages for behaviors such as aggression, "It is commonly acknowledged that decreases in responding under NCR may result from either (a) elimination of the motivating operation (MO) to engage in behavior (in the present case, deprivation) due to the delivery of reinforcers "for free" or (b) elimination of the response–reinforcer contingency that maintains behavior, which results in extinction. (Wallace, Iwata, Hanley, Thompson, & Roscoe, 2012). The use of NCR has been shown to have few side effects, however. Vollmer, Righdahl, Roane, and Marcus (1997) noted that the use of NCR can result in incidental reinforcement. They suggested that the use of omission training (DRO) in combination with NCR was beneficial in reducing potential side-effects.

In working with persons who have sexually offended, the use of NCR may be effective in setting the stage for the individual to receive reinforcement and build resiliency. As noted above, many individuals who offended in treatment have been subject to random acts of power within the agencies supporting them, to the point where there is little to lose by re-offending. An environment that is rich in non-contingent reinforcement throughout the course of daily routines, while extinguishing the inappropriate responses, can establish a reinforcement schedule that may satiate the need for desired outcomes that may be related to the sexual offense, such as social reinforcement. The use of NCR can be seen as an element in the *Good Lives Model*, in which the individuals who offended are provided a range of opportunities to engage in activities that will bring them both contingent (DRA), as well as non-contingent reinforcement (NCR).

The *Good Lives Model* bears logical merit in behavioral terms as well. That is, if an individual is not deprived of reinforcement but, alternatively, receives it by engaging in appropriate behaviors, the individual may not be in a deprivation state and may therefore be less likely to engage in inappropriate behaviors to receive it. This brings up a question, however, as to how this relates to the function of the target sexually inappropriate behavior. For example, if conditioned generalized reinforcement (i.e., attention) is what maintains the behavior, then generalized attention can be assumed to be effective in providing the individual with the desired interaction to fill the deprivation state. However, if the behavior is maintained by attention that is sexually based or based on a desire for attention from a desired person, then generalized attention will be unlikely to have the same reinforcing properties. The individual who offended may not have access to outlets for appropriate sexual behavior with another individual, because of personal circumstances or issues of safety, especially at early stages of treatment. In this situation, the individual who offended can be positively reinforced for engaging in appropriate social interactions (e.g., respecting privacy and space), for engaging in appropriate behaviors that would serve as competing behaviors (e.g., demonstrating coping skills), or self-satisfying sexual urges in an appropriate place and time.

Additionally, the authors suggest that it provides the provision of a dense schedule of reinforcement that many persons with intellectual disabilities have not received; especially those who have presented with challenging behaviors. As noted above, under these circumstances, the typically positive elements of life have been removed for many individuals following an offense in an attempt to restrict or punish them to manage the behavior, resulting in the loss of most reinforcing opportunities for the individual who offended not just those related to the sexual offending. The use of reinforcement approaches establishes a new history of reinforcement for the individual who offended that is based upon appropriate behavior. Establishing non-contingent reinforcement and building a better life creates a condition under which a re-offense would be costly for the individual in terms of loss of a range of reinforcing opportunities that are afforded for non-occurrence (e.g., a life worth keeping). This may also be described in terms of motivating operations. For example, by establishing an environment that is rich in reinforcement for appropriate behaviors, the value and frequency of appropriate behaviors may temporarily increase and create an abolishing operation for inappropriate behaviors, in that the value and frequency of the inappropriate behaviors may be temporarily decreased.

***Figure 10.2* Habilitative "Good Life Model" Paradigm Following a Sexual Offense**

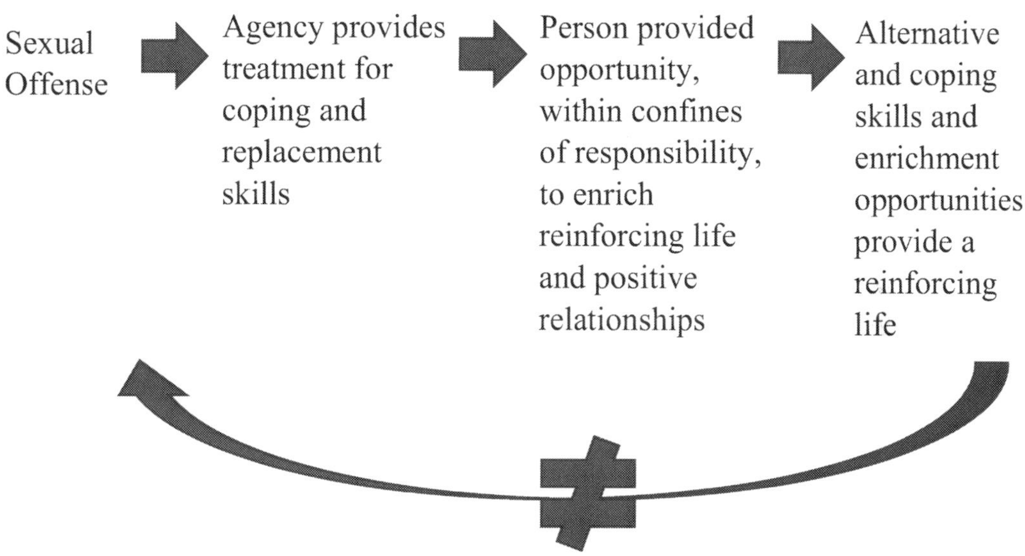

A rich life with reinforcement can provide an abative influence on future offenses.

As noted above, it is vital to "trap" the coping and management behaviors described above into the natural environment through building natural contingencies for other behaviors, such as assessing the presence of arousal to appropriate targets and activities and building reinforcement for appropriate sexuality. The efficacy of teaching functional skills to replace the inappropriate behavior depends upon whether there is functional replacement value that is of equal or greater reinforcement value (Favell & Reid, 1988). In addition, the replacement behavior must require less effort and be more readily available than the sexually offensive behavior. To ensure that the behavior will be trapped in the conditions of the natural environment, it is important to ensure that staff are trained to reinforce behavior initially as frequently, intensely, under the same conditions, and in as many variations as possible. If a behavior is subject to what Hingsburger (1996) termed *reinforcement trade-down*, where the replacement behavior has less reinforcement value in eliciting the same frequency, intensity, or quality of reinforcement than the inappropriate behavior, then the new behavior will not become trapped in the natural environment. With sexualized behavior, this can be difficult to achieve. As a result, Ward and Stewart (2003) suggested that providing a community of reinforcement for a range of other behaviors is important to attempt to reduce recidivism. They suggested that by establishing a reinforcing lifestyle, clinicians can set up competing reinforcement that may influence the offending behavior.

The Role of Pharmacological Treatment

Pharmacological treatment of persons who have sexually offended can be either hormonal (directed at affecting the part of the brain that are associated with sexual urges), or indirect treatment, including treatment of comorbid conditions (Sherak, 2000). Hormonal therapy that serves to curb ruminations that relate to sexual arousal has been recommended in some cases to reduce the impulsivity of the sexual drive among individuals who offended, such as we saw in the case of Scott in Chapter 7. Hormone therapies and medications that have similar effects have often been suggested as being helpful in supporting clinical approaches to curb the ruminations associated with sexual offending behavior, either as a temporary or long-term measure. Some treatments can have a dramatic effect on sex drive – most often using anti-androgens. Individuals with intellectual disabilities are significantly more likely to have certain psychiatric conditions. "[T]he rate of psychosis, particularly schizophrenia, and the rate of phobic disorder were significantly higher among adults with mild to moderate intellectual disability compared with those in the general population without intellectual disability" (Deb, Thomas, & Bright, 2001). It can then be assumed that psychiatric medications, specifically anti-psychotics, are prescribed disproportionately within the community of persons with intellectual disability. Several of these formulations, including anti-psychotics, also cause sexual dysfunction (Serretti & Chiesa, 2011), which can make sexual activity nearly impossible and, thus, reduce the reinforcing effectiveness. Anti-androgen drugs such as Lupron or Provera are prescribed to reduce the sex drives of individuals who have offended. These drugs do not completely eliminate all desires, either inappropriate or appropriate but, if used correctly, these medications can reduce an individual's sex drive to such a degree that they are able to manage and regulate their impulses and behavior. Chemically reducing the individual's sex drive using anti-androgen medications could have a similar effect to satiation and, as such, make sexual behavior less reinforcing (and serve as an abolishing operation) – the positive outcome being that sexually inappropriate behaviors are less likely to occur. For a comprehensive discussion on pharmacological treatment of sexually offending behavior see Sherak (2000).

To summarize, the use of medications to curb sexual arousal has been employed in many instances as either a temporary or management measure. For example, a person in therapy may be making great strides, but the therapeutic team is not fully confident that the person can control arousal in the community. This could result in denial of opportunities for the person to actively engage in a range of reinforcing opportunities in the community that could set up elements of a life rich with reinforcement of desirable behaviors. When prudently used, these medications can allow the person to potentially interact in ways that will build up resiliency by curbing impulsivity associated with the degree of arousal he is experiencing. Such decisions require careful evaluation by the clinical team to ensure that medications are being used in a therapeutic way and not just as a management strategy to substitute the obligation to provide active treatment. These ethical questions of treatment vs. management will be examined more fully in Chapter 13.

RECOMMENDED PRACTICE

Recommended practice models supported by empirical evidence for mainstream treatment and rehabilitation for people who have offended have led to a shift away from traditional punitive measures towards the application of human services to reduce recidivism. As noted above, the *Risk, Need, Responsivity Model* (Bonta & Andrews, 2017) has gained empirical support for reducing recidivism and poses three principles for effective rehabilitation: The *risk* principle states that the intensity of an intervention must match the offending person's level of risk. A high-risk individual should not be receiving minimal interventions and supervision and a low-risk individual should not be receiving intense interventions and supervision. According to this principle, a mismatching of intervention to the level of risk (e.g., a low risk individual who offended receiving intense interventions) can worsen an offending person's state and, consequently, increase risk (Andrews, Bonta, & Wormith, 2011). The *need* principle states that treatment programming must target those dynamic risk factors and criminogenic needs most related to offending. There must be a specific focus on lifestyle areas that led to the offending for treatment to be effective and to reduce the risk of re-offending (Andrews et al., 2011). The *responsivity* principle states that the style and type of interventions or supports must match the individual's personal characteristics such as learning style, cognitive ability, strengths, motivation, and "the individual's personal and interpersonal circumstances" (Wilson & Yates, 2009, p. 158).

Supervision (or, rather, adherence to the terms of "supervision") has been frequently cited in the literature as a fundamental dynamic risk factor. Hanson and Harris (2000; see also Hanson, Harris, Scott, & Helmus, 2007) conducted a comprehensive study comparing 208 persons who sexually re-offended to 201 persons who did not sexually re-offend on several variables through interviews and file reviews. They found that individuals who had not re-offended were more cooperative with supervision than the individuals who re-offended. Further, although both groups of individuals attended the same number of treatment programs, the persons who re-offended were more often disengaged from treatment and supervision, and they tended to miss scheduled appointments more than those who did not re-offend. This suggests that the amount of compliance with supervision was related to recidivism in sexual offending, while less supervision and lower compliance with supervision were related to an increase in the risk of re-offending (Hanson & Harris, 2000).

Ioannou (2013) explored management of risk in the context of a culture of rights in community-based treatment programs for persons with intellectual disabilities who sexually offend. She noted that the emerging and prevailing literature discussed that people with intellectual disability who sexually offend must be granted the same human rights as all people, while being cognizant of the public's right to safety and right to be free from harm (Birgden & Cucolo 2011; Ward et al., 2007; Ward & Salmon, 2011). In her research, Ioannou found that individuals who offended who were supported in three different community settings (treatment homes, residential or group homes, or transitional homes) demonstrated an unequal balance of rights and risk. She noted that the extent of the imbalance was more prominent in the residential settings than in the treatment and transitional settings. Specifically, in the treatment and transitional settings, there was more emphasis on risks than rights. In the residential settings, there was more emphasis on rights than risks. Although one could argue that this imbalance may represent a difference to the individual who offended and, as such, reflect some element of responsivity, there was no evidence presented to support this. The residential (group home) settings were typically indoctrinated by a philosophy of individual supports, autonomy, and rights that now rightly is ensconced in the field of intellectual disability with the recent advent of rights-based training and movements. Ioannou noted that the residential settings illustrated an over-exuberance in the application of this newly applied concept, often with inattention to the potential risks and responsibility to the community. She concluded that human rights must be enforced, and this is consistent with building resiliency in the GLM and quality of life research (Dewhurst & Nielsen, 1999; Felce & Perry, 1995; Ward et al., 2007), but these rights must be regarded in the context of risk. It is creating an extreme disservice to the individuals and the community if rights and risk are not viewed as equally important separate entities. In the absence of this kind of balanced approach, which also encompasses a lack of fidelity in the implementation of the responsivity principle, people with intellectual disability who sexually offend may be insufficiently supported.

SUMMARY

The type of contrived consequences for sexual offending behavior have shifted in the field to value the importance of not just putting sanctions and restrictions in place to manage or attempt to reduce problematic behavior, but also to focus on providing consequences for the use of prosocial appropriate behaviors both directly related to the targeted behaviors as coping skills and as a general enhancement of reinforcement in the life of the person to enhance resiliency. This shift is consistent with the changes that have occurred in ABA over the past few decades and have the potential to make significant differences in the effectiveness of treatment and the maintenance and generalizability of treatment gains over time. Further development of functional behavior assessment and function-based treatment is needed.

Davis et al. (2016) suggested that a treatment model for inappropriate sexual behaviors should includes identifying the function of behavior through a functional behavior assessment if possible, treating the behavior based on the function, implementing reinforcement-based interventions (e.g., DRO) if the function is unknown, and implementing punishment-based strategies only if reinforcement-based strategies were unsuccessful or if there is risk to the individual or others in the environment. The authors also emphasize that a Board-Certified Behavior Analyst (BCBA) with relevant and notable experience should supervise all aspects of the assessment and treatment, given the complexity of the behaviors and ethical considerations involved (discussed further in Ch. 13).

REFERENCES

Andrews, D. A., Bonta, J., & Wormith, S. J. (2011). The risk-need-responsivity (RNR) model. Does adding the good lives model contribute to effective crime prevention? *Criminal Justice and Behavior, 38,* 735-755.

Behavior Analysis Certification Board (2014). *Professional and Ethical Compliance Code for Behavior Analysts.* Retrieved from: https://bacb.com/wpcontent/uploads/2017/05/170525-compliance-code-english.pdf.

Birgden, A. & Cucolo, H. (2011). The treatment of sex offenders: evidence, ethics, and human rights. *Sexual Abuse, 23,* 2965-313,

Bonta, J. & Andrews, D.A. (2017). *The psychology of criminal conduct* (6th ed.). Cincinnati, OH: Anderson.

Cautela, J. R. & Kearnet, A. J. (1990). Behavior analysis: Cognitive therapy andcovert conditioning. *Journal of Behavior Therapy and ExperimentalPsychology, 21,* 83-90.

Davis, T. N., Machalicek, W., Scalzo, R., Kobylecky, A., Campbell, V., Pinkelman, S., ... Sigafoos, J. (2016). A review and treatment selection model for individuals with developmental disabilities who engage in inappropriate sexual behavior. *Behavior analysis in practice, 9*(4), 389-402.

Deb, S., Thomas, M., & Bright, C. (2001). Mental disorder in adults with intellectual-disability. 1: Prevalence of functional psychiatric illness among a community based population aged between 16 and 64 years. *Journal of IntellectualDisability Research, 45,* 495-505.

Dewhurst, A. M. & Nielsen, K. M. (1999). A resiliency-based approach to working with sexual offenders: Sexual addiction and compulsivity. *The Journal of Treatment and Prevention, 6,* 271-279.

Favell, J. E., & Reid, D. H. (1988). Generalizing and maintaining improvement in problem behavior. In R. H. Horner, G. Dunlap, & R. L. Koegel (Eds.), *Generalization and maintenance: lifestyle changes in applied settings* (pp. 171-199). Baltimore, MD: Paul H. Brookes.

Felce, D. & Perry, (1995). Quality of life: its definition and measurement. *Research in Developmental Disabilities, 16,* 51-74.

Gaither, G. A., Rosenkranz, R. R., & Plaud, J. J. (1998). Sexual disorders. In Plaud, J. J., & Elfert. G. H. (Eds.), *From Behavior Theory to Behavior Therapy* (pp. 152-171). Boston, MA: Allyn & Bacon.

Grant, L. & Evans, A. (1994). Principles of behavior analysis. New York, NY: Harper Collins.

Griffiths, D. M., Owen, F., Gosse, L., Stoner, K., Tardiff, C. Y., Watson, S., ... Vyrotsko, B. (2003). Human rights and persons with intellectual disabilities: An action-research approach for community-based organizational self-evaluation. *Journal on Developmental Disabilities, 10,* 25-42.

Griffiths, D. M., Quinsey, V. L., & Hingsburger, D. (1989). *Changing inappropriate sexual behavior: A community-based approach for persons with developmental disabilities.* Baltimore, MD: Paul H. Brookes Publishing.

Hanson, R. K., & Harris, A. J. R. (2000). Where should we intervene? Dynamic predictors of sex offense recidivism. *Criminal Justice and Behavior, 27,* 6-35.

Hanson, R. K., Harris, A. J. R., Scott, T.L., & Helmus, L. (2007). *Assessing the risk of sexual offenders on community supervision* (User Report No. 2007-05). Ottawa, Ontario, Canada: Public Safety and Emergency Preparedness Canada.

Hingsburger, D. (1996). *The ten commandments of reinforcement.* Algonquin, IL: Creative Core, New Orient Media.

Ioannou, S. (2013). *Managing risk in a culture of rights: Providing support and treatment for sex offenders with intellectual disability in community-basedsettings* (Master's Thesis). Brock University, St. Catharines, Ontario, Canada.

Ioannou, S. (September 2016). Restrictions on autopilot: Protecting people with intellectual disabilities from random acts of power. *Executive Functioning: A Newsletter for Senior Leadership in Organizations Providing Human Services, pp. 1-8.*

Iwata, B. A., Dorsey, M. F., Slifer, K. J., Bauman, K. E., & Richman, G. S. (1992). Toward a functional analysis of self-injury. *Analysis and Intervention in Developmental Disabilities, 2,* 1-20.

Kazdin, A. E. (1982). Symptom, substitution, generalization and response covariation: Implications for psychotherapy outcome. *Psychological Bulletin, 91,* 17-25.

Laws, D. L. R. & Marshall, W. L. (1990). A conditioning theory of the etiology and maintenance of deviant sexual preference and behavior. In W. L. Marshall, D. R. Laws and H. E. Barbaree (Eds.), *Handbook of sexual assault: Issues, theories and treatment of the offender* (pp. 209-229). New York: Plenum Press.

Lennox, D. B., Miltenberger, R. G., Spengler, P. & Erfanian, N. (1988). Decelerative treatment practices with person who have mental retardation: A review of fiveyears of the literature. *American Journal of Mental Retardation, 92,* 492-501.

Lindsay, W. R. (2007). *The treatment of sex offenders with developmental disabilities: A practice workbook.* West Sussex, UK: Wiley-Blackwell.

Maletzky, B. M. & McGovern, K. B. (1991). *Treating the sexual offender.* Thousand Oakes, CA: Sage Publications.

Marshall, W. L., Eccles, A., & Barbaree, H. E. (1991). The treatment of exhibitionists: A focus on sexual deviance versus cognitive and relationship features. *Behavior Research and Therapy, 29,* 129-135.

Marshall W. L. & Laws, D. L. R. (2003) A brief history of behavioral and cognitive behavioral approaches to sex offenders. Part II - The modern era. *Sexual Abuse, 15,* 93-120.

McGrath, R. J., Hoke, S. E., & Vojtisek, J. E. (1998). Cognitive-behavioral treatment of sex offenders: A treatment comparison and long-term follow-up study. *Criminal Justice and Behavior, 25,* 203-225.

Miltenberger, R. (1997). *Behavior modification: principles and practices.* Pacific Grove, CA: Brooks/Cole.

Plaud, J. J., Plaud, D. M., Kolstoe, P. E., & Orvedal, L. (2000). Behavioral treatment of sexually offending behavior. *Mental Health Aspects of Developmental Disabilities, 3,* 54-61.

Poling, A. E., & Ryan, C. (1982), Differential reinforcement of other behavior schedules: Therapeutic applications. *Behavior Modification, 6,* 3-21.

Quinsey, V. L. & Marshall, W. L. (1983). Procedures for reducing inappropriate sexual arousal: An evaluation review. In J. G. Greer and I. R. Stuart (Eds.), *The sexual aggressor: Current perspective son treatment* (pp. 267-289). New York: Van Nostrand Reinhold.

Rea, J. A., Williams, D., Saunders, K. J., Dixon, M., Wright, K., & Spradlin, J. E. (2003). Covert sensitization: A generalization analysis in the laboratory and natural environment through the use of a portable-penile plethysmograph. *The Behavior Analyst Today, 4,* 192-201.

Serretti, A., & Chiesa, A. (2011). A meta-analysis of sexual dysfunction in psychiatric patients taking antipsychotics. *International Clinical Psychopharmacology, 26,* 130-140.

Sherak, D. M. (2000). Pharmacological treatment of sexually offending behavior in people with mental retardation/developmental disabilities. *Mental Health Aspects of Developmental Disabilities, 3,* 62-74.

Singh, N. N., Lloyd, J. W., & Kendall, K. A. (1990). Non-aversive and aversive interventions: Introduction. In A. Repp & N. N. Singh, N. N. (Eds.) (1990). *Perspectives on the use of nonaversive and aversive interventions for persons with developmental disabilities* (pp. 3-16). Pacific Grove, California: Brooks/Cole Publishing.

Skinner, B. F. (1953). *Science and human behavior.* New York: MacMillan.

Smith, P., Goggin, C., & Gendreau, P. (2002). *The effects of prison sentences and intermediate sanctions on recidivism: General effects and individual differences.* (User Report 2002-01). Ottawa, ON: Solicitor General Canada.

Tarnowski, K. J., Rasnake, L. K., Mulick, J. A., & Kelly, P. A. (1989). Acceptability of behavioral interventions for self-injurious behavior. *American Journal on Mental Retardation, 93,* 575-580,

Tough, S. (2001). *Validation of two standard risk assessments (RRASOR, 1997; Static-99, 1999) on a sample of adult males who are developmentally disabled with significant cognitive deficits* (Master of Arts Dissertation). University of Toronto, Ontario.

Uhl, C. N. & Garcia, E. E. (1969). Comparison of omission with extinction in response elimination in rats. *Journal of Comparative and Physiological Psychology, 69,* 554-562.

Vollmer, T. R. & Iwata, B. A. (1992). Differential reinforcement as treatment of behavior disorders: procedural and functional variations. *Research in Developmental Disabilities, 13,* 393-417.

Vollmer, T. R., Ringdahl, J. E., Roane, H. S., & Marcus, B. A. (1997). Negative side effects of noncontingent reinforcement. *Journal of Applied Behavior Analysis, 30,* 161-164.

Wallace, M. D., Iwata, B. A., Hanley, G. P., Thompson, R. H., & Roscoe, E. M. (2012). Noncontingent reinforcement: a further examination of schedule effects during treatment. *Journal of Applied Behavior Analysis, 45,* 709-719.

Ward, T. & Gannon, T. A. (2006). Rehabilitation, etiology, and self-regulation: The comprehensive good lives model of treatment for sexual offenders. *Aggression and Violent Behavior, 11,* 77–94.

Ward, T., Mann, R. E., & Gannon, T. A. (2007). The good lives model of offender rehabilitation: Clinical implications. *Aggression and Violent Behavior, 12,* 87-107.

Ward, T. & Salmon, K. (2011). The ethics of care and treatment of sex offenders. *Sexual Abuse: A Journal of Research and Treatment, 23,* 397-413.

Ward, T., & Stewart, C. A. (2003). The treatment of sex offenders: Risk management and good lives. *Professional Psychology: Research and Practice, 34*, 353-360.

Wilson, R. J. & Yates, P. M. (2009). Effective interventions and the good lives model: Maximizing treatment gains for offenders. *Aggression & Violent Behavior, 14*, 157-161.

PART IV:

GENERALIZATION AND MAINTENANCE

Chapter Eleven

Long Term Management

In discussing behavioral treatment for persons with intellectual disabilities who have sexually offended, Plaud, Plaud, Kolstoe, and Orvedal (2000) suggested that:

> *The three tiers of quality behavioral programming: daily living skills, education, and specialized sexual offender behavioral services, should be interlocked. The ultimate goal of a behavioral treatment program is to achieve behavioral competency skills in all three areas simultaneously, and fade advances in each area to the other areas. For example, an individual's teaching in a classroom setting should be integrated with attaining appropriate sexual behavior skills through specialized behavioral programming and opportunities to practice appropriate expression of sexuality in an interpersonal situation.... In other words, it is a major function of a quality program to integrate ongoing daily living behavior skills with daily educational and specialized behavioral programming skills for sexual offending (Plaud et al., 2000, p 55).*

Studies of individuals without disabilities who have sexual offense histories have demonstrated the importance of maintenance components to treatment, in which clients are afforded the opportunity to practice new skills while receiving supervision and regular feedback (Wilson, Cortoni, Picheca, Stirpe, & Nunes, 2009; Wilson, Stewart, Stirpe, Barrett, & Cripps, 2000). However, to date, the research on individuals with intellectual disabilities who have sexually offended has not produced strong evidence to support the social validity of treatment, in that transfer of learned skills to the new environment appears to be limited. Hanson and Morton-Bourgon (2005) reported that skills learned by individuals with intellectual disabilities during treatment designed for typical individuals did not transfer out of treatment settings. Similarly, Rea, Dixon, and Zettle (2013) found that individuals with intellectual disabilities showed less generalization of learned replacement skills in the community when accompanied by non-treatment staff or community adults, compared to when with treatment staff. They noted that lower levels of generalization occurred if participants were older, presented with a wider range of paraphilias, and when the treatment consequences in the program were less severe.

Long-term change in behavior requires that the maintenance of change move from external monitoring to self-monitoring and from external reinforcement to self-reinforcement and reinforcement contingencies in the natural environment. The possibility of re-offense is a common concern in the treatment of people who have sexually offended. Hanson, Harris, Helmus and Thornton (2014) recently reported that most sexual offenders who are going to re-offend will do so within five years of release to the community. They noted that as greater stability in the community is established, the propensity for re-offending decreases. Thus, upon treatment completion, priority must be given to transferring treatment effects to the natural community to establish those elements of stability as soon as possible. Transferring treatment effects, although a logical and socially valid objective, poses both pragmatic and ethical concerns.

For individuals with intellectual disabilities who have sexually offended, there has been a lack of focus on generalization and maintenance of their skills across situations and time for various reasons. First, there still is a reliance on behavior management rather than function-informed and comprehensive treatment in the field. Second, even those who are responsive to treatment, often continue with intense management strategies in the form of supervision recommendations for the rest of their lives. Of course, for some individuals who do not respond to treatment, such intensive life-long risk management in the form of heavy supervision is necessary, but our experience is that the extent to which it is currently utilized is not always based on an evaluation of the reasonable and responsible supervision to protect the individual and others, but heightened levels of management and restrictiveness to protect the interests of the agency. Decisions regarding the degree of necessary supervision should be evaluated according to dynamic risk assessments.

The concept of a dynamic risk assessment is that variables affecting behavior are changeable and as such require repeated evaluation to determine if there are improvements in dynamic factors as a result of teaching or situational circumstances. Moreover, within the treatment protocols there needs to be an emphasis on embedding generalization strategies to maximize the potential that the person can eventually learn to use the skills in different settings and with less supervision, should appropriate progress and generalization be achieved.

Researchers have asserted that programs designed to develop skills to reduce anti-social behavior are more effective if delivered in a community-based settings rather than in institutions (Hayes, 2004; McGrath, Livingston, & Falk, 2007). One of the fundamental reasons for this is because persons with intellectual disabilities are often challenged when generalizing skills to different settings and with different people (Taylor, 2002). The generalization literature for persons with intellectual disabilities has long identified the basic principles on which generalization and maintenance can be enhanced (Stokes & Baer, 1977). As a result, optimal teaching environments are supervised settings in which the goals are individualized and where individuals gradually work towards the reduction in restrictions as appropriate to their learning outcomes (Hayes, 2007).

Plaud et al. (2000) have suggested six criteria to use to evaluate transitional programming. The following quality assurance questions have been adapted from their criteria to use as a guideline for making decisions regarding treatment effectiveness and the potential of transition to a less restrictive regime. First, has successful engagement in the treatment program produced an absence of the target behaviors for a minimum of three months? Second, have phallometric evaluations and risk management assessments shown a change or reduction in target areas of concern? Third, has the individual shown a lack of covert behaviors that may be preconditions to overt offending behavior (i.e., the use of child images to masturbate) and has the person acknowledged the inappropriateness of their past behavior? Fourth, has the cycle of offense been identified so that precursor behaviors or high-risk situations are known by the individual and the therapist? Fifth, has the individual clearly demonstrated that the required skills were learned and used in situations where they would be needed to prevent re-offense, based upon the understanding of factors that contributed to the previous offense? Sixth, under controlled and monitored conditions, has the person shown effective use of the learned skills in situations in the community and with natural supports?

In order to determine efficacy of skills and motivation to utilize them, Vollmer (2014) discussed creating experimental conditions where individuals with an intellectual disability, who have received treatment, are presented with a perceived opportunity to re-offend or engage in pre-offending risky behaviors, under highly controlled and risk managed scenarios. These scenarios would provide information on the degree to which external supervision is required and whether certain staff can serve as discriminative stimuli for pro-social, non-offending behavior. In order to do this, the individual would be presented with a perceived opportunity that puts themselves in a risky situation, such as a new staff telling the individual they are going to McDonalds for lunch (McDonalds being a high-risk place that should be avoided for this particular individual). The preferred response would be, given the individual's time in treatment, for them to tell the staff they should not go to McDonalds because it is a high-risk place for them to be. The non-preferred response would be for the individual to not say anything and go along with eating at McDonalds. The outcomes of creating these sorts of conditions would provide information on the individual's motivation and ability to use their learned treatment skills without the need for external controls.

For example, an offender who has previously offended when staff are diverted or lax in following the protocol might be placed in a situation where this is seemingly occurring to see if the person would use their learned self-management strategies or take the opportunity that appears that will put the person and a potential victim at risk. At no time, however, are either at risk, as the potential for the person to be placed in a real risk condition or in the presence of a potential victim (such as a child) would never be real. These situations provide valuable information regarding the likelihood of a re-offense, as the person has demonstrated whether the strategies that have been taught will be employed in the natural situations and the degree to which (experienced) staff served as discriminative stimuli for preventing a sexual re-offense.

Testing for generalization and maintenance of self-management skills requires objective measurement. The use of covert (undercover) observation represents a promising approach to test the effectiveness of learned coping strategies under evocative situations.

Two similar approaches to assess generalization while concurrently ensuring public safety have been used for the past thirty years within community-based treatment programs for persons with intellectual disabilities who have sexually offended. Griffiths has referred to one of these approaches in her work as the *Casper Effect*, as described in Griffiths and Fedoroff (2008). This approach, however, was likely based on the

Harvey Phenomenon developed in Alaska, although provenance is not fully clear (Ward et al., 1992). More recently, these techniques have evolved into community trust programs being utilized in treatment programs in Ontario (see Chapter 9; Stevenson, Lynn, Miller, & Hingsburger, 2010).

The basic concept of the Casper Effect is rooted in the use of known generalization strategies to transfer stimulus control from the presence of staff and highly controlled settings to natural stimuli in the general community. Following treatment, when the individual has learned the appropriate skills and has consistently shown the use of the skills under controlled conditions, the individual is systematically provided with increasing degrees of independence. The objective is to move towards community access – to whatever degree the individual's coping strategies will safely allow. Over a period of time and with multiple exposures, the individual gradually gains access to a variety of community venues with treatment staff. During community outings, appropriate skills are reinforced and non-adherence behaviors result in corrective consequences. Eventually, and assuming effective use of the self-management skills in the presence of staff in a variety of settings, the individual moves to engagement in a range of community activities with non-treatment staff (i.e., a family member) still employing a similar protocol for reinforcement for appropriate behavior and consequences for non-adherence. Then, assuming adherence, the individual is allowed to go to the community with non-staff, who must continue to follow the same protocol. Assuming all other steps have resulted in evidence that the self-management skills have been learned and applied, the last phase is when the individual is allowed to go into the community on a limited and controlled basis.

Vollmer, Reyes, & Walker (2012) noted that "undercover" measurements of treatment effects for sexual offenders may provide the most accurate and valid approach. In the approach taken by Reyes, Vollmer, and Whitehouse (in preparation, as cited by Vollmer 2014), covert observation is used to assess the influence of generalization under situations in which there is an establishing operation for offending behavior. In these situations, individuals are presented, unbeknownst to them, with previously-evoking situations while under surreptitious observation. In this way the application of learned self-management skills and observation of breaches in the use of those skills under high-risk simulated situations may be evaluated within a safe environment in which there is no risk to the public (Vollmer et al., 2012).

The objective of generalization training is to gradually move towards more community access in keeping with whatever degree the individual's coping strategies will safely allow. Eventually, and assuming effective use of the self-management skills in the presence of staff in a variety of settings, the individual progresses to engagement in a range of community activities with non-treatment staff, still employing a similar protocol for reinforcement for appropriate behavior and consequences for non-adherence. The protocol may allow the individual a half hour to go to the corner store, buy a chocolate bar, and return, with an understanding that someone unknown to the person will be watching. These experiences continue in multiple settings and over expanded periods, but always with the understanding that someone is or could be watching. The aim is to transfer stimulus control of self-management strategies in the treatment environment to a variety of other people and places, including a larger audience of strangers in the community, while fading the overt discriminative stimuli (e.g., treatment staff) over time. Obviously, the individual's ability to demonstrate the transfer of self-regulation skills to the community will play a significant role in determining the degree of supervision and external management necessary.

Vollmer (2014) suggested that the decision to use covert observation, to assess the risk an individual poses, is not binary (yes or no). He recommended a contextual evaluation of the risk and benefits and that a clinician should ask: Can the use of a covert approach be justified because of the potential risk that the behavior might pose to others? Additionally, does the potential benefit of the person engaging in appropriate skills in the natural environment, thereby increasing the potential for greater community integration, outweigh the potential challenges that this type of observation might pose? Moreover, if the use of covert observation is justified, the data obtained during the assessment can further be used to determine what skills an individual requires in order to keep the behavior from occurring in the future (Vollmer et al., 2012). Thus, the use of covert observation may have significant value as an assessment tool if carried-out systematically based on assessed high-risk situations and with protections to ensure that public safety is maintained. Additionally, because covert observation may be seen as a rights violation, it requires justification in terms of scientific, legal, applied, or educational value (Vollmer, 2014). It should be noted that such an approach is conducted with consent of the individual and fully outlined in their treatment protocol. The use of the procedure must also receive prior ethical review, involve informed consent, and enable opportunities for debriefing (Vollmer, 2014).

THE ROLE OF MOTIVATING OPERATIONS

The keys to generalization and maintenance may lie in the assessment of motivating operations, which have both abolishing and establishing effects in terms of frequency of behavior and reinforcing value of consequences. The abative and evocative influences within the natural environment that relate to sexually offending behaviors should be carefully assessed and altered to enhance treatment efficacy. It is important to consider motivation in combination with other antecedents and consequences that may be contributing to any treatment related behavior change, since motivating operations have temporary influences on behavior. Further, appropriate sexual behavior may come under the control of irrelevant antecedent stimuli (e.g., certain staff members or materials), which results in faulty stimulus control and, hence, lack of generalization to environments in which those stimuli or conditions are absent.

Abative Influences.

Abolishing operations (AO) refer to a decrease in behavior due to decreased reinforcing value of the consequence that follows the behavior. The classic example is if a person has just eaten a huge meal, food searching behaviors decrease due to lessened value of food as a reinforcer (satiation). In treating challenging behavior, including sexually offending behavior, the objective is to create an AO in which there is an abative effect for inappropriate or offensive sexual behaviors, and attempt to create an establishing operation (EO) for appropriate sexual behavior. For someone who is reinforced through coercive sex, a simplistic response would be to create an abolishing effect by allowing the individual to engage in coercive sex. Since this is not a desired, ethical, or realistic practice, an alternative goal is to weaken the reinforcing value of coercive sex and, therefore, the behaviors that lead to it.

Sexual arousal is an unconditioned motivating operation and, as such, the reinforcement can never be completely removed. Although the value-altering effect is unlearned, the behavior-altering effect of an MO is learned. Thus, alternative environmental restrictions can be put in place to ensure that coercive sex cannot occur (through extinction by removing the reinforcement). This alone, however, is not sufficient, and the person must also be provided with the opportunity to obtain the reinforcement in an acceptable way (perhaps, via masturbation). Thus, if the motivating operation involves unconditioned reinforcers (food, sex, warmth), then we can never remove the reinforcing properties altogether. Instead, we can weaken the reinforcers that follow the inappropriate behavior and attempt to provide the same reinforcers in response to appropriate behavior.

If the individual has the means to attain adequate reinforcement through appropriate behavior then the motivation to offend will likely be at least temporarily reduced (AO). For many persons with intellectual disabilities, there is minimal payoff for non-offending behavior and, therefore, the reinforcing value of offending outweighs that of non-offending. The use of non-contingent reinforcement as an intervention component may not only enhance opportunities for the individual to gain much needed and valuable reinforcement in their daily lives, it may also potentially decrease the likelihood of re-offense. Ward, Mann, and Gannon (2007) suggested that building a strong prosocial life that has meaningful relationships and activities leaves the individual little time or opportunity to commit an offense. This, of course, is an old and basic behavioral management adage that "there is only 100% of behavior" and if the individual is engaged in appropriate behavior 100% of the time, then inappropriate behavior will be at zero.

By using knowledge of the conditions that previously evoked or inhibited the behavior, the natural environment can be programd to produce conditions that will set the stage for success. Abative influences may involve variables in the environment that reduce the effectiveness/value of a stimulus, object, or event as a reinforcer. As noted above, the presence of treatment staff can produce conditions under which an individual may be less likely to respond to previously evoking situations. This does not lead to long term maintenance and generalization of treatment effects as the behavior is under faulty stimulus control (presence of a certain staff vs. stimuli that would be present in the natural environment). Employing known generalization strategies such as exposing the individual to diverse stimulus conditions with multiple trainers and situations will help to prevent faulty stimulus control.

Evocative Influences

A corollary to maximizing abative influences is to ensure that the environment is as free as possible of evocative influences for offending behavior. Establishing operations (EOs) lead to a temporary increase in behavior and increase the reinforcing value of a consequence. Again, the classic example is food. If a person is starving, the reinforcing value of food increases, and so behaviors that have previously led to food access (e.g., searching the house, checking the fridge, making a meal) will also increase. When dealing with sexually offensive behavior, deprivation of sexualized behavior may create an EO (i.e., increased reinforcement value of sexual interactions and increased behaviors that have led to reinforcing effects of sexual interaction in the past). Although motivating operations are an important component of treatment, the effect is temporary; therefore, firmly established discriminations of appropriate self-management behavior are needed.

McGrath et al. (2007) noted that "[t]houghtful community placement has advantages beyond cost savings. Services delivered to individuals in their natural environment, such as home, school, and community, are typically more effective than those delivered in congregate settings, where individuals are grouped together with other antisocial and sexually abusive individuals" (p. 396). This view is consistent with the findings of Andrews and Bonta (2010) who suggested recidivism is related to associations with peers who provide negative influence, by serving as discriminative stimuli (cues for offending) vs. prosocial behaviors.

From the perspective of managing risk of re-offense in the community, establishing operations can also be used to set up the individual for success during and following treatment by ensuring the presence of conditions that evoke self-management behaviors. From the perspective of managing risk to the community and risk of re-offense, the natural environment must provide optimal opportunity for offense-free interactions and activity, while providing appropriate levels of supervision that match the degree of risk posed. The treatment and post-treatment environments must: (a) not present conditions that are likely to evoke the previous behaviors (e.g., don't place an individual with sexual attraction to children next to a school) if possible ever or until the individual has demonstrated sufficient self-management strategies; (b) trap alternative appropriate self-management and sexual behaviors in natural contingencies in the environment; and (c) balance support and supervision against the potential risks.

As noted above, the pathway for offense and the individual's response to treatment will determine if, and under what levels of supervision, expanded opportunities for community integration are appropriate. The degree of supervision for the individual is dependent on the degree of risk balanced against the degree of self-control. It would be unethical to assume that all treatments will provide equal assurance of social validity for all individuals. Kazdin (1977) suggested that the social validity of outcomes depends upon both social comparison and subjective evaluation. Social comparison refers to how the individual would respond to others who were functioning typically (e.g., a comparison of the response of non-offending individuals in situations that had evoked an offensive response from the individual in question). Subjective evaluation refers to the importance of the behavior and its significance to the individual and others. Thus, for the treatment of an individual with an intellectual disability to be socially valid, the individual must be able to respond typically and not pose a risk to self or others.

In the past, individuals often provided self-report information as to long-term treatment and maintenance effects. However, Vollmer et al. (2012) noted that individuals who have sexually offended who have been reintegrated into the community may be reluctant to report sexual arousal or behaviors that were inappropriate because of fear of consequences, such as incarceration or return to a treatment setting. Thus, it has been suggested that reliance on self-report measures may be insufficient to assume social validity of treatment is achieved or maintained.

Generalization of Skills Across Time, Settings, and Behaviors

Programming for generalization of skills should occur as soon as treatment begins and should continue into post-treatment aftercare. Often, an individual with an intellectual disability is taught content or skills and then expected to use them outside of the instructional setting, when generalization was not imbedded into the teaching process. Preparation for the time when the individual will be responsible for managing his own must begin from the point of referral and be updated throughout the clinical and case management process. Generalization and maintenance strategies should be incorporated within treatment plans for individuals who have sexually offended, the same way they would be imbedded in other behavioral programs (Wilson et al., 2000; Wilson, Cortoni, Picheca et al., 2009). In a systematic review of behavioral interventions for individuals with intellectual disabilities who have sexually offended, Marotta (2017) found a consistent gap in incorporating generalization strategies and concluded that "the design of future treatment studies must hardwire relapse prevention and maintenance therapy to ensure skills are generalized and gains are maintained over time" (p. 182).

In order to promote generalized behavior change, the following elements must be incorporated in treatment (Cooper, Heron, & Heward, 2007):

- Teach the full range of relevant stimulus conditions and responses. For example, an individual where assessment has shown that issues with anger are associated with the offenses, would be taught anger management skills. However, general anger management training is likely insufficient. The training should be directed to situations that are known to be associated with stimuli/situations that evoke offending. Additionally, the person would need to learn to generalize anger management through opportunities to practice their management skills using a variety of responses specific to the situation. Strategies may include assertiveness, walking-away, or seeking someone with whom they can vent. Generally, the more examples used during instruction, the more likely the individual will use the proper skills in untrained circumstances.
- Make the instructional setting similar to the generalization setting. This includes teaching in vivo and providing immediate feedback as problematic situations occur. If an individual is working on prosocial behavior with peers and a situation occurs in which they become verbally abusive, caregivers or staff can intervene and provide immediate teaching on how else the situation could be handled.
- Maximize the reinforcement of the target behavior in the generalization setting. The skills that the individual is learning to generalize should be ones that evoke reinforcement through natural contingencies. Early in the teaching phase reinforcement may have to be contrived, but once the skill is in their repertoire the individual can learn to use the skill to access reinforcement appropriately in more natural community settings.
- Mediate generalization. Use something that can help the individual remember to use their skills (e.g. self-talk or deep breathing) outside of treatment in the community. These can be visual reminders through the use of key chains, wallet cards, or self-management skills. Self-monitoring is a self-management

strategy that can be introduced in treatment and have substantial post-treatment effects. The person can document their progress and continue to monitor any of the red flags or danger signs they learned in treatment. This method can help the individual to maintain and practice their treatment skills in new environments, in addition to holding themselves accountable.

- Train to generalize. The individual should be reinforced if they show a variety of appropriate responses to an antecedent. For example, a person learning to stay away from vulnerable people in the community may end up in a situation where vulnerable people are present. They may leave the area, call a trusted person or, if unable to leave, use various coping techniques until the situation is over.

As with other skills taught to persons with intellectual disabilities, successful transference of treatment effects from the treatment condition to the natural environment is dependent on the application of known generalization strategies, as elaborated in the classic paper by Stokes and Baer (1977). Applications of social skills training have shown that generalization can be enhanced by employing known strategies such as selecting relevant behaviors, use of common social and physical stimuli, providing multiple exemplars, providing reinforcement for unprompted generalization, and trapping to the natural environment of reinforcement examples (Griffiths, 1995; Griffiths, Feldman, & Tough, 1997). Griffiths et al. (1997) showed that social skills can be generalized outside the treatment setting to the natural environment using the Social Life Game, described earlier. To promote generalization, the game was played using common social and physical stimuli in the participants' natural environments with staff who frequently worked with the participants. Initially, the skills were taught using instruction, modeling, roleplay, and feedback. Generalization was enhanced through using immediate reinforcement for correct responses, using a variety of different scenarios for social skills, and tailoring the game to each participant's target skills (as opposed to a standardized curriculum). Further, participants were taught problem solving skills through group discussions of the circumstances in which certain responses may be correct or incorrect. Lastly, participants' caregivers were requested to set up situations outside of the game setting, in which the participant would have to use their skills and provide social reinforcement or corrective feedback. With these generalization strategies in place, the participants showed significant improvements in social skills acquisition over a control group (Griffiths et al., 1997). These generalization principles can also be employed in treatment programs for individuals who have sexually offended, as well for teaching various risk management and other necessary skills.

GENERALIZATION AND MAINTENANCE THROUGH A NATURAL COMMUNITY OF REINFORCEMENT

For behaviors to be maintained over time and across settings, they must be reinforced. According to the relevance of behavior rule, behaviors to change must produce reinforcers in real life settings (Ayllon & Azrin, 1968). Furthermore, a rule for practitioners is to not attempt behavior changes that will not meet natural communities of reinforcement (Stokes & Baer, 1977). By teaching the individual behaviors for which there is a natural community of reinforcement, the individual learns how to recruit their own reinforcement from the natural environment, thereby making them "prominent agents of their own behavior change, rather than being hapless pawns of more or less random environmental contingences" (Stokes & Baer, 1977, p. 354). This concept is evidence in the approach to changing problem drinking through the use of community resources such as in-person support groups or via the internet, in order to maintain learned skills and access reinforcement from the natural community.

Furthermore, it is reasonable to suggest that psychological wellbeing and risk are inversely related to one another (i.e., as wellbeing increases, risk decreases, and *vice versa* – see Yates, Prescott, & Ward, 2010). For many individuals, re-offending might indicate that the reinforcing value of the offense outweighed the reinforcing value of alternative self-management or appropriate sexual behaviors. A non-contingent reinforcement procedure (NCR; as described in Chapter 10) can help to create conditions rich in reinforcement, which may create an abolishing operation for re-offense.

These are the underlying tenants of the *Good Lives Model* that was explained in Chapter 6 and elsewhere. Essentially, "the best way to reduce risk is by helping offenders live more fulfilling lives" (Ward et al., 2007, p. 94), which includes a life that provides functional skills (e.g., coping skills, social skills), the opportunities to use these skills, and a dense schedule of reinforcement. These outcomes can be achieved through the creation of community activities such as church events, sports teams, volunteer groups, employment, regular community hobbies, and support groups. Equally important are positive relationships with peers and family and the opportunity to make and work towards life goals, so that the person has a sense of purpose and identity outside of their past offending behavior. However, it is important to recognize that "simply seeking to increase the well-being of an offender without regard for his level of risk may result in a happy, but dangerous individual" (Ward et al., 2007, pp. 92-93). Thus, there must be a functional balance between a reinforcement-rich life and risk management.

One technique to ensure the person has access to plenty of reinforcement while managing risk is through successive approximations. Safe community behavior including using learned treatment skills should be reinforced through close data collection and monitoring, so that certain risk management restrictions may be lessened. The community trust program that was described in Chapter 9 provides more detail on these carefully planned, data driven techniques. Sometimes, behavioral programs that are designed for the person to earn an incentive after showing "good behavior" are not properly monitored or are too drawn-out. The person's "good behavior" may not always be recognized, the time period to earn the incentive be too long, or the required steps to get the incentive be too complex. The same can be said for people who have sexually offended and who are trying to gain more independence in the community. Progress and results must be monitored, and appropriate reinforcement given so that the person is not waiting idly, the reinforcement still has its intended effect, and generalization is achieved.

TRANSITION, RISK MANAGEMENT AND GENERALIZATION AFTER TREATMENT

Hanson and associates have shown that most sexual recidivism occurs within the first five years after release to the community, but that with each passing year of offense-free existence, the more likely it is that individuals will be successful in *continuing* to be offense-free (Hanson et al., 2014; Hanson, Harris, Letourneau, Helmus, & Thornton, 2017). This demonstrates the critical need for enhanced generalization strategies throughout treatment and for follow-up and aftercare in the community.

The concept of resilience also plays a role in decreasing risk of re-offense. Resilience speaks to the ability of an individual to encounter situations in which they have had difficulty in the past and to respond more appropriately in the present. There are often "transferable skills" involved, in that people learn to cope with problems and to "soldier on," as it were. One such skill is the ability to develop and maintain new, prosocial, and supportive relationships in spite of the many impediments to forming new relationships that many individuals with sex offense histories may encounter (e.g., public notification, residency restrictions, and other aspects of public intolerance of "sex offenders" in the community).

In harkening back to an earlier statement, there is a body of literature suggesting that access to relationships can play a role in protecting the individual against sexual offending behavior, such as being part of a peer group, family, or community that can serve as a protective influence or having access to someone supportive who can act as a confidante (Borowsky, Hogan, & Ireland, 1997; Bremer, 2006; Gilgun, 1990; Wilson, McWhinnie, Picheca, Prinzo, & Cortoni, 2007a). Being resilient in the face of problems establishing and maintaining supportive relationships is an important factor in remaining offense-free.

Critical to the maintenance of skills in the community after treatment is that individuals are not left on their own in a community without supports, follow up, or accountability. In a study of 24 males with sex offense histories who had just been released from prison, 67% found it challenging to be out of prison and alone, while another 56% experienced a lack of supports (Wilson et al., 2007a). Circles of Support and Accountability (CoSA) is a community-driven response that has become an integral component in preventing sexual offenses in Canada (Wilson, McWhinnie, & Wilson, 2008). Based on positive results showing significant decreases in post-release re-offending, the model has since been adopted in the United Kingdom, Europe, and the United States, among other jurisdictions. CoSA is a "community response to sexual violence prevention" (Wilson et al., 2008, p. 28) that brings together persons with sexual offense histories (known as "core members"), volunteers, and community professionals. Community volunteers are provided with training (albeit, not enough to be considered experts) and may consist of church members, former support staff, school personnel, sports coaches, and so forth. Professionals consist of people who can help to support the volunteers and who have expert knowledge in sexual violence prevention, such as police officers, social workers, psychologists, and other correctional/case management staff. The idea is that the volunteers play a crucial role in helping the individual to remain offense free, by building a tight circle of support around them. Ideally, the relationship between core member and volunteers should be established at least six months before the core member will be discharged as this helps to ensure that community relationships are in place prior to release (Wilson et al., 2008).

This method has been shown to reduce the amount and severity of re-offenses after being integrated into the community compared to individuals who did not have a circle of support (Wilson, Picheca, & Prinzo, 2007b). Sixty high-risk individuals who had sexually offended in the typical population received CoSA after being released from prison, and another sixty high-risk individuals did not (i.e., matched comparison subjects). Sexual re-offending was 70% lower in the group that had CoSA than in the control group, and, in those situations in which a sexual re-offense occurred, the CoSA participants engaged in re-offenses that were significantly less severe than the comparison group (e.g., an obscene phone call versus a violent rape – see Wilson, Picheca, & Prinzo, 2007c). Overall, CoSA has helped core members to feel more supported and less isolated (thereby reducing risk) prior to re-entering the community; approximately 67% of people who received CoSA stated that they would have re-offended had they not received this support (Wilson et al., 2007b). Although CoSA is not without its critics (see Clarke, Brown, & Vollm, 2017), further research in Canada (Wilson, Cortoni, & McWhinnie, 2009), in addition to findings in the US (Duwe, 2018) and UK (Bates, Williams, Wilson, & Wilson, 2013), underpins CoSA's contribution to sexual violence prevention in those communities that employ the model. It is important to note that the CoSA model alone, or others like it, does not *eliminate* re-offending; CoSA has been shown to be a potentially critical piece for some individuals with respect to sexual violence risk management and community-based maintenance after treatment.

Transferring to the Natural Environment

Plaud and colleagues (2000) have suggested that treatment of sexual offending behavior from a behavioral analytic approach must include investigation of the environmental influences that impact the person's behavior. Thus, there needs to be careful attention given to the environment to which a person could be transferred post-treatment. One way of accomplishing this is to conduct a thorough discrepancy analysis.

A discrepancy analysis examines the socioenvironmental factors that need to be present in the environment to ensure that a re-offense is unlikely to occur (e.g., trained staff, appropriate supervision levels, established routines, set expectations, and selection of an environment that does not present situations with which offending behavior has been associated). Further, from the perspective of desistence and protection against offending, it is also important to assess the conditions in which the person is likely to engage in activities, interactions and behaviors that promote a prosocial and valued life. In behavioral terms, this is similar to establishing environmental stimulus control, similar to that proposed by Touchette, MacDonald, and Langer (1985). In their stimulus control approach to managing behavior, Touchette and colleagues were able to reduce high-risk behaviors, such as self-injury, by removal of the conditions associated with self-injury and introducing only conditions where self-injury did not occur.

A careful assessment of the conditions associated with either sexual offending or a lack thereof provides the basis for creating a socio-environmental template by which decisions for placement and support should be based.

Table 11.1 ***Template for Completing a Discrepancy Analysis***

Assessment of Required Conditions for Placement and Support	**Assessment of Proposed Placement and Supports for Community Living**	**Discrepancy Between Required Conditions and Proposed Placement and Supports**
Reduce Evocative Conditions for sexual offending: Assess conditions that need to be avoided to reduce risk of re-offending (i.e., known as setting events, or antecedents that are discriminative stimuli for offending behaviors). Examples: • *Placement should not be near schools or playgrounds or involve community activities where the individual would be alone with children.* • *Expectations should be established regarding family visitation, such that visiting brother's family consists of full supervision ensuring that he is never alone with the children.* • *Skills for avoiding high-risk situations must be demonstrated by the individual and be deemed effective by support and treatment staff.*	Compare the selection criteria and protocol for establishing an environment for the individual in the community regarding assessed conditions to determine if all criteria are met to avoid situations associated with the offending behavior. If the criteria and protocol have not been met, then the community setting would be deemed inappropriate. Examples: • *Future placement is next to a playground.* • *Individual does not display self-management skills in high-risk situations or settings.*	Given that the future placement is next to a playground and the individual has not shown the skills to avoid high-risk settings, this placement would not be deemed suitable.

Maximize Abative Conditions for sexual offending: Assess conditions that are essential to instill the appropriate socio-environmental circumstances in which offending is less likely to occur (i.e., conditions serve as ess-deltas or abolishing operations for offending behaviors). Examples: • *Highly trained staff (describe type of staff and required training)* • *Supervision levels (provide detailed description of needed supervision in all appropriate settings)* • *Established routines that provide enriched activity and interactions* • *Set expectations* • *Enriched environment* • *Valued relationships*	Compare the proposed placement and supports to ensure that all conditions known to have abative influences are present in the environment prior to placement. If all possible abative influences have not been established, then the community setting would not be deemed appropriate. Examples: • *The future placement has other individuals living there who are significantly older than the individual with nothing in common to establish a relationship* • *The future placement has 4:1 (individual to staff) ratio and the individual requires 2:1*	The discrepancy in the individual's environmental support needs and the current disposition of the future placement indicate that it would not be a fit for a suitable place to live.

Supportive treatment environments for persons who have sexually offended were discussed in Chapter 8. In addition to methods described previously, another way to ensure maintenance of skills and protections in the community is to conduct ongoing risk assessments using scales like the ARMIDILO-S (described in Chapter 8). To recap, the ARMIDILO-S contains 27 dynamic factors (changeable through treatment and other interventions; also known as criminogenic needs) that have been shown to impact risk of re-offending, such as the presence/absence of deep-seated sexually inappropriate urges and fantasies, emotional coping skills, consistent supervision, and changes in victim-related behaviors. These indicators are trackable with data and can be monitored over time to determine the degree to which individuals are able to establish maintenance of skills acquired in treatment. The main purpose of risk assessments is to promote public safety; however, they also guide case management of the individual in the community (Boer, McVilly, & Lambrick, 2007). The ARMIDILO-S should be conducted every 6-12 months, or whenever a major change occurs in the person's life (e.g., a move, a loss, or other important changes in circumstances), or if the person is showing red flags in behavior that could lead to a re-offense. Through use of the dynamic risk factors in the ARMIDILO-S, we are contextualizing risk; in other words, looking at behavior within a context.

The purpose of these follow-up strategies through self-monitoring, Circles of Support and Accountability, and risk assessment is to determine signs that the person is not doing well and to intervene early, rather than responding after a crisis or re-offense has happened. It is an almost universal truth that early identification of potential problems provides more time and opportunity to intervene than simply leaving inopportune circumstances to fester while options dwindle. If there are behavioral indicators present that highlight increased risk, then supports should be tightened until the person is back on track. Additional supports may include environmental changes, supervision, and booster treatment sessions, which may include reviewing safety plans and brushing up on treatment skills.

When considering the type of environment into which the person with offending behaviors will move, the process of discrepancy analysis described previously is an important tool to help correct implementation deficiencies. However, critically important for maintenance and generalization of treatment skills and behaviors is that the supports, risk management strategies, and levels of independence be based on data showing the individual's progress and risk factors. You may remember that Ioannou, Griffiths, Owen, Condillac, & Wilson (2014) found that consideration of rights and risk were not necessarily based on the individual and their support needs but on the setting in which they lived. In other words, the type of setting where the individual with sex offending behaviors resided determined the level of weighing of rights versus risks, rather than the individual's static and dynamic risk factors.

When transitioning out of treatment, the individual's level of supervision and community independence must match their risk (in keeping with the risk principle of the RNR model we discussed earlier – see Bonta & Andrews, 2016), and the environment must also be reflective of this. For example, someone with a history of targeting vulnerable individuals should not move into the basement of a dwelling with vulnerable individuals living upstairs. In the example used earlier, someone who has a history of offending against children and is triggered by child-related items should not move next to a playground, no matter how many staff they have supervising them.

These may seem like obvious examples of inappropriate living placements post-treatment. However, decisions to transition individuals to inappropriate and high-risk environments are often made under pressures of funding, space availability, and needing to move people through the system, rather than what is clinically necessary to maintain individual and community safety. Under these circumstances, it is important to work collaboratively to problem-solve funding or other pressures without sacrificing what the individual needs to be safe and successful.

WHEN GENERALIZATION AND MAINTENANCE ARE NOT EFFECTIVE

A critical element of effective generalization and maintenance is ensuring that the natural environment supports the treatment goals. Despite best attempts to apply behavioral approaches, there can be complications in transitioning some individuals who sexually offend to less restrictive environments: "With regard to persons with developmental disabilities (DD) who also exhibit sexually offending behavior, special concerns arise due to the adaptive skill deficits that may hinder attempts at shaping new, more socially appropriate sexual behavior repertoires" (Plaud et al., 2000, p. 54).

A critical decision following treatment is to determine if the individual will be able to live without external controls in place or if the person will always require a level of restriction in their lives, due to their lack of motivation or skills, and the extent of the restriction required. Some individuals, particularly those who historically followed the "approach/explicit" pathway (see Ward & Hudson, 1998) may never receive that degree of self-control to move through the phases of the Casper Effect successfully. For a person with this level of risk, management of environment may be necessary in order for the person to maintain self-control. Conversely, others who have offended may be able to earn increasing community access if they historically followed a different pathway (i.e., approach/automatic, avoidant/active, or avoidant/passive). Ioannou and colleagues (2014) identified that community protection varies depending on the pathway of offense, the level of assessed risk, the density of criminogenic needs, and other pertinent individual characteristics. For people deemed high-risk, their motivation to offend may override other factors and be insufficient to inhibit re-offense, despite other factors supporting quality of life. As with all individuals who have offended, there remains an ethical duty to support the individual while ensuring that the community is not at risk. People should not be placed in situations that will be potentially dangerous to self or others; however the level of resources allocated to an individual must match their level of risk.

A second complication of moving to less restrictions where warranted by treatment effects can be created by the person's support network. Not only can the individual become dependent on the external controls, so can the agencies that support them. Transferring learned skills for sexual behaviors from treatment to a natural environment can come with risks to both the person and the agency. As a result, the supporting agency may demonstrate resistance and lack confidence in how to effectively create a program to fade external supports with the patience and immense detail that would be required. Thus, failure to generalize and to fade external controls that may have been in place for years may not always be about the individual's failure to respond to treatment. This failure to progress may be more about the reliance on external controls that the agency has developed over time; the end result being that treatment generalization strategies are not effectively employed because the agency is not willing to reduce controls. Indeed, our collective experience has illuminated a tendency for case managers to take a decidedly conservative approach (e.g., residency restrictions, electronic monitoring, and polygraph examinations for some individuals, among other measures) when working with persons who have engaged in sexually offensive conduct (see Levenson & D'Amora, 2007). Further, this tendency is often exacerbated when the individuals in question present with special needs profiles (e.g., intellectual disability, autism spectrum, fetal alcohol syndrome). It seems that despite years of research showing exactly how best to provide treatment and supervision in a variety of settings (see review in Wilson & Sandler, in press), the default is to either consider all persons with sex offense histories to be at high risk *or* to ignore those individuals who are indeed high risk and act complacent through inadequate supports and supervision.

SUMMARY

A solid generalization plan is based on integration of the assessment of antecedents, maintaining consequences, motivating operations, function, and the approaches to treatment, including teaching of alternative and coping skills and provision of remedial consequences. In generalization, all elements of the assessment and intervention plan combine to develop a plan that will provide antecedents for prosocial behavior and capitalize on motivating operations to create an abative effect for sexual offending and an establishing effect for self-management strategies and appropriate sexual behavior. To maintain positive treatment outcomes, the generalization plan will also provide opportunity for and reinforcement of the use of alternative and coping skills and ensure that the maintaining consequences for the inappropriate behavior do not pay off, while instituting remedial consequences to ensure that there is an ongoing deterrent for the inappropriate behavior. Such a plan also requires a carefully selected and prepared transitional setting with staff who are appropriately trained and monitored. It is important that the evaluation of whether skills have maintained and are transferrable to a less restrictive setting be based on a thorough evaluation of the potential risk to the community and the individual. If the combined factors do not produce a high degree of confidence that risk has been minimized (if not eliminated), then there must be reevaluation of the need for supervision and risk management strategies so as to appropriately match intervention intensity to the potential risk.

REFERENCES

Andrews, D. A. & Bonta, J. (2010). *The psychology of criminal conduct* (5th ed.). Cincinnati, OH: Anderson.

Ayllon, T., & Azrin, N. (1968). *The token economy: A motivational system for therapy and rehabilitation.* Englewood Cliffs, NJ: Prentice-Hall.Bates, A.,

Bates, A., Williams, D., Wilson, C., & Wilson, R. J. (2013). Circles South East: The first 10 years 2002-2012. *International Journal of Offender Therapy and Comparative Criminology, 58,* 861–885.

Boer, D. P., McVilly, K. R., & Lambrick, F. (2007). Contextualizing risk in the assessment of intellectually disabled individuals. *Sexual Offender Treatment, 2,* 1-5.

Bonta, J. & Andrews, D.A. (2016). *The psychology of criminal conduct* (6th ed.). Cincinnati, OH: Anderson.

Borowsky, I. W., Hogan, M., & Ireland M. (1997). Adolescent sexual aggression: risk and protective factors. *Pediatrics, 100,* 7-14.

Bremer, J. (2006). Building resilience: An ally in assessment and treatment. In D.S. Prescott (Ed.), *Risk assessment of youth who have sexually abused: Theory, controversy, and emerging issues* (pp. 222–238). Oklahoma City, OK: Wood'N' Barnes.

Clarke, M., Brown, S., & Vollm, B. (2017). Circles of support and accountability for sex offenders: A systematic review of outcomes. *Sexual Abuse, 29,* 446-478.

Cooper, J. O., Heron, T. E., & Heward, W. L. (2007). *Applied behavior analysis* (2nd ed.). Upper Saddle River, NJ: Pearson Education Inc.

Duwe, G. (2018). *Minnesota circles of support and accountability (MnCoSA) at 50: Updated results from a randomized controlled trial.* St. Paul, MN: Minnesota Department of Corrections.

Gilgun, J. (1990). Factors mediating the effects of childhood maltreatment. In M. Hunter (Ed.), *The sexually abused male: Prevalence, impact and treatment* (pp.177-190), Lexington. MA: Lexington Books.

Griffiths, D. (1995). Teaching for generalization of social skills for persons who have a developmental disability. *Developmental Disabilities Bulletin, 23,* 43-58.

Griffiths, D., & Fedoroff, P. (2008) Persons with intellectual disabilities who sexually offend. In F.M. Saleh, A.J. Grudzinskas, J.M., Bradford, & D.J. Brodsky (Eds.), *Sex offenders: Identification, risk, assessment, treatment, and legal issues (pp. 352-374).* New York: Oxford University Press.

Griffiths, D., Feldman, M., & Tough, S. (1997). Programming generalization when teaching social skills to adults with mental retardation: Effects on generalization, social validity and self-report. *Behavior Therapy, 28,* 253-269.

Hanson, R. K., Harris, A. J. R., Helmus, L., & Thornton, D. (2014). High risk sex offenders may not be high risk forever. *Journal of Interpersonal Violence, 29,* 2792-2813.

Hanson, R. K., Harris, A. J. R., Letourneau, E., Helmus, L. M., & Thornton, D. (2017). Reductions in risk based on time offense free in the community: Once a sexual offender, not always a sexual offender. *Psychology, Public Policy and Law.*

Hanson, R. K., & Morton-Bourgon, K. E. (2005). The characteristics of persistent sexual offenders: A meta-analysis of recidivism studies. *Journal of Consulting and Clinical Psychology, 7,* 1154–1163.

Hayes S. (2004) Pathways for offenders with intellectual disabilities. In W.R. Lindsay, J. Taylor, & P. Sturmey (eds.), *Offenders with developmental disabilities* (pp.67-90). Chichester, UK: John Wiley and Sons Ltd.

Hayes, S. (2007). Missing out: Offenders with learning disabilities and the criminal justice system. *British Journal of Learning Disabilities, 35,*146-153.

Ioannou, S., Griffiths, D., Owen, F., Condillac, R., & Wilson, R. J. (2014). Managing risk in a culture of rights: Providing support and treatment in community-based settings for persons with intellectual disabilities who sexually offend. *ATSA Forum, 26,* online

Kazdin, A. E. (1977). *The token economy.* New York: Plenum Press.

Levenson, J.S., & D'Amora, D.A. (2007). Social policies designed to prevent sexual violence: The emperor's new clothes? *Criminal Justice Policy Review, 18,* 168-199.

Marotta, P. L. (2017). A systematic review of behavioral health interventions for sex offenders with intellectual disabilities. *Sex Abuse, 29*(2), 148-185.

McGrath, R. J., Livingston, J. A., & Falk, G. (2007). Community management of sex offenders with intellectual disabilities: Characteristics, services, and outcome of a state-wide program. *Intellectual and Developmental Disabilities, 45,* 391-398.

Plaud, J. J., Plaud, D. M., Kolstoe, P. D., & Orvedal, L. (2000). Behavioral treatment of sexually offending behavior. *Mental Health Aspects of Developmental Disabilities, 3,* 54-61.

Rea, J. A., Dixon, M. R., & Zettle, R. D. (2013). Assessing the generalization of relapse-prevention behaviors of sexual offenders diagnosed with an intellectual disability, *Behavior Modification, 38, 25-44.*

Stevenson, B., Lynn, L., Miller, K., & Hingsburger, D. (2010). The way back: A reasoned and data-based approach to increasing community access for sex offenders during and post treatment. *Journal of Learning Disabilities and Offending Behavior, 2,* 63-71.

Stokes, T. F., & Baer, D.M. (1977). An explicit technology of generalization. *Journal of Applied Behavior Analysis, 10,* 349-367.

Taylor, J. L. (2002). A review of the assessment and treatment of anger and aggression in offenders with intellectual disability. *Journal of Intellectual Disability Research, 46,* 57–73.

Touchette, P. E., MacDonald, R. F., & Langer, S. N. (1985). A scatterplot for identifying stimulus control of problem behavior. *Journal of Applied Behavior Analysis, 18,* 343-351.

Vollmer, T. R. (2014, June). Ethical issues for applied behavior analysts: Covert observation. *Severe and Challenging Behavior of Persons with Intellectual Disabilities or Autism: Supporting Individuals in the Community.* Dual Diagnosis Certificate Program, Brock University, St. Catharines, ON.

Vollmer, T. R., Reyes, J. R., & Walker, S. F. (2012). Behavioral assessment and intervention for sex offenders with intellectual and developmental disabilities. In. J.K. Luiselli (Ed.), *A handbook of high-risk challenging behaviors in people with intellectual and developmental disabilities (pp. 121-144).* Baltimore, MD: Paul H. Brookes.

Ward, K. M., Heffern, S. J., Wilcox, D. A., McElwee, D., Dowrick, P., Brown, T. D, ... Johnson, C. L. (1992). *Managing inappropriate sexual behavior: Supporting individuals with developmental disabilities in the community.* Anchorage: Alaska Specialized Education and Training Services, Inc. (ASSETS Inc.).

Ward, T., & Hudson, S. M. (1998). The construction and development of theory in the sexual offending area: A meta-theoretical framework. *Sexual Abuse, 10,* 47 - 63.

Ward, T., Mann, R.E., & Gannon, T.A. (2007). The good lives model of offender rehabilitation: Clinical implications. *Aggression and Violent Behavior, 12,* 87-107.

Wilson, R.J., Cortoni, F., & McWhinnie, A.J. (2009). Circles of support & accountability: A Canadian national replication of outcome findings. *Sexual Abuse: A Journal of Research & Treatment, 21,* 412-430.

Wilson, R. J., Cortoni, F., Picheca, J. E., Stirpe, T. S., & Nunes, K. (2009). *Community-based sexual offender maintenance treatment programming: An evaluation.* [Research Report R-188] Ottawa, ON: Correctional Service of Canada.

Wilson, R. J., McWhinnie, A. J., & Wilson, C. (2008). Circles of support and accountability: An international partnership in reducing sexual offender recidivism. *Prison Service Journal, 178,* 26-36.

Wilson, R. J., McWhinnie, A. J., Picheca, J. E., Prinzo, M., & Cortoni, F. (2007a). Circles of support & accountability: Engaging community volunteers in the management of high-risk sexual offenders. *Howard Journal of Criminal Justice, 46,* 1-15.

Wilson, R. J., Picheca, J. E., & Prinzo, M. (2007b). Evaluating the effectiveness of professionally-facilitated volunteerism in the community-based management of high-risk sexual offenders: Part one – Effects on participants and stakeholders. *Howard Journal of Criminal Justice, 46,* 289-302.

Wilson, R. J., Picheca, J. E., & Prinzo, M. (2007c). Evaluating the effectiveness of professionally-facilitated volunteerism in the community-based management of high-risk sexual offenders: Part two – A comparison of recidivism rates. *Howard Journal of Criminal Justice, 46,* 327-337.

Wilson, R. J. & Sandler, J. C. (in press). What works (or does not) in community risk management for persons convicted of sexual offenses? A contemporary perspective. *International Journal of Offender Therapy and Comparative Criminology.*

Wilson, R. J., Stewart, L., Stirpe, T., Barrett, M., & Cripps, J. E. (2000). Community-based sex offender management: Combining parole supervision and treatment to reduce recidivism. *Canadian Journal of Criminology, 42*, 177-188.

Yates, P. M., Prescott, D. S., & Ward, T. (2010). *Applying the good lives and self-regulation models to sex offender treatment: A practical guide for clinicians.* Brandon, VT: Safer Society Press.

Chapter Twelve

Pulling It All Together

There are eight basic questions that behavior analysts should ask themselves when applying a logical functional model to the treatment of persons with intellectual disabilities and histories of engaging in sexual offending.

1. Have the setting events and motivating operations that set occasion for the offense been identified? Have these setting events/motivating operations been altered or prevented where possible?
2. Have other antecedent events that preceded the offense been identified? Were these antecedent events altered?
3. Has it been identified what function the offense serves for this person?
4. Has the person been set up for success?
5. Have the replacement or coping skills to achieve personal goals in appropriate ways been identified and incorporated into the treatment?
6. Have elements been added to the person's life that will provide reinforcing and positive qualities and enhance quality of life?
7. Have consequences been put in place to ensure positive behaviors occur more frequently and inappropriate expressions are discouraged?
8. Have strategies been put in place to ensure generalization across settings and people to "trap" the behaviors in the natural environments, while minimizing risks?

Let's do a brief review:

1. Setting Events and Motivating Operations: Have the setting events and motivating operations that set occasion for the offense been identified? Have these setting events/motivating operations been altered or prevented where possible?

Setting events are stimulus conditions or events that occur before antecedent events that increase the likelihood of behavior. Setting events can be conceptualized as slower acting "triggers" for behavior and can be both public (observable) or private (unobservable) events, including emotional or physical distress, lack of sleep, illness, medications, etc. Something as innocuous as a change in routine can serve as a setting event for behavior, so it is imperative that risk be assessed and managed. Conditions that can serve as setting events can also be more serious such as loss of a job or end of a relationship. These events interact with respondent components of emotion and together increase or decrease the likelihood of various behaviors.

As described in Chapter 5, motivating operations (MOs), commonly referred to as the "fourth term" of the behavioral contingency, are closely related to setting events. MOs momentarily alter the reinforcing value of a stimulus or event and increase or decrease the frequency of behaviors relevant to that stimulus or event and, thus, can have both an establishing and abolishing effect on behavior. For example, if a person is deprived of water, the reinforcing value of water increases, as do the behaviors that have been associated with obtaining water in the past, such as going to the fridge for a drink (establishing operation; EO). Whereas, if the person just consumed a lot of water (i.e., is satiated), the reinforcing value of water decreases and behaviors associated with finding and drinking water also decrease (abolishing operation; AO).

It is critical to have a fulsome understanding of both setting events and motivating operations to appropriately assess and treat sexual offending behavior given the important impact both have on the likelihood of behavior occurring. For example, if negative moods such as anger or depression are setting events for sexual offenses, treatment may include emotion management strategies. If an individual is in a deprivation state and is hyper-aroused by way of deprivation, drugs/alcohol, or mania, sexual behavior is more reinforcing and thus offenses may be more likely to occur as there is an EO present. Whereas, if the individual is under-aroused through sexual satiation or anti-androgen medication, sexual behaviors are less-reinforcing and offenses may be less likely to occur (there is an AO present). When used ethically, medication can be used to decrease the likelihood of offending behavior so that an individual can practice self-management strategies and/or more appropriate adaptive sexual behaviors.

2. ***Antecedents: Have other antecedent events that preceded the offense been identified? Were these antecedent events altered?***

The contingencies of sexual behavior can be broken down the same as any other operant behavior: the events or stimuli that preceded the behavior (antecedents/setting events/MOs), the behavior, and the events that follow the behavior (consequences). Understanding the antecedents to sexual offending is particularly important since manipulating antecedents can reduce risk before the opportunity to offend arises. The antecedents that evoke sexual offending behavior, *discriminative stimuli*, are established due to history of being followed by a reinforcing consequence and vary across individuals, and when antecedents reliably evoke behaviors, *stimulus control* is established. For example, if the absence of staff supervision has led to an individual offending against a person in their group home in the past, staff presence should be appropriately managed until the individual has developed appropriate coping or self-management skills.

Some sexual offending behaviors may occur when individuals engage in the behavior in inappropriate places, at inappropriate times, or with inappropriate people (*faulty stimulus control*). That is, a behavior that is appropriate in one setting may be inappropriate in another (e.g., masturbating in the bedroom vs. playground). In treatment, it is important for the individual's appropriate behavior to be under the control of variables or stimuli that will always be present (e.g., self-control strategies) versus variables that may be inconsistent or not always present in the individual's environment (e.g., staff supervision).

As indicated in Chapter 4, respondent conditioning may combine with operant conditioning to influence offending behavior. For example, previously neutral stimuli (e.g., children) paired with unconditioned stimulus-response relationships (i.e., arousal and physiological sexual gratification) can become conditioned stimuli for sexual responding. Understanding these processes will assist in developing appropriate assessment and treatment strategies.

3. ***Function: Has the function that the offense serves for the person been determined?***

As described in Chapter 6, functional behavior assessment (FBA) is composed of experimental functional analyses, direct observation or descriptive assessment, and indirect assessment. The FBA process is imperative to understanding the function of behavior (i.e., why it is occurring) to help inform effective treatment and risk prevention strategies. Function-based treatment is considered best practice and more ethical than hypothesizing function, which may potentially waste valuable treatment resources. Despite many years of empirical support, experimental functional analyses are lacking in the realm of sexually offending behavior for ethical and practical reasons. That is, it is difficult and inherently risky to construct a situation in which there is an opportunity to offend. Further research is needed to determine the utility of modified functional analyses such as those conducted on precursor behaviors, arousal to various stimuli, latency to response, etc. One such alternative may be structural analyses, which focus on the antecedent-response relationship versus the response-reinforcer relationship (Carr & Durand, 1985; Dozier, Iwata & Wordsdell, 2011). Until then, other sources of information must often be used to try to determine function. For example, although sexual offending behaviors are typically private, can occur infrequently, and without any observation, there are occasions when the behavior will be either attempted or observed. In these situations, staff and authorities will likely provide immediate intervention and management of immediate risk. It is also critical to fully document what was observed and provide objective information on the circumstances. Police reports can also be valuable sources of potential indirect measures of behavior and help to identify the antecedents and consequences of the offending behavior. Certain non-contact behaviors, such as exhibitionism or public masturbation, may be more readily directly observed and information may be available on these offenses given their lower risk. As described in Chapter 4, risk assessments (that include both static and dynamic variables) are also useful for providing a framework to gather information, assess and monitor risk over time, and begin a treatment and risk management plan that matches risk and need. Ultimately, the goal of assessment and treatment is for the individual to access whatever reinforcement is maintaining the offending behavior in a more appropriate way.

4. ***Has the person been set up for success?***

There are many variables that may contribute to increase the risk of a re-offense. These vulnerabilities may be biological, psychological, or social. As described in Chapter 8, setting the stage for success involves four areas: (1) establishing an environment that creates conditions under which the offending behavior is less likely to occur and appropriate, alternative, prosocial behaviors are taught and reinforced; (2) selecting and training staff members to ensure that appropriate supervision, therapeutic interactions, and support are provided; (3) developing an individualized plan of activities and programming to provide skill building opportunities and access to reinforcement; and (4) providing opportunities for social relationships and interactions that promote motivation for appropriate engagement and non-offending behavior.

Preventative steps can be taken to maintain behavior change in the natural environment through the manipulation of abative and evocative influences. Functional analysis of offenses can reveal what stimuli evoke and maintain sexual offending behavior. Deprivation of appropriate sexual behavior, through lack of privacy or prohibition from staff, increases the value of the reinforcing properties of offending. Allowing for appropriate sexual expression can reduce this effect and, correspondingly, the reinforcing value of offending, so as to potentially lower the risk of future offending. Stimuli in the environment can evoke behaviors through history of reinforcement. Conditions under which offending had previously been successful or reinforcing will evoke future occasions, such as the absence of supervision around potential targets. Victims themselves can serve as an evocative influence, especially if specific features (or idiosyncratic variables) contribute to offending (e.g., lower functioning or non-verbal individuals). These influences should be considered and minimized through appropriate planning and problem solving. Likewise, abative influences, those factors that decrease likelihood of offending, can be implemented to lower risk.

A fundamental issue to examine with persons with intellectual disabilities who have committed a sexual offense relates to the opportunity afforded them for appropriate sexuality. As discussed previously, the lack of opportunity for appropriate sexual expression can increase the reinforcing value of any sexual behavior and make it more likely to occur, as you will see in the case of Porter described later in this chapter. Once risk has been managed and skills have been taught to engage in appropriate sexual behavior, the opportunity to do so must be provided. For sexual behavior such as masturbation, the environment must provide privacy and teach the individual where and when this is appropriate (stimulus control). For engaging in sexual behavior with a partner, once relevant relationship skills have been taught and there is confidence that consenting relationships are possible, then the opportunity to engage in such relationships should be provided if possible. These opportunities could be natural (e.g., meeting someone at day program) or more contrived (e.g., planned social events, dances). It is important to emphasize that staff attitudes are critical in that clients watch staff very closely, attend to what they say (both positive and negative), and, ultimately, at times, tend to model themselves after certain staff members. As such, staff need to be very careful what they say and do and under what circumstances. In all situations, support must be provided to ensure that quality of life improves while risk is managed.

Lastly, without a reason to remain offense-free in the community, sexual offending behavior may be reinforcing enough that it is worth the potential risk. If the environment in which the person resides provides a low quality of life with little reinforcement, it can create a significant risk factor that should be addressed, which can be done in a structured, clinical manner.

5. ***Replacement/Coping Skills: Have the replacement or coping skills to achieve personal goals in appropriate ways been identified and incorporated into the treatment?***

To recap from Chapter 9, the replacement behaviors being taught must be functionally equivalent to the problematic behavior. Further, when teaching replacement behaviors, they must follow these recommendations in order to be effective:

i. ***Serve the same function as the problem behavior***

ii. ***Access a reinforcer that is just as valuable or of higher value than the reinforcement received from problematic behavior***

iii. ***Access the reinforcer more efficiently than the problem behavior***

iv. ***Access the reinforcer with less effort than the problem behavior***

v. ***Access the reinforcer reliably and consistently***

Finding appropriate and powerful replacement behavior for sexual behavior can be challenging, especially if the behavior is rooted in inappropriate sexual fantasies and urges. Therefore, a critical component of assessment is determining if the inappropriate sexual behavior stems from deep-seated or non-sexual social contingencies. Some persons who engage in sexually inappropriate conduct do so for reasons linked to their sexual interest or preference profile, which refers to any sexual behavior that is based in an inappropriate sexual pathology, such as attraction to children or forced sexual intimacy (i.e., coercion). Differentiating between the two provides important information for which replacement behavior will be effective and how it will be taught.

Once upon a time, the field referred to interventions as being "sex offender specific." However, with time and through trial and error, we have come to understand that the difficulties encountered by individuals are rarely that focused – it is much more likely to be a confluence of different contributing factors, only some of which may be specifically sexual in nature. So, when inappropriate sexual behaviors are present, assessment will show that the individual has a host of skill deficits that are contributing to the behavior. In order to have effective long-lasting change, the individual must be taught pivotal behaviors that will not only replace the problem behavior(s) but will also open doors to achievement of personal goals with access to more natural and appropriate reinforcement in the future. Not all individuals will require the same level of skills training, so an individualized treatment program must be tailored to their specific needs (recall our discussion of the ARMIDILO-S). A list of some areas that may need to be targeted in a comprehensive treatment program was discussed in Chapter 9. These included both socio-sexual skills and coping skills that may be needed to replace the inappropriate behavior.

Also discussed in Chapter 9, throughout the teaching component of treatment, the clinical needs of the individual must be taken into consideration from the perspective of providing trauma-informed care. Traumatic experiences in one's life have been shown to have an impact on behavior across the lifespan (Levenson, Willis, & Prescott, 2014), even more so for individuals with intellectual disabilities who are likely to have experienced complex trauma (e.g., sexual abuse themselves – see Sobsey & Doe, 1991). This must be an active component throughout the teaching process; early experiences and histories of reinforcement are necessary pieces of information that must guide the treatment approach.

In line with the basic principles of applied behavior analysis (ABA), every component of treatment must be objectively defined and measured to determine if the intervention is having an effect. No treatment approach should occur without consistent and accurate data collection to monitor effectiveness. Prior to starting treatment, a target goal or mastery criteria must be outlined as well as the behavioral indicators showing when the target goal has been achieved. This can be done through pre-post and descriptive assessment (ABC recording), self-evaluations, informant reports, and community trust programs. This is not an exhaustive list of behavioral data collection methods, as the measurement system used will be tailored to the individual, the specific target behavior(s), and who is collecting the data. However, through ongoing data collection, analysis, and monitoring the effects of treatment can be determined, and any necessary changes to the treatment protocol can be made.

6. ***Enriched quality of life: Have elements been added to the person's life that will provide reinforcing and positive qualities and enhance quality of life?***

A key element to build motivation and establish a foundation for sustained change is ensuring that the individual has a positive and reinforcing lifestyle. As described throughout this book, the *Good Lives Model* (GLM; Ward, 2002 a,b; Yates, Prescott & Ward, 2010) has been proposed as a means to ensure that personal goals are appropriately met and that the individual realizes an enhanced quality of life. This model posits that offenses are often influenced by unmet needs that are then met by inappropriate means. Building long-term quality of life includes addressing these unmet needs to improve overall wellbeing while at the same time addressing those specific needs met by offending. By addressing those goals which have been implicated in offending, clinicians can attempt to determine the function and find suitable replacement behaviors. Among the goals that may contribute to offending are a need for intimacy.

Given the stigma attached to sexual offending behavior, persons who have offended are often the recipients of significant negative social consequences. It is worth noting that these consequences are often more severe than for other types of crimes and, as such, provide ample reason to avoid re-offense. Thus, part of treatment involves establishing motivation to remain offense free, both in regard to the positive reinforcement gained from having access to desired goals and the potential loss of reinforcement if re-offense occurs. It is akin to setting up a cost/benefit ratio that leans strongly in favor of non-offending.

If an individual has no reinforcement in his day-to-day life and if appropriate behavior and community integration offer no goals worth protecting, then the individual may find that offending is worth the risk. As such, part of long-term maintenance includes increasing quality of life. A full *Good Lives Model* assessment will determine what goals are of value to the individual and what goals are absent from his/her life. Providing access and opportunity to achieve these goals can increase motivation to remain offense free and clinically targeting these goals can reduce risk of re-offense.

The *Good Lives Model* can also be used to target those specific gaps and unmet needs which set the stage for offending. In many cases a desire for intimacy may be the goal that is directly tied into the offenses; setting the stage for successful replacement means providing not only the skills but also the opportunity to engage in appropriate sexual behavior, which may mean self-gratification and, if treatment is successful, a reciprocal sexual relationship.

7. ***Consequences: Have consequences been put in place to ensure positive behaviors occur more frequently and inappropriate expressions are discouraged?***

Sexual offending behavior comes with natural and logical consequences that are enshrined in the law and social mores. It is important that these consequences be clearly understood by the person who has offended and the implications that these consequences will have to their freedom, their social interactions, and their access to desired reinforcement. These outcomes can be extremely aversive and have served as the justification for treatment approaches such as covert sensitization (Quinsey & Marshall, 1983). Contrived aversive behavioral therapies, such as faradic stimulation, were traditionally used to decrease sexually inappropriate behaviors suggestive of paraphilic interests, with limited long-term success. As a result, consequences that are non-aversive, such as differential reinforcement strategies, have been employed increasingly in more recent treatment approaches.

Miltenberger (1997) noted that differential reinforcement involves either reinforcing zero or low rates of the inappropriate behavior (differential reinforcement of zero or low rates, DRO) or reinforcing any alternative behavior (differential reinforcement of alternative behavior, DRA) or incompatible appropriate behavior (differential reinforcement of incompatible behavior, DRI) in attempt to reduce/replace inappropriate behavior. Antecedent manipulations to the environment reduce the likelihood of the inappropriate behavior, while at the same time increasing the likelihood of desirable behavior.

Initially, alternate and appropriate sexual expression may be less reinforcing or even more difficult to obtain than sexual offending behavior. Clinicians should plan for the use of differential reinforcement in an effort to create a stronger association with appropriate behaviors and reduce the reinforcing properties of inappropriate behavior. Masturbation using age-appropriate, nonpornographic erotica is an appropriate alternative; reinforcing such behavior can occur by providing easier access to pornography and erotica, as well as increased privacy and opportunity to engage in such behavior.

Additionally, the *Good Lives Model* can function as a differential reinforcement of alternate or incompatible behavior (DRA/DRI) and can be incorporated into a contingency management program. The goals established in the model are designed to be more appropriate alternatives to offending and may be potentially similarly motivated as the offending behavior. Goals such as engagement, participation, and having relationships can give the individual access to valued reinforcement and avenues for natural reinforcement. The overall good lives plan represents a "life worth living" and attaining those goals is likely incompatible with sexual offending behavior, given the consequences and sanctions that can result from conviction.

As with any treatment, effects may take time to emerge. Access to appropriate opportunities to gain reinforcement may require a degree of safety that is not readily available, or for some may never be achieved. In such cases psychopharmacological management may be required to allow the person to move forward in other areas of life, while treatment is in place, or in some cases, on a long-term basis. As described at length in Chapter 10, the goal, however, must be one of treatment (i.e., prevention), and not only one of ongoing management.

8. ***Generalization: Have strategies been put in place to ensure generalization across settings and people to "trap" the behaviors into the natural environments, while minimizing risks?***

Maintenance and generalization strategies must be imbedded in every treatment plan from the beginning. The successful generalization and maintenance of skills outside of the treatment setting has not been reported in the literature on treatment for persons with intellectual disabilities and sexual offense histories. In fact, Lindsay and colleagues (2002) found that re-offense rates can increase over time, suggesting the need for generalization and maintenance strategies post-treatment.

The generalization principles outlined by Cooper, Heron, and Heward (2007) for generalized behavior change can also be applied to sexual behavior. These were outlined in more detail in Chapter 11 but include components of teaching a variety of potential conditions and appropriate responses, making the instructional setting similar to the generalization setting, and ensuring that reinforcement of the appropriate behavior is readily available in the natural environment.

A noteworthy generalization principle for people with intellectual disabilities is promoting a natural community of reinforcement, as this can so often be dismissed or minimized due to safety restrictions, systemic issues, or false assumptions of cognitive functioning. Reinforcement increases the future occurrence of behavior, and if an individual with a sex offending history has a bereft reinforcement schedule in their lives appropriate behaviors will decrease and inappropriate behaviors will increase. Therefore, by teaching skills and behaviors to the levels that are required by natural contingencies, the person can access their own reinforcement, thereby establishing a strong base for natural reinforcement and building a better life where a sexual offense is less rewarding and less likely to occur.

As noted earlier, part of long-term maintenance should include increasing quality of life. A full *Good Lives Model* assessment (Chapter 6) will determine what goals are of value to the individual and what goals are missing from his life. Providing access to and opportunity for achieving these goals can increase motivation to remain offense free and increase the reinforcement and natural supports in his life, thereby extinguishing the value and opportunity of offending.

Furthermore, determining where an individual will live after treatment must be carefully considered and planned for from the start of treatment. Careful planning with the individual's needs in mind will help to avoid the 'revolving door' in which the person keeps moving in and out of different systems and environments because they do not meet his support needs, which consequently increases risk of re-offending. Conducting a discrepancy analysis is a useful tool when assessing potential environments. This analysis highlights what the person needs in order to make an offense less likely to occur, including both risk management techniques and conditions that promote a valuable life for the person. These conditions and criteria should be compared to the potential environment that is being considered for the individual, and, if any of the criteria are missing, then there would be a discrepancy and the setting in its current state would not be considered appropriate.

LET'S DO A QUALITY CHECK ON OUR THREE CASES!

In the Preface, we introduced you to three cases: Scott, Jerry, and Porter. Later in Chapter 7, on integrating assessment components into an integrated treatment plan, we discussed the nature of the assessments that were conducted on each individual to identify the setting events and motivating operations that could set occasion for this person to offend, identify the antecedents that preceded the offense, the consequences that followed, and, if possible, to determine the function as well as any vulnerabilities that might leave the person at risk to re-offend. In this chapter, it is now important to use that information to determine a treatment plan for each of the three individuals. This will involve using the information gathered from the functional behavior assessment to create an individualized plan that includes altering or preventing factors that served as setting events or motivating operations, altering the antecedents that preceded the offense, addressing consequences, and developing a plan to overcome the vulnerabilities that may have originally contributed to the behavior. This can include providing the individual with new skills to achieve their goals in an appropriate way based on the function of their behavior or to cope with situations that previously resulted in an offense and establishing consequences that will ensure that positive behaviors are enhanced and inappropriate expressions are discouraged. Additionally, for each person, individualized elements will be added to their life to allow an enriched and reinforcing lifestyle, which will provide a foundation for a future without offense. Lastly, the program would be incomplete unless there was a carefully established plan put in place to generalize the new skills to the least restrictive environment possible, while maintaining a level of scaffolded support or supervision for the individual to whatever degree is needed to ensure the safety of all.

Now we will talk about some of the treatment issues that were addressed for each individual in terms of background, assessment, antecedent modifications, other treatment components and generalization and maintenance of treatment gains.

Case I: The Case of Jerry

Background

Jerry was the 21-year-old male, diagnosed with mild intellectual disability, oppositional defiant disorder, and attention deficit hyperactivity disorder. Jerry had a long history of sexual assaults. The first was when he was 16 and fondled a five-year-old girl in his neighborhood, and there were no charges laid. The next offense was when Jerry invited a 7-year old neighborhood boy into his home and rubbed on top of him in the basement. There were no charges laid in this offense either. The latest offense that prompted involvement with a behavior analyst was when Jerry was 19 and living in a group home with 24/7 staffing and four other similarly aged males. Jerry entered all the bedrooms of the male peers at night, while staff were sleeping, and fondled the men without their consent. As before, no charges were laid.

Assessment

The following is a recap of the assessment results from this case in Chapter 7:

- During phallometric assessment, Jerry showed inappropriate levels of arousal to forced sex, male and female prepubescents, and female adults

- All four bedrooms were on the upper floor with no preventative safety systems (i.e., no locks or alarms on the bedroom doors)
- The overall set up of the home was vacant and bare due to an individual's previous property damage, and therefore there was a lack of opportunity for appropriate activity
- There was little to no social engagement in the home
- The offenses occurred during states of boredom and arousal
- The two staff members were asleep on the main floor during the offenses
- Jerry has never received any socio-sexual education
- There were no aversive consequences for his actions (i.e., no charges were laid in any of his offenses)

Environmental (Antecedent) Modifications

Jerry was removed from the group home where his offenses occurred, as it was deemed unsafe and inappropriate for Jerry to continue living with his victims. His behavior analyst made several recommendations on what his future home must consist of.

To start, it was imperative that Jerry's future staff team be trained on his previous offenses, including his risk factors and conditions that make offenses more likely to occur. Well-trained staff, who are able to alter antecedents and intervene early if risk factors are present (e.g., boredom), will attempt to use strategies to decrease the risk of offending.

In his most recent offense, Jerry's behavior was influenced by both socially mediated and automatic reinforcement. Jerry's arousal, combined with a lack of activity and social engagement, made him more likely to offend. His lack of sexual education put him at a disadvantage with respect to addressing and contextualizing these urges. As well, this lack of education meant Jerry might not have been aware of any prosocial alternatives. Jerry's offenses occurred at night in the residence. All resident rooms were on the same floor, and he had close proximity to potential victims; two asleep staff were located on the floor below.

Because of property damage caused by one of the residents, the environment was rather barren with very little in the way of materials or activities for people to do unless staff engaged them. Aside from arousal, Jerry discussed feeling bored and it appears that his offenses were at least partially motivated by a desire to engage in some type of stimulation. It was notable that there was little staff engagement in the time prior to the offenses, and a lack of attention likely played a role as well. A lack of both stimulation and staff attention served as potential setting events and motivating operations for his offenses. As noted, Jerry's environment was relatively barren, and he had very little stimuli, especially at night time.

Other Treatment Components

An important part of Jerry's program was to keep him actively engaged, partly because his behaviors are influenced by drive states. The lack of stimuli, lack of attention, and increased arousal all made the offending behaviors more reinforcing. Jerry responded to being bored or isolated by engaging in an offense, which would alleviate these conditions. For Jerry, offending was not just driven sexually, but also by a need for stimulation. His level of arousal also played a factor in his offenses, notably at times during previous offenses when he was going through puberty. Therefore, it was a crucial part of his treatment to be given ample access to hobbies and activities that he enjoyed. Though this was alone insufficient to address the specific topographical stimulation of the sexual behavior, it was hypothesized that it would decrease the motivation for stimulation in general. The isolation and boredom, as previously discussed, was dealt with by altering antecedents through creating an enriched environment and increasing opportunities for interaction. Also, teaching Jerry to initiate interactions with staff when he is feeling bored was also encouraged to help him alleviate his boredom in appropriate ways. In order for this to be effective, staff were advised to be available for conversations and engagement upon request.

At the time of the most recent offenses, there were two overnight staff asleep in the residence. While Jerry was in the psychiatric unit, he required at least one overnight awake staff at all times as a risk management strategy. This was important for two reasons: First, it enabled staff to provide sweeps of the unit throughout the night to ensure no inappropriate behaviors were occurring, and second, this provided Jerry with access to staff engagement during his most high-risk periods. The behavior analyst made recommendations for risk management strategies in Jerry's future residence. Jerry could not return back to his old residence where the offenses occurred because returning him to live with his victims would be morally and ethically unacceptable. In his future residence, the behavior analyst recommended that he have chimes on his bedroom door as an added preventative measure until such time that Jerry had developed the necessary self-regulation skills to consistently manage his own behavior. The chime would be a cue for staff to do a sweep and confirm everyone's location. Further, in his future residence, Jerry's room should be on a separate floor from other residents in order to create distance and natural barriers between his room and others.

Jerry had received virtually no socio-sexual education growing up. This lack of education may have partially contributed to Jerry's poor understanding of boundaries and consent. As part of the intervention, sexual education occurred before any future relationships could be explored to ensure any potential risk would be minimized. The goal of this education was to prevent any potential sexual risky behavior that could arise from Jerry's lack of knowledge and experience in normative sexual behavior. The rationale was based on the findings from his responses on the SSKAAT-R (Griffiths & Lunsky, 2003), in which he scored significantly below the normative sample across all topics.

Increasing Jerry's understanding of consent was specifically targeted in training to provide him with skills to engage in a mutual and intimate relationship with an appropriate partner. In addition to targeted education around consent, Jerry received education about which sexual acts were against the law, what constituted healthy relationships, and how to establish boundaries. Consent education included discussions of who can and who cannot provide consent and how it is established. This was directly tied to discussions about sexual acts that are against the law and what can happen if consent is not established or not possible.

Socio-sexual education was also provided to give Jerry prosocial ways to gain interactions with others and develop appropriate intimate relationships with peers. This was also considered to be an important element going forward as an aid in generalization so he might have the skills to develop prosocial relationships in the future.

Jerry's assessment revealed that his behaviors often served multiple functions. The behaviors served a sensory function in that they were automatically reinforced through sexual gratification. Negative reinforcement contingencies were also at play by acting in a way that reduced his boredom. The behaviors were also preceded by periods where Jerry received little to no interaction with staff, and attention appeared to be a key motivating factor. Functional replacement skills were essential to eliminate behaviors that were maintained by positive and negative reinforcement. Jerry's phallometric assessment results showed paraphilic interests to forced sex and male and female prepubescents, as well as to female adults. Therefore, all opportunities for sexual acts against prepubescents must be eliminated and replaced by opportunities for Jerry to have intimate relationships with female adults. This preference was shaped through gradual and phased-in ease of access, in addition to providing Jerry with the social opportunities and relationship skills needed to engage with female adults.

Jerry's most recent offenses suggested an approach-automatic pathway. He had not planned his offenses far in advance, instead setting events and motivating operations due to boredom, arousal, lack of access to appropriate mutual partners, and lack of attention may have influenced his behavior. As such, the assessment determined that his offenses followed an approach pathway, and he had poor regulation. The keys to treatment were building up motivation to engage in appropriate sexual behavior and providing him with the skills and opportunities to do so. Since Jerry's offenses indicated poor self-regulation and an inability to manage his arousal, Jerry participated in Adapted Dialectical Behavior Therapy (ADBT) to teach him how to get what he wants in prosocial ways, how to cope with stressful or distressing situations, and to help him develop emotional regulation skills. Simple, concrete teaching strategies were used, including modelling, repetition, and role-play, which were adapted based on his specific learning needs.

Along with providing functional replacements to Jerry's offending behavior as already discussed, there was also a need to ensure that there was sufficient motivation to engage in alternative functional behaviors. Targeting motivation was achieved by providing him with the elements outlined in the *Good Lives Model* (GLM; Ward, 2002 a,b).

In utilizing the GLM and by providing more rich reinforcement for various alternative appropriate behaviors, Jerry had less opportunity to offend and decreased motivation to offend due to an enriched environment that was more rewarding than engaging in offending behaviors. For example, in sticking with GLM terminology, Jerry's boredom and lack of stimulation demonstrated a lack of excellence in work and play. Engaging in leisure and recreation were important to him; therefore, suitable and reinforcing recreation activities were introduced to enrich his life in this aspect.

Furthermore, the automatically reinforcing properties of Jerry's offenses fell under the goal of happiness. This goal is the pursuit of pleasure and activities that are automatically reinforcing. In the meantime, while Jerry's arousal to female adults was being shaped and prosocial opportunities sought, Jerry was provided with education and ample privacy for masturbation and self-stimulatory behavior. The goal of excellence in work and play was implicated through an absence of recreational activities and stimuli prior to the offenses. By providing Jerry with a more enriched environment and choice of activities, reduction in the drive state of boredom, and the MO for offenses were targeted. Additionally, by providing Jerry with increased opportunity for independence and autonomy, within the parameters of safety, his overall quality of life was enhanced by allowing him increased opportunity to find prosocial means of achieving pleasure or stimulation. Teaching Jerry appropriate ways to achieve his goals in natural settings also sets the stage for generalization and maintenance of his skills and encouraged a whole host of positive behaviors. For example, engaging in socio-sexual education gave him the skills to form healthy relationships which, in turn, opened doors for more social and recreational opportunities in the community, even though these opportunities were still under careful scrutiny as confidence was being built that he was utilizing his safety skills.

Generalization/Maintenance

Jerry's treatment was focused on teaching him functional replacement skills while simultaneously employing risk management techniques to ensure extinction (i.e., the consequences that followed his previous offenses were prevented/withheld) and therefore, no other people were at risk of harm. Functional replacement skills were targeted to increase generalization of appropriate sexual behaviors. For instance, Jerry learning and practicing socio-sexual knowledge skills increased opportunities to develop prosocial relationships and meeting an age-appropriate partner. Although his offenses included sexually inappropriate fantasies and urges, assessment results showed that he also had sexual interest in same aged women, so function-based intervention also focused on shaping these preferences. From the onset, Jerry's offenses were minimized by his parents, who dealt with the matters privately or shifted blame onto the victim. They expressed the opinion that despite his age, Jerry was more like a child himself, and since no charges were laid in his early offenses, no early intervention was sought. As a result, he had a history marked by reinforcing consequences (sexual gratification, terminating boredom, etc.) versus aversive consequences. More recently, a response-cost protocol was introduced in which Jerry would lose a highly reinforcing outing if he displayed any precursor behaviors indicative of risk for future offending behavior. The rationale was based on the level of risk that his behaviors posed as precursors to a re-offense.

Jerry's behavior analyst will continue to work with him in his current and future setting and track his progress. Emphasis will be placed on ensuring his future home is an environment in which he can be successful, with appropriate staff supervision, staff training, activities and social engagement, socio-sexual skill building, no victim access to minimize risk of offending, and ensuring the maintenance and generalization of his skills.

Let us see how we did in following the logical functional model for Jerry in Table 12.1.

Table 12.1 ***Logical Functional Model: Quality Checklist for Jerry***

Questions	Yes/No
Have the setting events and motivating operations that set occasion for the offense been identified? Have these setting events/motivating operations been altered or prevented where possible?	Yes
Have other antecedent events that preceded the offense been identified? Were these antecedent events altered?	Yes
Have we identified what function the offense achieved for this person?	Yes*
Has the stage been set for success?	Yes
Have replacement or coping skills to achieve personal goals in appropriate ways been identified and incorporated into treatment?	Yes
Have elements been added to the person's life that will provide reinforcing and positive qualities and, ultimately, enhance quality of life?	Yes
Have consequences been put in place to ensure positive behaviors occur more frequently and inappropriate expressions are discouraged?	Yes
Have strategies been put in place to ensure generalization across settings and have people been identified to "trap" the behaviors into the natural environments, while minimizing risks?	Yes

*Based on descriptive assessment results (not confirmed in a functional analysis)

Case II: The Case of Porter

Background

At the time of the index offense, Porter was a 21-year-old man who lived in a large multi-bed setting. The staff reported that he was placed there by his family for sexual behavior reasons. While residing at that setting, three known episodes of alleged sexual offending behavior occurred. The first two involved someone who he had courted, and the alleged offense turned out to be consenting; the latter sexual encounter involved a person who was new to the facility and with whom Porter had no relationship prior to the offense. This woman, named Sally, had limited cognitive abilities and would not be deemed to have capacity to consent to sexual contact.

Assessment

Investigation into the background of the alleged history of offending through extensive review of the records and interviews with staff and family revealed that one, and not three, offenses had occurred. Rather, the environment and conditions Porter lived in set him up for failure; he was systematically denied the opportunity for consensual and appropriate sexual expression and received aversive consequences, which potentially served as punishment. The assessment of his background was important because his only offense was ultimately viewed as being one more of opportunity than planned. Because staff had misinterpreted his prior relationships as inappropriate, he was denied opportunity for consenting relationships with women and was on a 1-to-1 watch at all times. Once he had engaged in any sexually questionable behavior, all sexual behavior thereafter was viewed through a lens of sexual impropriety, regardless of whether or not that was a fair assessment. This likely created a situation in which relationships and, as such, sexual interactions were denied creating a deprivation state that impacted the motivating operations involved with the sexual behavior. It was hypothesized that the deprivation may have set a condition wherein any sexual behaviors (including inappropriate) were more valuable/reinforcing and therefore more likely to occur (establishing operation). Combined with the fact that appropriate and consenting behavior had previously been followed by aversive consequences (and potentially punished), and there was a potential abolishing operation for appropriate sexual behavior, the inappropriate behaviors were more likely to occur.

Environmental (Antecedent) Modifications

Initially, all incidents occurred with individuals who were consenting and often in an established relationship with Porter. He showed no evidence of a preference for forced or non-consensual sexual interaction until the latest offense. His preference was for consensual sex, which had been (potentially) punished through prohibition of any sexual behavior by the agency. Thus, the agency may have created contingencies that punished age-appropriate sexual interaction and set up conditions in which either Porter was to deny his sexual urges (thereby setting up a deprivation state) or he was put in a position to seek quick sexual interaction, with whomever was available, when staff were otherwise engaged. The key to long-term appropriate treatment for Porter was to find him an alternative agency that understood and promoted healthy sexual practices for individuals who resided in their homes, thereby reversing the contingencies for sexual interaction. The setting events and motivating operations that set occasion for the offense were identified and steps were in place to alter the stimulus conditions. Although imperative, moving Porter to a new residence operated by a different agency was not sufficient to be called effective treatment. Porter had engaged in a non-consenting relationship and had done so in a public venue.

The immediate antecedents to the assault on the woman at the day program, Sally, were: (i) that staff attention was diverted away from him, giving him a chance to elude his 1-1 watch, and (ii) the presence of Sally and her location in or near the washroom where he could sequester her without being seen.

The function of his offense was hypothesized to be physiologic (automatic) reinforcement in the form of sexual gratification. In his current setting, not only were relationships prohibited, but masturbation and the use of erotica were strongly discouraged. As well, he lacked privacy, in that he shared a bedroom with another man.

The sociosexual assessment showed that Porter had learned that all sex was "bad," both through his experience of receiving aversive consequences and through the formal and informal sex education he received from his parents and staff. This created a vulnerability that could have contributed to his offense behavior. He had learned that intimacy was bad, not allowed, and would be sanctioned. He had also learned from his interactions with consenting women in the past that relationships that were intimate were positive and reinforcing. He, therefore, due to his reinforcement history, was conflicted in his views of what appropriate sexual interaction would be because in his world all sexual encounters were deemed inappropriate by others. Additionally, his offense against Sally, albeit legally non-consensual, was not forced. Sally had gone along with it thinking he wanted to be her boyfriend. As well, his lack of a private place to engage in sexual contact meant that any sexual act would be lacking in privacy (i.e., a public washroom was inappropriate).

Other Treatment Components

A major focus of Porter's treatment was teaching appropriate skills, both in terms of functional replacement behaviors and coping. His socio-sexual education focused clearly on what appropriate and inappropriate sexual contact involved. In addition, he was educated on moral and legal aspects of sexual contact, to understand the ramifications of any future inappropriate behavior. Porter engaged in sexual activity with someone who could not provide legal consent. The behavior analyst had administered the *Tool for the Assessment of Levels of Knowledge: Sexuality and Consent* (TALK-SC; Hingsburger et al., 2015), a specialized tool developed to measure sexual knowledge, specifically regarding consent. Based on the results, the behavior analyst and a sex educator commenced discrimination training to teach him when consent must be gained, when it cannot be gained, and how to do so. The behavior analyst arranged to have a sex educator work with her on the case, as she had not previously conducted sexual education and wanted to be trained in doing this by a qualified professional. As well, Porter was taught the legal consequences for sexual behavior and the importance of established consent. This training was important to conduct before Porter engaged in any sexual activity. His post-treatment assessments suggested that he could provide appropriate responses when asked questions about appropriate vs. inappropriate sexual behavior.

Porter was also taught about appropriate sexual contact. The *Socio-Sexual Knowledge and Attitude Assessment Tool- Revised* (SSKAAT-R; Griffiths & Lunsky, 2003) was used as a tool to identify his areas of confusion and eventually as a post-assessment. The sex educator worked with him alongside the behavior analyst to help him understand that there was nothing wrong with appropriate sexual contact as defined by "age appropriate, consenting partner in a private location." As such, his experiences with the two women he had courted earlier were used as examples, helping him to discriminate that his earlier behavior was not "wrong" and should not have been met with the consequences it did. However, in order to ensure that this could occur and that he no longer received conflicting contingencies, he had to be moved to a new agency.

Environmental Modifications

The new agency was selected based on their policies and practices regarding sexual activity and human intimacy: namely, that both were natural processes that should be available to all persons, disabled or not. Although it was not an easy task to shift individuals between agencies, the behavior analyst and the sexual educator advocated for the change to a more appropriate agency that would respond respectfully and responsibly to Porter's right to be a sexual person. They could not in good conscience teach him about appropriate sexuality when the messages he would be receiving from agency staff would be opposing. Secondly, in order to help him understand that the original agency staff were incorrect in attempting to punish his earlier relationships, he would first have to move.

Porter also needed to be provided with the opportunity and encouragement to engage in consensual sexual relationships or self-satisfying sex. This meant affording him privacy in appropriate locations and relationship training as needed (specifically looking at public/private behaviors). The lack of both had led Porter to meet his needs in inappropriate ways that were more a product of environment than deep-seated inappropriate sexual thoughts and urges. The behavior analyst also taught Porter to address his sexual urges through masturbation. Because of the index offense, it was important to help him learn how to appropriately gain sexual satisfaction, even when a partner was not available. In his previous home, masturbation had been discouraged. In his new home, he was afforded his own room and provided erotica (a poster on the back of his bedroom door) so that he could masturbate in private. He was encouraged to masturbate prior to going out in public to ensure that he had been sexually satisfied before going out with staff or his friends (in an attempt to create an abolishing operation for inappropriate behaviors). He was also provided with access to non-pornographic erotica to have in his room to provide visual aids to enhance his arousal.

Once Porter was moved to an appropriate agency, it was important to build elements into his life that would provide reinforcing and positive qualities and enhance his quality of life. Porter's *Good Lives Plan* focused on those goals that may have contributed to offending. The primary maintaining reinforcers associated with his offending were hypothesized to be sexual gratification and intimacy, with a preference shown for reciprocal sexual relationships. Another thing he identified as important was to be free of 24/7 surveillance by staff. To accommodate this, and until treatment had been completed and he could demonstrate that he learned skills, he was placed in an all-male residence. There was no one in the home with a history of sexual offending, and two of the three other men were actively involved in positive relationships with women who lived elsewhere. At the end of his training, the data showed that he had learned the skills he needed to avoid re-offense and had demonstrated over and over again that he was at low risk to re-offend. For Porter, it was important to utilize a *Good Lives Plan* to establish valued 'goods' in his daily life and to establish goals to achieve that good life as motivation to prevent future offenses.

Generalization and Maintenance

Porter demonstrated previously that he had the social skills necessary to begin and maintain an intimate relationship, as evidenced by his earlier encounters. His expressed goal was to have the opportunity to become involved with a woman in a mutually satisfying relationship. In order to facilitate this, he began to participate in social activities in the community and got a job. In both of these situations, staff accompanied him. In the former agency, staff were in the social activity and were observing his behavior but were not hovering over him. His offending behavior may have initially been under the stimulus control of the diverted staff attention. In the new agency, stimulus control in the form of staff presence was established temporarily. Their presence served to ensure Porter regulated his behavior in public and only engaged in sexual activity with consenting adults. This type of close supervision with external stimulus control was required until such time as an appropriate level of confidence was achieved that a re-offense would not occur. At such time, a fading approach similar to the Casper Effect described in the generalization chapter was introduced.

Porter was given clear rules about not leaving social activities without a staff member; however, he was able to interact with the other men and women without interference. The staff member was instructed about what to watch for and how to intervene if anything inappropriate seemed imminent. Porter also knew the consequences of doing anything inappropriate; his privileges would be revoked and, if an offense occurred, the police would be called. Similarly, in his work placement, he was with a staff member for six months learning a new job. The staff member was also Porter's instructor and, as such, worked side-by-side with him. Again, rules were in place so that he knew he could not leave his staff without permission.

Over the course of the year, Porter did extremely well in his new home. He made friends with his male peers. They engaged in social activities together and earned the trust of the therapist, sex educator, and staff of the agency sufficient enough that he began going out with his housemates without staff accompaniment. Initially, a staff member from another house was shadowing him, and he knew that that might happen and he agreed to this. Eventually, the shadow was discontinued. He also met a woman at one of the social meetings and over the course of the year they developed a strong friendship and eventually began to date.

An important element of the treatment protocol was to ensure that Porter had the skills and knowledge necessary to engage in appropriate sexual contact only (i.e., not re-offend), not the least of which was to make sure he was aware of what natural and legal consequences would follow if he re-offended, as well as what he would lose. Pivotal to that, of course, was providing a life worth keeping. At Porter's previous residence, he had all positive elements in his life taken away or restricted, such that he virtually had nothing to lose, perhaps creating an abolishing operation for appropriate behavior.

The obvious goal for intervention for Porter was to reduce his sexually inappropriate behavior to zero, with sexually inappropriate behavior defined as any sexual contact that involves an age-inappropriate partner, is not consensual, or lacks privacy. The concept of zero tolerance for any re-offense sets a very high but socially valid benchmark for this type of behavior. Unlike any other behavior for which an ABA program is designed, reduction in behavior is considered success. However, as Lindsay (2014) noted when discussing sexual offending anything but zero would be deemed a failure. Although the careful history taken on Porter and the assessments conducted all pointed to the hypothesis that this was likely a case of counterfeit deviance (Griffiths, Hingsburger, Hoath, & Ioannou, 2013), data collection of generalized effects, the key to building confidence that treatment effects had taken place, was required over a sustained period and in different settings with different people. The careful generalization strategy described above was monitored closely by the behavior analyst to ensure that fading of staff monitoring and increased access to social opportunities and community occurred in a carefully constructed manner with feedback and data collection. Porter's success and, potentially, to his move into a setting including the presence of women (or development of a lasting relationship with a woman) also depended on establishing the skills and knowledge necessary to help him to appropriately cope with his sexual urges, and to understand the consequences of not doing so.

Finally, let's evaluate how we did in following the logical functional model for Porter in Table 12.2.

Table 12.2 ***Logical Functional Model: Quality Checklist for Porter***

Questions	Yes/No
Have the setting events and motivating operations that set occasion for the offense been identified? Have these setting events/motivating operations been altered or prevented where possible?	Yes
Have other antecedent events that preceded the offense been identified? Were these antecedent events altered?	Yes
Have we identified what function the offense achieved for this person?	Yes*
Has the stage been set for success?	Yes
Have replacement or coping skills that can be taught to achieve personal goals in an appropriate way been identified and incorporated into treatment?	Yes
Have elements been added to Porter's life that will provide reinforcing and positive qualities and, ultimately, enhance quality of life?	Yes
Have consequences been put in place to ensure positive behaviors occur more frequently while inappropriate expressions are discouraged?	Yes
Have strategies been put in place to ensure generalization across settings, and have people been identified to "trap" the behaviors into their natural environments while minimizing risks?	Yes

*Based on descriptive assessment results (not confirmed in a functional analysis)

Case 3: The Case of Scott

Background

At the time of offending, Scott was a 25-year-old man with high functioning cognitive challenges (IQ 68). He had an unremarkable early history and moved to supported living at age 18. Due to his abilities, he took on many extra chores and referred to himself as "junior staff" in his day program, which staff encouraged. He eventually started to assert control over other residents, assigning them tasks that he often supervised alone. Across settings, he engaged in five separate instances of offending behavior, ranging from touching the genitals of a female peer to coercive anal penetration. Staff viewed these behaviors as accidental and were reluctant to report the instances believing that Scott would be unfairly restricted. The first-time staff notified authorities, police refused to press charges for similar reasons – they felt that Scott was not aware of any wrongdoing. Supervision was enhanced in his residence; however, staff members who did not believe that his actions were intentional were inconsistent in their supervision. Scott continued the offending behaviors and attempted to hide them by only assaulting non-verbal individuals, especially when he was moved to a different group home with more vulnerable peers. Police were called again when a staff member witnessed Scott engaging in non-consensual anal penetration with an individual. He was angry and confused about why he was arrested and charged with sexual assault, which eventually became simple assault. He received no prison time and was placed on probation with no conditions, apart from a treatment protocol.

The prosecutor told Scott that he was "a fine young man who was the victim of a misunderstanding. He needs support and compassion, not a sentence." The logical model of a functional behavior assessment and treatment plan is outlined below.

Assessment

The results of the SSKAAT-R (Griffiths & Lunsky, 2003) indicated that Scott had a higher overall score than other individuals who presented with the same intellectual functioning (e.g., T-score of 83 for Anatomy) and even higher than some of the typically developing population. Scott received education from his agency in relationships and social skills, abuse prevention, and personal boundaries and understood physical and emotional boundaries quite well (e.g., he could describe what consent was and some means of how to obtain it). However, he also had cognitive distortions regarding consent, in that he believed it could be obtained non-verbally, that if his victims did not want to have sex they should have fought back harder, and that his offenses did not impact the victims and they were likely to forget about it. He revealed to a therapist that he preferred coercive sex and was homosexual but did not want a consenting relationship. He had sufficient knowledge to understand the impact of his actions and how he orchestrated them. A Good Lives/self-regulation assessment (Yates et al., 2010) illuminated the explicit and planned nature of his offenses and that Scott possessed intact self-regulation; so, he could conceivably manage his behavior. However, Scott indicated an intention to re-offend and stated a belief that if his actions had been wrong, he would already be in jail. In essence, Scott had never been afforded an opportunity for consequential learning regarding his sexually inappropriate conduct.

Environmental (Antecedent) Modifications

According to direct assessments of the incidents, there was no clear pattern of setting events. In one instance, there was indication of sexual deprivation (i.e. being aroused, but not being able to masturbate), but in other instances it was unclear what setting events, if any, were present (e.g., ranging from potential depressed mood – wanting to stay in bed, to having a productive morning). Indirect assessment by a therapist indicated that Scott was highly sexual and hyper-aroused, which may have created an establishing operation for any sexual activity. For example, Scott would watch pornography on his phone before work but would not have an opportunity to masturbate, which increased the reinforcing value of any sexual behavior and actions that would lead to obtaining sexual gratification. As such, Scott would often go to day program extremely aroused with no chance for appropriate sexual behavior, which may have increased the likelihood and value of inappropriate sexual behavior.

Scott's treatment plan included strategies to reduce risk by altering the setting events/motivation operations, including: (i) Scott masturbated before work to attempt to reduce his arousal (i.e., temporarily alter the establishing operation by making sexual activity less reinforcing); (ii) Scott was prescribed a trial of Lupron, an antiandrogen medication used to decrease libido, which led to near-immediate improvement (i.e., Scott reported that he felt more in control and less urges for sexual offending behavior when in the community).

The most common antecedents for Scott's offenses were lack of supervision, lack of activity, and access to victims (e.g., "supervising" peers without staff present). These antecedent variables paired with Scott's high state of arousal with little opportunity for sexually appropriate behaviors, may have created ideal conditions for inappropriate sexual behaviors. Given Scott's motivation to re-offend, it was critical to provide external risk management until he learned new skills that would allow him to engage in appropriate sexual behavior.

Scott's treatment plan included: (i) one-on-one "eyes on" supervision at all times; (ii) Scott was never allowed alone with any client, at home or in the community; (iii) Scott was given his own room and access to privacy at all times; (iv) Scott's schedule was altered to give him private time in the morning before work (and free access whenever he wanted); and (v) he could view approved erotica when he wanted.

Other Treatment Components

Due to ethical and practical concerns with performing an experimental functional analysis to confirm the function of Scott's behaviors, function can only be inferred from the available evidence. His behavior appeared to be maintained by automatic reinforcement (i.e., sexual gratification), resulting from coercive sexual behaviors. In future cases, a modified functional analysis (e.g., of precursor behaviors) could be considered, but may not be appropriate due to risk. Scott had orchestrated situations at day program in which he could isolate the other individuals and under the guise of "supervising" them he could abuse them. When Scott was in the presence of vulnerable individuals he would become aroused, leading him be motivated to isolate potential victims. He would ensure his victims were non-verbal and the lack of supervision allowed him to offend. Scott would offend and then continue his day at work. The immediate consequences for his behavior were positive; he often achieved ejaculation and there were no aversive sanctions or other consequences imposed.

Given that Scott's sexually inappropriate and coercive thoughts were automatically reinforcing, it was challenging to find functional replacement behaviors. It is generally a straightforward process to program appropriate means of attaining sexual gratification, but it can be significantly more difficult to replace the coercive nature of the behavior when the coercion is strongly reinforcing. Therefore, the replacement behavior must be as much or more reinforcing, but easier (and safer) to obtain. Although masturbation may not serve the same automatic sensory function as an intimate relationship, Scott indicated no desire to engage in a relationship of any kind. As noted above, Scott's environment was restructured so he had his own room and access to privacy at all times; consequently, he had easy access to sexual gratification without aversive consequences.

Scott's treatment plan attempted to set him up for success through the following:

(1) Establishing an environment that creates conditions under which the offending behavior is unable to occur while appropriate, alternative, prosocial behaviors are taught and reinforced;
(2) Selecting and training staff members to ensure that appropriate supervision, therapeutic interactions, and support are consistently provided;
(3) Developing an individualized plan of activities and programming to provide skill building opportunities and access to reinforcement; and
(4) Providing opportunities for supervised social interactions that promote motivation for appropriate engagement and non-offending behavior.

Although Scott possessed intact self-regulation and was able to manage his behavior, he was not motivated to use these skills to avoid re-offense. Scott's treatment plan included: 1) teaching Scott skills and strategies to avoid re-offense; 2) teaching Scott what his risk areas were and how to manage arousal in the community; and 3) once he began regaining some independence, teaching him how to rely on external supports, such as staff and family, in situations where there were targets or heightened risk. Scott's motivation to offend was extremely high, and his desire to avoid recidivism very low. Functionally-equivalent replacement behaviors, such as obtaining sexual gratification through appropriate means, may be insufficient to sustain long lasting change.

However pivotal to his success was educating him on the realities of a re-offense. Considerable time was spent ensuring that he understood the real consequences that would likely follow if he re-offended. He now had a criminal file where his previous offense had been documented. The nature of a future trial and the consequence of jail or prison time were elaborated, explaining clearly what this would be like and how much he would dislike this experience. Additionally, a cost benefit analysis was laid out that clearly identified what he would lose if this occurred. All the things that he loved about his life (access to family, his television shows, his favorite foods, his special hobbies) would be lost while in prison. He kept this list with him at all times. Daily he would record the positive things in his life that he would miss if he re-offended. This list became longer over time as Scott's treatment plan was based on the *Good Lives Model,* in which a plan was created for him to highlight positive aspects of his life and future goals. The idea was for Scott to build a life worth keeping with the understanding that he may want to avoid re-offense in order to protect it. Scott's parents were an invaluable resource in supporting the positive and appropriate goals, ensuring that they were both realistic and highly motivating.

In assessment, Scott appeared as an *approach-explicit* individual; therefore, risk management needed special attention. Although building a good life in which he could feel successful in other ways was an important element in creating competing contingencies, the focus was always on keeping Scott and those with whom he interacts safe, especially those who are most vulnerable.

As noted above, Scott had an affinity for coercive sexual activity. However, over a long period of time with no offense behavior, he expressed an interest in pursuing a consensual relationship with a male friend, who also wished to have a relationship. However, despite Scott's level of functioning he had very immature social skills and had not been in an intimate relationship for years. As well, his knowledge of consent was strong but his ability to apply the concept was quite weak. The well-being of his partner was important to consider; therefore, part of his treatment program involved addressing these deficits while teaching him relationship skills and, importantly, providing him the opportunity to engage in an appropriate and consensual relationship. This was difficult for both staff and Scott's parents as they feared this could create an opportunity for re-offense, and as such considerable time was spent with both Scott and his partner in discussing mutual issues of intimacy. It was critical to provide a supportive attitude to Scott while managing the potential risks and allowing him to find more appropriate means of achieving his goals.

However, during the assessment he noted some arousal to older males.

Scott's overall treatment plan included: (i) addressing his cognitive distortions and issues of control while teaching him relationship skills, (ii) providing him the opportunity to engage in consensual relationships, and (iii) providing support to Scott while managing the potential risks and allowing him to find and be in control of means of achieving his goals in appropriate ways.

Scott's behavior represented an offense pattern that was unlikely to produce treatment outcomes that alone would be sufficient to reduce recidivism. As such, his case continued to be managed through both environmental and pharmacological management strategies, in addition to habilitative approaches.

Now let's review in Table 12.3 to see whether we have completed the checklist for Scott.

Table 12.3 ***Logical Functional Model: Quality Checklist for Scott***

Questions	Yes/No
Have the setting events and motivating operations that set occasion for the offense been identified? Have these setting events/motivating operations been altered or prevented where possible?	Yes
Have other antecedent events that preceded the offense been identified? Were these antecedent events altered?	Yes
Have we identified what function the offense achieved for this person?	Yes*
Has the stage been set for success?	Yes
Have the replacement or coping skills to achieve personal goals in appropriate ways been identified and incorporated into treatment?	Yes
Have elements been added to the person's life that will provide reinforcing and positive qualities and, ultimately, enhance quality of life?	Yes
Have consequences been put in place to ensure positive behaviors occur more frequently while inappropriate expressions are discouraged?	Yes
Have strategies been put in place to ensure generalization across settings and have people been identified to "trap" the behaviors into the natural environments, while minimizing risks?	Yes

*Based on descriptive assessment results (not confirmed in a functional analysis)

CONCLUSION

The plans for Jerry, Porter, and Scott were developed by following a set protocol based on the logical functional behavior assessment model. There are ten basic steps to this model. First, identify the setting events and motivating operations that set occasion for the person to offend. Second, determine how those can be altered or modified. Third, isolate the antecedents that preceded the behavior. Fourth, explore how they can be altered to prevent an offense. Fifth, establish the function(s) that the offense served (confirmed in an experimental functional analysis or variation if possible). Sixth, investigate vulnerabilities that could leave the person at risk to re-offend or interfere with effective learning of new skills. Seventh, determine the replacement or coping skills that could be taught to achieve personal goals in an appropriate way. Eighth, explore elements that can be added to allow the person to gain a rich life that will provide reinforcing and positive qualities to enhance quality of life. Ninth, establish consequences to ensure positive behaviors are augmented and inappropriate expressions are discouraged. And lastly, systematically build in strategies to increase the likelihood of generalization of the appropriate behaviors across settings (e.g., employ others to help trap the behaviors to the natural environment as much as possible, while minimizing risks of re-offense). These 10 steps can be translated into quality assurance questions that can be used to evaluate if the elements of the logical functional model have been fully explored.

REFERENCES

Carr, E. G., & Durand, V. M. (1985). Reducing behavior problems through functional communication training. *Journal of Applied Behavior Analysis, 18,* 111-126.

Cooper, J. O., Heron, T. E., & Heward, W. L. (2007). *Applied behavior analysis* (2nd ed.). Upper Saddle River, NJ: Pearson Education Inc.

Dozier, C., Iwata, B., & Worsdell, A. (2011). Assessment and treatment of foot-shoe fetish displayed by a man with autism. *Journal of Applied Behavior Analysis, 44,* 133–137.

Griffiths, D., Hingsburger, D., Hoath, J., & Ioannou, S. (2013). Counterfeit deviance revisited. *Journal of Applied Research in Intellectual Disabilities, 26,* 471-480.

Griffiths, D. & Lunsky, Y. (2003). *The socio-sexual knowledge and attitude assessment tool-Revised.* Wood Dale, Illinois: Stoelting.

Hingsburger, D., Beattie, K., Charbonneau, T., Hoath, J., Ioannou, S., King, S., ... Woodhead, S. (2015). *Tool for the Assessment of Levels of Knowledge: Sexuality and Consent (TALK-SC).* Unpublished assessment tool, Vita and Mackenzie Health Centre for Behavior Health Sciences: York Region, ON.

Levenson, J. S., Willis, G. M., & Prescott, D. S. (2014). Adverse childhood experiences in the lives of male sex offenders: Implications for trauma-informed care. *Sexual Abuse: A Journal of Research and Treatment, 28,* 1-20.

Lindsay, W. R. (2014). *Behavioral assessment and treatment of sex offenders with intellectual disabilities and autism.* International Dual Diagnosis Certificate Program, Brock University, St. Catharines, ON, CA.

Lindsay, W. R., Smith, A. H. W., Law, J., Quinn, K., Anderson, A., Smith, A., ... Allan, R. (2002). A treatment service for sex offenders and abusers with intellectual disability: Characteristics of referral and evaluation. *Journal of Applied Research in Intellectual Disabilities, 15,* 166-174.

Miltenberger, R. (1997). *Behavior modification: Principles and practices.* Pacific Grove, CA: Brooks/Cole.

Quinsey, V. L. & Marshall, W. L. (1983). Procedures for reducing inappropriate sexual arousal: An evaluation review. In J. G. Greer and I. R. Stuart (Eds.), *The sexual aggressor: Current perspective son treatment* (pp. 267-289). New York: Van Nostrand Reinhold.

Sobsey, R. & Doe, T. (1991). Patterns of sexual abuse and assault. *Sexuality and Disability, 9,* 243-259.

Ward, T. (2002a). Good lives and the rehabilitation of offenders: Promises and problems. *Aggression and Violent Behavior, 7,* 513 – 528.

Ward, T. (2002b). The management of risk and the design of good lives.
Australian Psychologist, 37, 172 - 179.

Yates, P. M., Prescott, D. S., & Ward, T. (2010). *Applying the good lives and self-regulation models to sex offender treatment: A practical guide for clinicians.* Brandon, VT: Safer Society Press.

PART V:

ETHICAL DILEMMAS

Chapter Thirteen

Ethical Dilemmas in Treating Persons with Intellectual Disabilities Who Have Sexually Offended

Dorothy Griffiths, Kendra Thomson, Jan Frijters, Stephanie Ioannou, Jordan Hoath & Robin Wilson

The treatment of persons with intellectual disabilities is often fraught with many ethical challenges. One reason for this is that the sexuality of persons with intellectual disabilities, both historically and currently, is still the subject of much debate within society and the developmental service sector. As Griffiths, Richards, Fedoroff, and Watson (2002, p. 11) noted:

> *Research-oriented clinicians are guided by ethics committees to ensure individual rights are not being violated. Social workers are governed by a code of ethics that guides treatment of people in different social environments. Scientists have to consider the bio-ethics of their research and the effects it may have on humans. Ethics are recognized in many professions, yet when it comes to what is ethical regarding sexuality and persons who have a developmental disability, there are no standards or practices. Basically, each case is treated differently, depending on who is in the position to make decisions.*

In exploring this issue, many ethical questions emerge. In the chapter that follows we will attempt to address some of these.

HOW DO HUMAN RIGHTS FIT INTO TREATMENT OF PERSONS WITH INTELLECTUAL DISABILITIES WHO SEXUALLY OFFEND?

In 1999, the World Association for Sexology adopted a consensus declaration on sexual rights during their 14th World Congress that was later adopted by the UN General Assembly. It stated:

> *Sexuality is an integral part of the personality of every human being. Its full development depends upon the satisfaction of basic human needs such as the desire for contact, intimacy, emotional expression, pleasure, tenderness and love. Sexuality is constructed through the interaction between the individual and social structures. Full development of sexuality is essential for individual, interpersonal, and societal well-being. Sexual rights are universal human*

> *rights, so must sexual health be a basic human right. In order to ensure that human beings and societies develop healthy sexuality, the following sexual rights must be recognized, promoted, respected and defended by all societies through all means. Sexual health is the result of an environment that recognizes, respects, and exercises those rights. (Coleman, 2002, p. 8).*

As mentioned throughout this book, the settings and culture in which many individuals with intellectual disabilities live have routinely not recognized nor respected their sexual rights. In contrast, their sexuality has been met with oppression, castration, institutionalization, restrictions, and punishment. As such, the foundation to establish healthy sexuality has not existed for many persons with intellectual disability. In the past, when a person with an intellectual disability exhibited a sexual behavior, there was little discriminative difference in the response received, whether the behavior was an attempt at sexuality that was non-offensive to a sexual act that was of an offending nature. Both were often treated the same and treated with some form of sanction or aversive consequence.

Although there have been significant strides made in recent years toward recognizing the sexual rights of persons with intellectual disabilities, these cultural shifts are slow and not universal. Therefore, as clinicians undertaking the task of providing treatment for persons with intellectual disabilities who have committed an act deemed sexually inappropriate or offensive, the nature of the environment in which the person resides and interacts is an important element for examination. It is important to remember that where there is no respect for healthy sexuality, there is no foundation for the person who has offended to learn appropriate sexuality. Appropriate sexuality is defined as a sexual interaction that is consensual (or self-arousing), age-appropriate (involving an age-appropriate partner), private (in place and time), and within the bounds of what is legally allowed within the culture.

HOW DO YOU BALANCE RIGHTS AND RISKS WITH RESPONSIBILITY?

In recent years, there has been an emergent interest in the rights of persons with intellectual disabilities, heightened by the adoption of the United Nations Convention on the Rights of Persons with Disabilities (United Nations, 2006). A challenge to the recognition of rights is ensuring that persons with intellectual disabilities and those who support them are not only aware of those rights but respect them and the rights of others and further are responsible in their use of those rights. Montenegro and Greenhill (2015) have suggested that the 3Rs (Rights, Respect, and Responsibility) approach to training is the most internationally recognized rights training program for staff and individuals with intellectual disabilities. This program adopts the perspective that persons with intellectual disabilities must not only learn about their rights and the fact that their rights are to be respected by others, but also that with rights comes responsibility which includes respecting the rights of others. Correspondingly, those who support a person with an intellectual disability must also abide by this perspective: that persons with intellectual disabilities have rights and that within their methods of support, the full range of human rights must be respected. However, in doing so they also must adhere to procedures that ensure that the rights of others are respected. When the discussion is about persons with intellectual disabilities who have committed a sexual offense, this involves the obligation to ensure the safety of others. As Ward and Salmon (2011) noted, "every aspect of practice is shot through with value commitments and each of us is obligated to think deeply about our responsibilities to sex offenders, victims, the community and ourselves" (p. 398).

All human beings are granted rights, and this includes individuals who have offended. Ioannou (2013) noted that most of the literature on persons who have sexually offended pertains to assessment, treatment, and risk factors associated with reducing the rate of recidivism, with very little discussion on the rights of these individuals. Ward, Gannon, and Birgden (2007) noted that many members of the community and those in the corrective system believe that people who have offended give up their rights because of the criminal acts they committed (e.g., Lippke, 2002). Brown and Thompson (1997) suggested that offenders with intellectual disabilities who cannot or choose not to give consent may be still subjected to research if the need to advance the research justifies their participation. Historically, these views on individuals with intellectual disabilities have led to exploitative research practices (Iacano & Murray, 2003) and ethics breaches, including forced sterilization (Aunos & Feldman, 2002; Tilley, Walmsley, Earle, & Atkinson, 2012). More advocacy-based thinking has been proposed by Ward and colleagues (2007) who recommended that human rights can be integrated into the assessment and treatment model for persons who have sexually offended. Their work, which was conducted with the general population of individuals with sexual offenses, identified that "there are ethical, pragmatic, and therapeutic reasons for respecting offenders' human rights," while still recognizing the ultimate importance of respecting and protecting the rights and safety of the community and past or potential victims (Ward et al., 2007, p. 204). They further noted that, "offenders have entitlements of their own that ought to be actively considered." Birgden and Cucolo (2011) also supported this view and argued that clinicians should focus on the supports needed to enhance community inclusion rather than resort to restriction and social exclusion and point to the need to achieve a community-offender balance.

Ward and Salmon (2011) elaborated on the ethical issues associated with risk management and community protection. They suggested a balance based on ethical treatment, "to ensure that sex offenders and non-offenders have the essential capabilities to live better lives, and this necessarily involves paying attention to offenders' needs as well as containing and reducing their risk" (Ward & Salmon, 2011, p. 401). However, "sex offenders also have obligations not to harm others" (Ward et al., 2007, p. 204).

Birgden (2009) undertakes the following argument regarding the balancing of rights and responsibilities:

> *Offender rehabilitation necessarily considers two complementary ethical positions - deontological and consequentialist. On the one hand, deontologists look to past conduct and state of mind at the time of offending. Deontologists appeal to the dignity of human beings and argue that it is never appropriate to violate human rights, and that individuals should not be treated as a means to achieve the ends of others. Deontologists maintain that the State and individuals have a duty to recognize the inherent value and worth of rights-holders. This position appeals to principles such as fairness, equality, or just deserts. On the other hand, consequentialists look to the future and ponder how to reduce the likelihood of*

> *re-offending. Consequentialists respect the utility of human rights in appealing to both individual and community rights and believe that the ends justify the means, utilizing whichever strategy - deterrence, incapacitation, or rehabilitation. A problem with a consequential position is that it justifies punishment and suspension of human rights if a cost-benefit analysis indicates that this will result in a greater amount of the value in question. That is, if the State overrides the offender's autonomy in the name of community protection, the deontological value for autonomy (e.g., never violate human rights) is overridden by the consequentialist value for autonomy (e.g., violate human rights on a cost-benefit basis). A normative framework can balance the deontological and consequential positions, and offender rehabilitation can aim to manage risk through control (justice for the community) and meet need through care (therapy for the offender). Therapeutic jurisprudence can assist in this balance (pp. 46-47).*

A key to examining issues of rights lies in the distinction between citizenship rights and human rights. All individuals have human rights guaranteed and unalterable by virtue of being human; citizenship rights, however, are those which one has by virtue of membership in a country or a community (Miller, 2007). Citizenship rights can, under certain circumstances, such as a legal violation, be removed or reduced.

However, for persons who have sexually offended, research has focused primarily on assessment, management, and treatment of risk for recidivism (Ward et al., 2007). Justification for this is based on protecting society from further victimization. Ward and colleagues (2007) suggested that persons who have sexually offended are often looked upon not as individuals who require treatment and support, but as being in need of management, which often takes the form of incarceration and punishment. In contrast, Glaser (2009) has suggested that:

> *It is no good trying to make decisions about treatment interventions if what you are offering is not treatment at all. It is also hypocritical for professionals to make a public commitment to an ethical code which stresses the primacy of the client when, all along their true concerns may be anything but the client's welfare (p. 254).*

WHAT IS THE DIFFERENCE BETWEEN TREATMENT AND MANAGEMENT?

Treatment is a designed approach that is developed to increase positive, functional skills and to reduce or alleviate a particular problem. Management, in contrast, is a reactive response aimed at controlling the behavior, responding to crises as they happen and 'putting out fires.' In a functional behavioral treatment program, the goal is to not only reduce the problem behavior but to provide the individual with the skills and abilities to control their own behavior, thereby allowing the individual as much control as possible over their own life and ultimately to enhance their quality of life. A functional behavioral approach also makes modifications to the environment to set the individual up for success. Whereas, management involves environmental engineering to control the behavior through sanctions, location or supervision. In the latter, the control remains largely with others. Unfortunately, once a person with an intellectual disability has committed a sexual offense, an agency supporting the individual often falls into management mode. Sometimes, if the management approach results in control of the behavior, the agency may not move forward on developing an active treatment program, because the problem is not causing imminent risk. However, management programs often can waiver over time, and inconsistent approaches may lead to recidivism. For example, in a case in which one of the authors was involved, a person was accused of a sexual offense. No active treatment program was put in place; instead the agency put the person on a 1-to-1, eyes-on supervision at all times. This strategy was effective for some time, but on many occasions the individual eluded staff supervision, and in one instance a second sexual offense occurred.

Management approaches are an important part of a comprehensive treatment package for persons who have sexually offended. However, in isolation they become repressive, restrictive, and, over time, are often ineffective. When used in combination with a treatment approach, management becomes part of a dynamic and fluid process that can change in relation to the risk factors present and, if treatment is effective, be reduced or even eliminated over time (see Wilson, Cortoni, Picheca, Stirpe, & Nunes, 2009).

In some programs, reducing risk to the community rather than rehabilitation is prioritized (Glaser, 2009). These programs are often court ordered, disregard human rights, and impose harsh restrictions and punishment as "treatment" (or, rather, treatment as punishment). Birgden and Cucolo (2011) championed this issue, asserted that treatment-as-management is unethical and ineffective, and argued that persons who offend often experience legal pressure to comply with forced treatment through processes like civil commitment that may not represent quality treatment with qualified professionals - offering minimal therapeutic benefits. In contrast, Ioannou (2013) noted that persons with intellectual disabilities who have offended may be living in community-based residential settings run by agencies that have embraced a rights-based approach to supporting individuals with intellectual disabilities. In these settings, balancing rights and risks may be skewed more towards the protection of rights of the individual, including the right to community living (Owen & MacKinnon, 2012), the right to consent to treatment (Watson, Richards, Hayes, Lecomte, & Taua, 2012), and rights within the justice system (Hamelin, Marinos, Robinson, & Griffiths, 2011). However, the literature on the rights of persons with intellectual disability is based on the cornerstone of the right of choice and decision-making within service delivery (Griffiths, Watson, Lewis, & Stoner, 2004). The cultural transformation towards rights has introduced a new dynamic of interacting with high-risk behaviors when exhibited by persons with intellectual disabilities, not just those who have offended. For example, does someone with Prader-Willi syndrome have the right to choose to consume large amounts of food and consequently put their health at risk? Does an individual with poor street safety skills have the right to choose to go into the community on their own and get injured? Does a person with an intellectual disability who has sexually offended against children have the right to choose to go to areas with children present and increase their risk of offending against a child? Owen and colleagues (2003) noted that community agencies that provide support for persons with intellectual disabilities must not only respect the rights of the people they support, they must also demonstrate responsibility for protecting the safety of those individuals who are considered vulnerable and who display high-risk behaviors (Owen et al., 2003).

Let us introduce some parallel issues that can inform the discussion of the potential paradox between ensuring rights while managing risk by examining the difficulties faced by persons supporting individuals with Prader-Willi syndrome. Prader-Willi syndrome is accompanied by severe overeating behavior that, if left unmanaged, can lead to life-threatening obesity and other serious health implications. Staff providing care to this population must manage two conflicting duties outlined in their agency policy: protecting the individuals by providing their duty of care, and respecting individual autonomy (Hawkins, Redley, & Holland, 2011). Through observations, semi-structured interviews, and file reviews, Hawkins and colleagues (2011) explored the balancing of these two competing demands. They found that although clearly identified risk management protocols had been established and areas were identified in which independence could be fostered, some staff elected to deviate from the established plan to incorporate unauthorized independence into the individual's care plan. This study illustrated that tension emerged between duty of care and autonomy but at the same time identified a valuable strategy of promoting independence where it is feasible without jeopardizing safety. Hawkins and colleagues (2011) illustrated a parallel discourse regarding balancing rights and risk. However, there is an exacerbated responsibility regarding this balance when referring to an individual who may pose a risk not only to themselves, but to others who may be very vulnerable. As such, a key factor in selecting an environment is maintaining a balance of both risk management and rights.

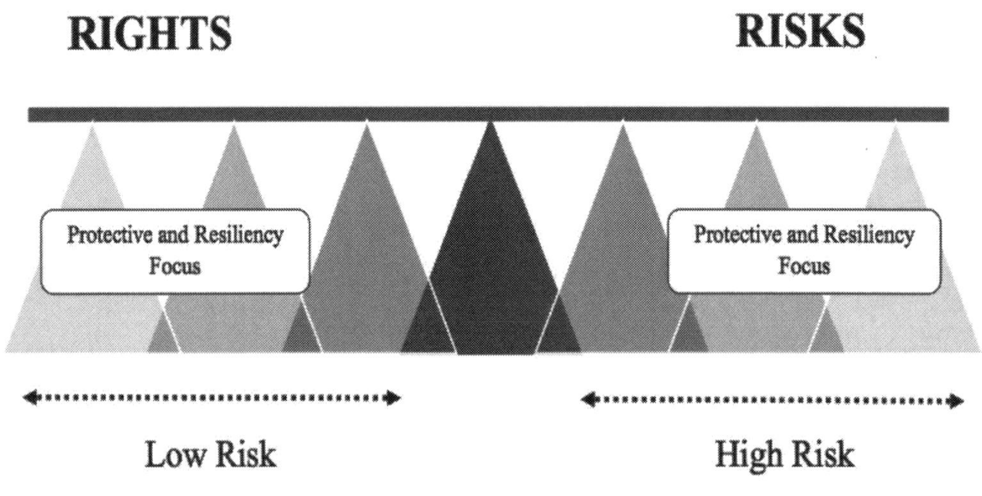

Figure 13.1. **Balancing rights with risks requires a shifting fulcrum depending on the needs, risk, and responsivity factors of the individual offender, but there should always be a focus on reinforcement (protection/ resiliency) Reproduced with permission from Ioannou (2013)**

Ioannou (2013) reported that there is often an unequal balance depending on the type of community setting. She noted that in residential settings, such as community group homes that are not designed for people who have offended, there was a greater emphasis on protecting rights than on reducing risks and community protection. In contrast, community-based treatment and transitional settings emphasized risks and community protection over rights. It could be argued simply that higher risk individuals resided in treatment and transitional homes and that lower risk individuals lived in residential homes. However, it could also mean that these different approaches are only based on the type of setting and not the individual's support needs and level of risk posed. This was the case in a meta-analysis of studies involving men with an intellectual disability who had sexually offended; levels of supervision were not consistent with their level of risk, where low risk offenders were receiving intensive supervision (Tough, 2001). Ioannou (2013) cautioned that the imbalance in some community settings could represent that rights and risk are not being considered as equally important but as separate entities. She suggested that "in the absence of this kind of balanced approach…sex offenders with intellectual disability may be insufficiently supported" (Ioannou, 2013, p. 104). As a result, she concluded that balancing the rights and risks requires a shifting fulcrum depending on the risk, needs, and responsivity factors of the individual in question (see Figure 13.1). Thus, regardless of setting, persons who have offended require an appropriate balance between protection and resiliency based on the needs of the individual who has the capacity to change over time. The balance must be adjusted as individual needs change. A unidimensional focus only on rights or risks does not ensure that individual needs are being appropriately met, nor that balance is alterable as the needs of the individual change in response to treatment.

HOW DOES THE BEHAVIOR ANALYSIS CERTIFICATION BOARD® (BACB) PROFESSIONAL AND ETHICAL CODE OF CONDUCT FOR BEHAVIOR ANALYSTS (2014) APPLY TO THE PRACTICE OF BEHAVIOR ANALYSIS WITH PERSONS WITH INTELLECTUAL DISABILITIES WHO HAVE COMMITTED A SEXUAL OFFENSE?

Persons with intellectual disabilities who display inappropriate sexual behavior are often referred to, or come into contact with, agencies and clinicians who provide behavioral services. Like other professions, when applying behavior analytic interventions with any client, there are specific guidelines that behavior analysts must follow, and the same considerations apply when working with individuals with intellectual disabilities who have sexually offended. The BACB® *Professional and Ethical Compliance Code for Behavior Analysts* (BACB, 2014), which will hereafter be referred to as "the Code," is composed of ten sections. The first four sections of the Code are particularly pertinent to practice: *1.0 – Responsible Conduct of Behavior Analysts; 2.0 – Behavior Analysts' Responsibility to Clients; 3.0 – Assessing Behavior; and 4.0 – Behavior Analysts and the Behavior - Change Program* (BACB, 2014). Although not every clinician working with persons with intellectual disabilities and sexual offending behavior will be certified by the BACB®, the Code still represents best practice for those providing behavioral assessment and intervention, regardless of their title or population served. Items in each section of the Code that are particularly relevant to assessment and treatment of individuals who have sexually offended will be discussed later in this chapter. The remaining sections of the Code include: Behavior Analysts as Supervisors –

5.0, Behavior Analysts' Ethical Responsibility to the Profession of Behavior Analysis – 6.0, Behavior Analysts' Ethical Responsibility to Colleagues – 7.0, Public Statements – 8.0, Behavior Analysts and Research – 9.0, and Behavior Analysts' Ethical Responsibility to the BACB – 10. When behavior analysts become certified by the BACB®, as a Board Certified Behavior Analyst (BCBA®), Board Certified Behavior Analyst-Doctoral (BCBA-D™), a Board Certified Assistant Behavior Analyst (BCaBA®), or a Registered Behavior Technician (RBT®) they are responsible for being familiar with and abiding by the Code (BACB, 2014). The information that follows does not replace the need for behavior analytic practitioners to review the Code in detail: (http://bacb.com/ethics-code/).

Section 1 of the Code (BACB, 2014), *1.0 - Responsible Conduct of Behavior Analysts,* attempts to ensure that "behavior analysts maintain the high standards of behavior of the profession" (p. 4). This includes relying on the best available scientific evidence when providing services (1.01), being aware of competency boundaries in all that they do (1.02), maintaining their competence through professional development (1.03), maintaining integrity (1.04), maintaining sound professional and scientific relationships (1.05), avoiding multiple relationships and conflicts of interest (1.06), and avoiding exploitative relationships (1.06 – BACB, 2014, pp. 4-6).

One clause regarding integrity (1.04) may be encountered when a clinician is working with individuals who have been in the criminal justice system:

> *1.04 (e) If behavior analysts' ethical responsibilities conflict with law or any policy of an organization with which they are affiliated, behavior analysts make known their commitment to this Code and take steps to resolve the conflict in a responsible manner in accordance with law.*

People with sexual offense histories may have probation orders or restrictions from the courts that interfere with the ethical standards outlined in the Code. Behavior analysts must abide by these orders and provide services that adhere to the Code within these parameters that have been dictated by law.

Two clauses with respect to maintaining professional and scientific relationships (1.05) that may be particularly relevant when working with individuals with intellectual disabilities and sexual offending behavior include:

> *1.05 (c) Where differences of age, gender, race, culture, ethnicity, national origin, religion, sexual orientation, disability, language, or socioeconomic status significantly affect behavior analysts' work concerning particular individuals or groups, behavior analysts obtain the training, experience, consultation, and/or supervision necessary to ensure the competence of their services, or they make appropriate referrals.* (BACB, 2014, p. 5)

> *1.05 (d) In their work-related activities, behavior analysts do not engage in discrimination against individuals or groups based on age, gender, race, culture, ethnicity, national origin, religion, sexual orientation, disability, language, socioeconomic status, or any basis proscribed by law.* (BACB, 2014, p. 5)

Clinicians undertaking this type of work must ask themselves about their own attitudes and biases. Someone who is uncomfortable discussing sexual topics for personal or religious reasons may experience great challenges acclimatizing to work involving persons who sexually offend. Additionally, the clinician's attitudes toward the sexuality or sexual rights of persons with intellectual disabilities is also important to consider, as are attitudes towards someone who has sexually offended. These attitudes are important to consider prior to undertaking this type of treatment commitment. The nature of this work means that it may not be possible for all clinicians to effectively or ethically undertake such duties. As such, this type of work should only be done by those who feel that they can be effective and ethical change agents. As a very wise supervisor from a Christian organization serving persons with intellectual disabilities once explained to a colleague years ago when asked if the lecture just given about sexuality was in her opinion morally sound, her reply was that working with sex offenders with intellectual disabilities is not about morality it is about ethics. Morality is how she chose to live her own life; ethics is what she did in her professional life to ensure the appropriate treatment of the persons she was entrusted to support.

Operating in the best interests of the client includes careful consideration of the client's rights which, as mentioned previously, can be complex and often misunderstood when treating those with sexual offending behavior. Section 2 of the Code (BACB, 2014), *2.0 - Behavior Analysts' Responsibility to Clients,* specifies that, "Behavior analysts have a responsibility to operate in the best interest of clients" (p. 6) and includes responsibilities common to providing any treatment, such as maintaining confidentiality (2.06, 2.08, described later), maintaining appropriate records (2.07, 2.10, 2.11, 2.12, 2.13), conducting appropriate referrals and fee schedules (2.14), and discontinuation or termination of services (2.15). Section 2 also includes clauses that may be particularly relevant to those practitioners who work with individuals with sexual offending behavior, including only accepting clients to whom the behavior analysts is qualified to provide services (2.01), arranging for appropriate consultations with other professionals (2.02), and "cooperating with other professionals, in a manner that is consistent with the philosophical assumptions and principles of behavior analysis, in order to effectively and appropriately serve their clients" (2.03, p. 6). Section 2 also describes the responsibility to clients when there is third party involvement (2.04). This is especially relevant since behavior analysts will often be working with individuals who reside in forensic mental health institutions or community agencies that have sought behavior analytic services. In working with third-parties:

> *2.04 (d) Behavior analysts put the client's care above all others and, should the third party make requirements for services that are contraindicated by the behavior analyst's recommendations, behavior analysts are obligated to resolve such conflicts in the best interest of the client. If said conflict cannot be resolved, that behavior analyst's services to the client may be discontinued following appropriate transition.*

Forensic mental health settings and support agencies may have strict policies that contradict standards in the Code, which can include restrictions or punitive measures decided by the agency that have not been directed by law. An agency supporting an individual may have policies that are against healthy sexuality or that may refuse reinforcement procedures due to staffing and operational issues. In these circumstances, behavior analysts need to make every effort to adhere to the Code, despite pressures from operational sources or third-parties.

Regarding treatment and client rights, the Code (BACB, 2014) specifies that all behavior analytic treatments should be based in science:

> *2.09. (a) Clients have a right to effective treatment (i.e., based on the research literature and adapted to the individual client). Behavior analysts always have the obligation to advocate for and educate the client about scientifically supported, most-effective treatment procedures. Effective treatment procedures have been validated as having both long-term and short-term benefits to clients and society. (b) Behavior analysts have the responsibility to advocate for the appropriate amount and level of service provision and oversight required to meet the defined behavior-change program goals. (c) In those instances where more than one scientifically supported treatment has been established, additional factors may be considered in selecting interventions, including, but not limited to, efficiency and cost-effectiveness, risks and side-effects of the interventions, client preference, and practitioner experience and training. (d) Behavior analysts review and appraise the effects of any treatments about which they are aware that might impact the goals of the behavior-change program, and their possible impact on the behavior change program, to the extent possible.* (p. 8)

This particular section of the Code has several implications for behavior analysts undertaking this type of work. First, it implies that treatment should be empirically-validated or supported through experimentation and found to produce significant and positive outcomes (Chamless et al., 1988). Psychology has long been a strong proponent of practice that is evidence-based (APA Presidential Task Force, 2006). One method of evaluating evidence-based practice is through the development of guidelines for best practice, such as those developed by the *Association for the Treatment of Sexual Abusers* (Blasingame, Boer, Guidry, Haaven, & Wilson, 2014). Second, the viability of implementation of recommended practice must be evaluated. Various jurisdictions or agencies may not have the supports or finances necessary to provide certain approaches. Ethical practice must ensure not only that the approach that best matches the person's needs is selected but that the practitioner is able to carry it out responsibly.

As mentioned in Chapter 4, before appropriate and effective interventions can be developed, a functional assessment of behavior is necessary and must be objectively conducted. Section three of the Code (BACB, 2014), *3.0 - Assessing Behavior,* asserts that "Behavior analysts using behavior-analytic assessment techniques do so for purposes that are appropriate given current research" (p. 10):

> *3.01 (a) Behavior analysts conduct current assessments prior to making recommendations or developing behavior-change programs. The type of assessment used is determined by client's needs and consent, environmental parameters, and other contextual variables. When behavior analysts are developing a behavior-reduction program, they must first conduct a functional assessment. (b) Behavior analysts have an obligation to collect and graphically display data, using behavior-analytic conventions, in a manner that allows for decisions and recommendations for behavior-change program development.* (p. 10)

In addition, when conducting assessments, behavior analysts should seek medical consultation to rule out behaviors being due to medical or biological causes (3.02);

ensure that appropriate consent is obtained; describe the assessment in full, including how the results will be used (3.03); explain the assessment in a way that makes sense to the client using supports if needed (3.04); and receive informed consent before sharing assessment results with other parties (3.05 - BACB, 2014, p. 11).

After the functional behavior assessment is completed (as described in Chapter 4), interventions should be based on the assessment results, taking into consideration all important variables (e.g., medical, contextual, richness of the environment, history of childhood trauma, etc.). The behavior analyst who was involved in the assessment should also be involved in the intervention planning and take responsibility for all aspects of implementation. Section 4 of the Code, *4.0 - Behavior Analysts and the Behavior-Change Program*, specifies that, "Behavior analysts are responsible for all aspects of the behavior-change program from conceptualization to implementation and ultimately to discontinuation" (p. 11). The program should be consistent with behavior analytic principles (4.01), clients should be involved in the planning of the program (4.02) the program should be individualized to the clients' needs and goals, and the program should be unique (i.e., not copied from a previous case, or clinician) (4.03). The client should provide written approval of the program before implementation or modification where possible (4.04) and the behavior analyst should describe the program risk-benefit analysis in detail and continue to do so throughout the duration of the relationship (4.05). The behavior analyst is also responsible for describing to the client the environmental conditions that are necessary for program success (4.06), as well as the conditions that may interfere with the program (4.07) and describing measurable criteria for program termination, in addition to how such services would be terminated (4.11). Section 4 also contains information regarding punishment procedures (4.08), least restrictive procedures (4.09), and avoiding harmful reinforcers (4.10) that are described later.

WHAT ARE THE ETHICS OF PUNISHMENT WHEN DEALING WITH PERSONS WITH INTELLECTUAL DISABILITIES?

Ward and Salmon (2011) have suggested that clinicians need to be clear about their opinions regarding punishment; without careful examination, there runs a risk that offenders may be treated in methods that are demeaning, create deprivation, or use unjustifiable sanctions. According to the Code (BACB, 2014):

> *4.08 (a) Behavior analysts recommend reinforcement rather than punishment whenever possible. (b) If punishment procedures are necessary, behavior analysts always include reinforcement procedures for alternative behavior in the behavior-change program. (c) Before implementing punishment-based procedures, behavior analysts ensure that appropriate steps have been taken to implement reinforcement-based procedures unless the severity or dangerousness of the behavior necessitates immediate use of aversive procedures. (d) Behavior analysts ensure that aversive procedures are accompanied by an increased level of training, supervision, and oversight. Behavior analysts must evaluate the effectiveness of aversive procedures in a timely manner and modify the behavior-change program if it is ineffective. Behavior analysts always include a plan to discontinue the use of aversive procedures when no longer needed.*

> *4.09 Least Restrictive Procedures. Behavior analysts review and appraise the restrictiveness of procedures and always recommend the least restrictive procedures likely to be effective.*
>
> *4.10 Avoiding Harmful Reinforcers. Behavior analysts minimize the use of items as potential reinforcers that may be harmful to the health and development of the client, or that may require excessive motivating operations to be effective.*

When consulting to agencies that support persons with sexual offending behavior, punishment-based procedures are often used first because they have immediate effects and require less response effort by the caregivers or staffing team when there is a lack of resources and if other operational issues are present. This approach may be justified if the individual is at high risk to harm others and when agency liability is on the line. However, in these circumstances, implementing reinforcement-based procedures does not become a priority and the sole focus becomes management, violating the client's right to effective treatment.

WHY HAS THERE BEEN SO LITTLE ABA RESEARCH ON THE TREATMENT OF PERSONS WITH INTELLECTUAL DISABILITIES WHO HAVE SEXUALLY OFFENDED? HOW DOES ONE RESEARCH THE EFFECTIVENESS OF TREATMENT WITH THIS POPULATION USING ABA PRACTICES?

The BACB Code (2014) clearly identifies that evidence-based practice must be followed. As noted in Chapter 1, early research on treatment for people with sexual offending histories was based on behavioral principles; however, the type of research that was conducted then typically involved punitive and unifactorial approaches. This approach failed to produce lasting changes and fell into disuse. More recently, as discussed in the Preface of this book, Vollmer (2014) and Lindsay (2015) posed rival hypotheses regarding the lack of current behaviorally-based research regarding persons with intellectual disabilities who have committed sexual offenses. Vollmer (2014) hypothesized that a lack of evidence-based research may be associated with the clandestine and infrequent nature of the behaviors. Lindsay (2015) proposed that the lack of empirical ABA research on persons who have sexually offended might be because it was tried and did not work. As noted, the authors of this book respect the logic of both hypotheses but have posited an alternative hypothesis. Our hypothesis, based on years of clinical experience, is that the challenge in producing empirically-supported ABA research with persons with intellectual disabilities who have sexually offended stems from the traditional methods of analysis. We believe that by using the logical functional model, discussed by Wulfert, Greenway, and Dougher (1996), and functional behavioral assessment widely used in other areas of ABA and elaborated in this text, that a clear protocol and testable analysis and treatment can be validated.

The key to effective and ethical treatment for people who have offended depends on being able to provide an individualized program that allows for habilitative opportunities, as well as learning and application to reduce dynamic risk factors such as self-management and regulation that serve as contributing conditions for an offense (Griffiths, in press). Some authors have suggested that treatment should follow a set manual (e.g., Newsom & Hovanitz, 2005) to ensure therapeutic integrity (Laws & Marshall, 2003; see also Bonta & Andrews, 2017). However, other authors (e.g., Marshall, 2009) have cautioned that following a highly prescriptive manual can produce a rigidity that will lose the individuality of treatment by producing a one-size-fits-all approach. The same consideration is evident in ABA, which takes a highly individualized treatment approach based on assessment results.

Marshall (2009) noted that guidelines, as opposed to prescribed manuals, provide valuable information that can inform treatment without running the risk of prescribing treatment goals or approaches, which should be dependent on individual needs based on assessment outcomes. An example of this is Lindsay's (2009) workbook on assessment and treatment of individuals with intellectual disabilities who have offended; the workbook was not prescriptive, rather it affords the reader with both the theoretical and research developments in the field and provided examples of how these are applied in his work with people who have offended.

Griffiths (2002) suggested that state of the art interventions for sexual offenses involve multi-component assessment and treatment. Although some earlier research has seen the application of functional assessment (e.g., Fredericks & Nishioka-Evans, 1999), few studies have evaluated multi-component treatment that would constitute best practice. One exception is Lund (1992), who reported on the effectiveness of a multi-component program involving individual counselling, socio-sexual training, and individualized behavioral programs. Although the study lacked tight empirical rigour, Lund reported that following treatment, individuals were able to be discharged to the community in less restrictive settings, experienced reduced restrictive procedures, and demonstrated generalization and maintenance of gains for up to two years.

Despite a lack of empirical demonstration of the outcomes of a comprehensive ABA approach to the treatment of sexual offenders with intellectual disabilities, the authors of this book propose that the principles of ABA can be appropriately applied to this population with adaptations, such as the type of research that is conducted to demonstrate the effects of multi-factorial treatment.

The traditional approach to research in the broader social sciences has revolved around variables as abstractions of constructs. For example, to study social skills, a group of individuals are measured on social skills and a person receives a score that places them within a rank order or, at best, a position on an interval scale. Consistent with Vollmer's (2014) reasons for the lack of research in this area, the clandestine and infrequent nature of the behaviors do not lend themselves to scaling on a normal distribution, an intransigent assumption of traditional methods. In addition, the strongly contextual nature of offenses is not easily characterized by a single construct measured at the individual level. For a detailed explanation of these weaknesses of the 'variable-centric' research approach, see Magnusson (2003). A final characteristic of traditional research models is that inferences can only be made from construct-to-construct. That is, knowing something about 'social skills' when measured across individuals only tells us something about the distribution of social skills and only allows us to compare groups on mean social skills, or correlate social skills with some other dimension. What it does *not* allow for are inferences back to a particular individual. These may be some of the reasons why research in this area has not worked, as has been noted by Lindsay (2015).

Noted behavior analysts have long been commenting on the limitations of our current research approaches to study complex phenomenon in the field of intellectual disability. Baumeister (1997, p. 9) suggested that the field of research regarding intellectual disability was experiencing "paradigm paralysis", indicating that our methods of research have been inadequate and inappropriate both conceptually and methodologically. Similarly, Risley (1999) noted that there is a need for researchers to adopt methodologies that are more innovative and that focus on goals that have more social validity. This was echoed by Holburn (2002), in citing Skinner's (1953) idea of social contingencies and Glenn's (1988) concepts of metacontingencies. In this latter theory "interlocking social contingencies can be linked to aggregate consequences." In some respects, this perspective echoes assertions by researchers like Cullen and Gendreau (2000) who suggest that a rigid adherence to traditional statistical significance ($p <$ .05) may not always fully appreciate the social significance of findings at the $p < .10$ level. This is particularly true of research seeking to establish the importance of treatment participation (i.e., efficacy).

Bergman and Magnusson (1997) have suggested a person-oriented approach to research that is both holistic and dynamic. In a holistic-interactional approach, the individual is studied in context, based on their patterns of individual characteristics that are relevant to the problem under consideration. Adapting their approach to the investigation of person-oriented outcomes for persons with intellectual disabilities who have sexually offended would have many advantages. First the process would be specific to an individual. Second, examination of a process allows for complex and multiple factors to be integrated. Third, each intervention is coherent and follows a logical and functionally organized structure. Fourth, the process follows the same operating patterns and allows for interaction with other factors. Lastly, although each individual obtains a different intervention plan geared to their needs as determined through assessment, globally, all individuals have followed the same process to obtain their individualized goals. A specific methodology is needed to address person-oriented assessment and treatment. Single-case experimental designs (SCED), first described by Murray Sidman in 1960, assess how certain systematic manipulations of the independent variable (e.g., specific interventions) impact changes in the dependent variable (e.g., outcomes of intervention). SCEDs differ from case studies in that experimental control is demonstrated and more than one individual can be involved. SCEDs differ from group designs in that important individual variability can be observed across time and is not "washed out" in group averages.

WHAT WOULD A PERSON-ORIENTED APPROACH TO RESEARCH WITH INDIVIDUALS WITH INTELLECTUAL DISABILITIES WHO HAVE OFFENDED ACTUALLY LOOK LIKE?

In this model, the inference space, which is the limits on how broadly a particular result applies (Lorenzen & Anderson 1993), is defined by the problem under consideration. This may include dimensions relating to personal and/or developmental characteristics (e.g., social skills or impulse control), contextual factors (e.g., experience of rights training, presence of risky environments), or behaviors (e.g., the number and type of sex offenses). Each person is represented by their position on each of these dimensions, such that several individuals who appear to be similar on one dimension may be quite dissimilar depending on their position on other dimensions. Figure 13.2 depicts this in schematic form. Persons A, B, and C have all committed the same number or type of sexual offenses, but the 'psychological/contextual significance' (adapted from Figure 1.1b in Magnusson, 2003, p. 15) of these offenses differ dramatically according to their position on the other constructs.

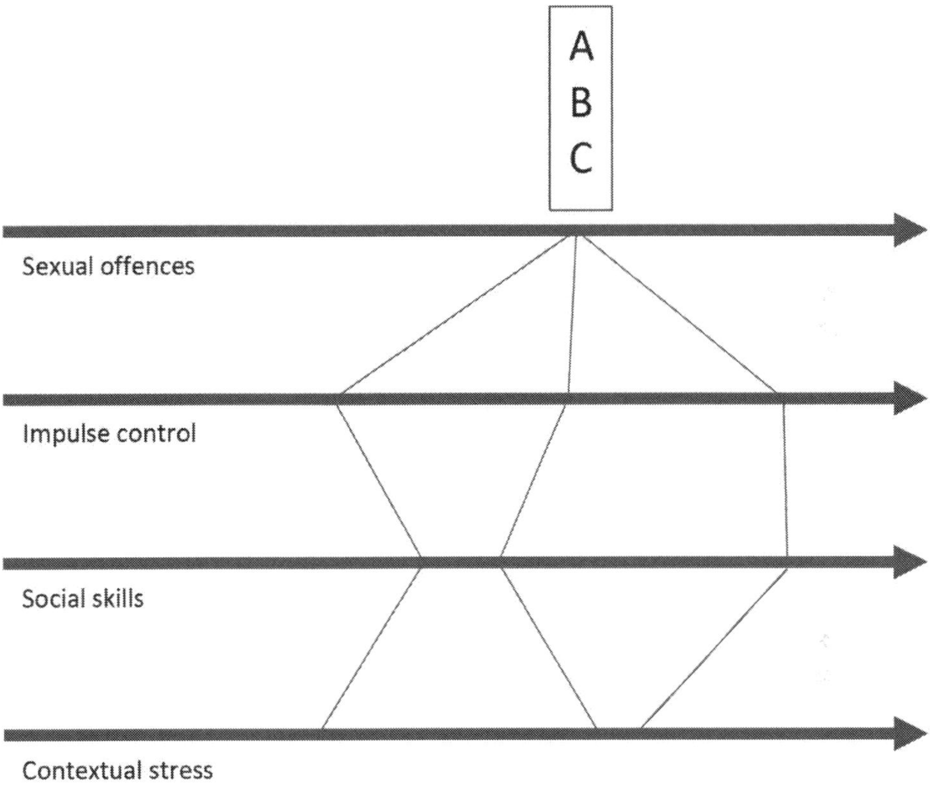

Figure 13.2. **A schematic representing how the person-centered approach characterizes across, rather than within, constructs that define a research problem. Person A, B, and C are all equivalent in the measure of sexual offense, but the developmental interpretation is dramatically different based on each person's profile across the constructs in the problem space.**

The purpose of a person-centered approach is two-fold. First, because the inference space is the *research problem,* individuals may be similar in their pattern across the dimensions, and inferences can be drawn to groups of individuals who cluster together. For example, higher risk individuals with greater socio-sexual knowledge and an awareness of social norms may be contrasted with individuals who commit sexual offenses with greatly reduced socio-sexual knowledge and familiarity with social norms, the so-called "counterfeit deviants" (Lunsky, Frijters, Griffiths, Watson, &

Williston, 2007). Second, developmental or personal change factors can be characterized in terms of relative movement on one dimension of the problem space. This may be particularly relevant to individuals who shift from one group to another due, for example, to rights training or a shift in context from more to less risky. In either case, the person-oriented approach allows for inferences back to the individual, while taking a strongly contextual approach to the research issue.

A person-oriented approach to research has been demonstrated in relation to other challenging behaviors. For example, Feldman, Condillac, Tough, Hunt, and Griffiths (2002) demonstrated the effectiveness of following a behavioral protocol for assessment and design of individually-based treatment for persons with intellectual disabilities and severe challenging behaviors (such as self-injury and aggression). Each participant received a comprehensive multi-component assessment of medical and environmental factors that may be maintaining behavior (function). Individualized intervention packages were derived from the assessment findings and included antecedent- and consequence-based strategies and mediator training. Using a multiple-baseline design across 20 participants, they reported decreases in problem behavior and increases in functional replacement skills in all participants, as well as notable improvement in quality of life.

The SCED approach used by Feldman and colleagues (2002) allowed for several critical areas to be integrated into the research design. First, the multiple baseline approach allows for effects of the treatment approach to be evaluated. Second, the design was not only able to measure reduction in challenging behavior, but also the correlated increase in replacement behaviors, which are critical for generalization and maintenance. Third, their study monitored the long-term effectiveness of treatment and impact on quality of life. And, last but not least, it allowed for the individualization of treatment for the specific needs of each individual through ongoing observation and documents of the individuals' behavior.

This latter point is perhaps critical to the design of current research on effective treatment for sexual offenders with intellectual disabilities. Previous studies have attempted "one-size-fits-all" approaches to treatment to determine efficacy. The challenge with selecting one component of treatment to explore is that it may not be the needed component for that individual, or it may be that that component will not be effective unless it is part of the multi-component package.

WHAT WOULD CONSTITUTE RECOMMENDED PRACTICE IN MEASURING EFFECTIVENESS OF PRACTICE OF TREATMENT USING ABA APPROACHES? WHAT ARE THE OUTCOME GOALS?

To ensure that intervention is meeting appropriate standards, it must be carefully evaluated. Much of the early work in the field was based on evaluation of frequency of occurrence (Polvinale & Lutzker, 1980), readmission rates (Dial, 1968), observation of precursor behaviors (Wong, Gaydos & Fuqua, 1982), response latency (Shaw & Walker, 1979), and self-report (Rosenthal, 1973). The reliance on relapse or readmission rates as the dependent measure may not represent accurate pictures of the re-offense rates because they depend on detection. It is a well-known phenomenon that a majority of persons who are sexually victimized fail to make a report of their experiences to authorities, resulting in difficulties in establishing both incidence and prevalence for sexual offending and re-offending. Self-report measures may suffer from report bias, as the individual who offended attempts to elude punishment. The use of analogue functional assessment, while valuable, may be subject to concern regarding treatment generalization. Due to the dangerousness and low frequency of the behaviors, some have argued for the use of precursor behaviors both as treatment targets and dependent measures.

Without a doubt, zero recidivism is the ultimate goal of treatment of persons with intellectual disabilities who have sexually offended although it is unlikely that this goal will ever be achieved. However, using an individualized approach, it may be more reasonable to employ a perspective like that advocated by Circles of Support and Accountability (discussed in Chapter 11). The principal motto of CoSA is "no more victims;" however, this is individually focused, in that the goal is to ensure no more victims for this particular core member, rather than no more victims as a global construct (Wilson & McWhinnie, 2017).

Interventions are focused on reducing dynamic risk factors (Beech & Ward, 2004). However, recommended practice suggests that it is not sufficient to evaluate just a lack of recidivism or even the lack of precursor behaviors. Recommended practice would suggest that concurrent to measuring the reduction of the problem behaviors, practitioners should also measure the development of positive skills or replacement behaviors that serve to allow the individual to maintain a level of positive engagement and activities to enhance the probability that the challenging behaviors will not re-emerge. As Ward (2007) notes, matters arising from risk management also include whether treatment programs are attentive to the interests and wellbeing of the offender.

In more recent years there has been an emphasis on the establishment of personal goals within treatment programs for persons who have sexually offended. Although some studies such as Swanson and Garwick (1990), evaluated effectiveness of their group training based on re-arrest rates, they also measured the impact on personal goals. However, the personal goals were not demonstrated to relate directly to recidivism. Recommended practice in the field would dictate that effectiveness should be measured as both the reduction in the target offending behavior and its precursors, as well as the concurrent increase in replacement and coping behaviors that have been individually determined to relate to offending. In addition, global skills and life enriching improvements in relationships, activities, and interests (which may serve to enhance the person's overall quality of life) should be evaluated to ensure that the program is providing a direct impact on the person's well-being and personal satisfaction.

To restate: "Current programs would benefit from evaluation of not just the reduction in challenging behavior, but also a concurrent demonstrating of increased coping and skill development and an improvement in quality of life" (Griffiths, Watson, Stoner, & Lewis, 2004, p. 324). As Ward and Salman (2011) suggest, "A caring clinician is obligated to ensure that sex offenders in treatment acquire the capabilities to function independently when released into the community. This obligation should encourage them to think beyond simply implementing a set of treatment protocols and instead inquire into the well-being and basic living skills an offender presents with" (p. 408).

In the field of intellectual disabilities, person-centered planning has been adopted as the preferred and often mandatory method to determine goals for the individual and to put in place supports needed to achieve those goals to enhance quality of life; however this approach is directed by the individual and based on self-directed goals.

HOW DOES PERSON CENTERED PLANNING FIT INTO A TREATMENT AND SUPPORT PLAN FOR PERSONS WITH INTELLECTUAL DISABILITIES WHO SEXUALLY OFFEND?

Challenging and adaptive behaviors have been linked to personal control and self-determination (see Schalock, 1994; Stancliffe & Wehmeyer, 1995). When individuals have limited means to assert themselves and reach their goals, either because of a lack of skill or because of a lack of agency, the person may use behavior that is inappropriate however potentially effective, to make desired change or reach a goal. Thus, it is important that the goals that are determined are those that coincide with those of the individual.

Decisions made in developing a person-centered plan are made by the individual with input from significant others who the individual chooses to be part of the plan. The goals of the individual are vital in providing direction for the person's plan, and, because they are the individual's goals, they are ones for which the person is more likely to be motivated to achieve. Not all goals selected may be possible or, perhaps, immediately available. However, working towards the goals or a possible variation thereof can be instrumental in moving forward on a person's plan. Let us take, for example, the person who has sexually offended against children and who wishes to work at McDonalds. The goal of work is one that could be planned for by the group; however, McDonalds represents a high-risk environment for someone who has offended against a child and would place the person and potentially vulnerable children at risk. Thus, through a process of creative discussion they find out that the individual wanted that job because he loved to cook. An alternative type of restaurant setting may therefore be possible for him to achieve his goal consistent with Good Lives principles we discussed in Chapters 6 and 12. Moreover, understanding the goal allows the support agency to begin a process in which he can learn to cook, start watching cooking shows on television, learn to read cookbooks, and, if appropriate, take a course at a community college. This plan may take some time to achieve, but because it is the person's goal and steps are being put in place to make it a reality the individual is likely to be motivated to work towards it. Moreover, this goal is one that has both immediate reinforcement (people get to eat) and can, if successful, be tied into the natural contingencies of reinforcement (people praise people who cook good food).

Obviously, because of the nature of the offense that was committed, the individual in the preceding paragraph will concurrently be in an active treatment program for the offending behaviors and may not have choice about where to live at this stage. However, the idea of planning *with* the person for long term goals sets a stage where the potential for success is enhanced and responsivity is maximized.

Using the SMART goal acronym can assist in goal development for persons who sexually offend (see Peel Behavioral Service & Wilson, 2017). When helping the individual come up with goals, it is important that the goal is Specific, Measurable, Attainable,

Realistic, and Timely. As outlined in the previous example of working at McDonalds, if a goal that the individual decides on is not attainable or realistic for risk purposes, it is the supporting group's responsibility to not dismiss the goal but gather more information to come up with an alternative goal that serves the same purpose.

As stated previously, the goal of offender treatment is to create a Good Life (Ward & Stewart, 2003). In the field of intellectual disabilities, we often refer to this as measured by quality of life.

HOW DOES THE CONCEPT OF QUALITY OF LIFE FIT IN WITH TREATMENT OF PERSONS WITH INTELLECTUAL DISABILITIES WHO HAVE COMMITTED A SEXUAL OFFENSE?

Steptoe, Lindsay, Forest, and Power (2008) have shown that persons with intellectual disabilities and sexual offense histories have poorer relationships and demonstrate less integration and involvement within society than persons with intellectual disabilities who have not sexually offended. They found that individuals who have offended had less support from parents and other relationships and reported being content with these more impoverished relationships. Additionally, they reported less involvement in the community and fewer leisure activities, such as hobbies. Lindsay and colleagues (2004) similarly reported more problems in relationships among persons with intellectual disabilities and sexual behavior problems.

Lindsay (2005) suggested that engagement in society may be a key element in treatment of persons with intellectual disabilities and sexual behavior problems by providing appropriate activities and social relationships. When discussing the importance of engagement in society, Lindsay (2005) emphasized the importance of not re-offending and the value of providing community opportunities. He suggested that we remember the Bob Dylan line, "When you ain't got nothing, you got nothing to lose." As discussed throughout this book, many persons with intellectual disabilities who have sexually offended have seemingly nothing to lose. They have barren relationships with others, and, because of their behaviors, they have typically lost all privileges and opportunities. Thus, another re-offense can have little impact on their already dismal existence.

There are several ways to move towards a richer existence in which the person has value that would be worth keeping one from re-offending. As well, these value-added elements of life make it less likely the person will re-offend because engagement in meaningful relationships and activities takes up time that may have previously been used to engage in inappropriate behavior. It may also potentially fill a reinforcement void that previously existed; in particular, if treatment has provided the individual with skills hooked into the natural contingencies of society.

The first way that treatment strategies can begin to build a life worth keeping is to begin by providing an environment in which the person is treated with dignity and respect and is provided opportunities to engage in life enriching activities. The concept of treating individuals who have offended with dignity and respect has been widely heralded by Ward (2011). Notwithstanding the fact that the person has committed a serious offense, the staff and therapists who elect to work with such an individual must be fundamentally understanding of the fact that this person has human value and, therefore, must be treated with respect. This means providing an optimal program for growth and engagement, in which the person can receive reinforcement within their daily life, both contingent and non-contingent.

Secondly, as relationship skills are modeled and taught, the individual needs to have opportunities to begin to build a network of positive social influence. Lindsay (2009) suggested that as an individual who offended progresses in treatment, there is a need to be transitioned into community activities by reaching out to other agencies, such as colleges or leisure activities in which the person can begin to expand their relationship pool. The caveat to this is, however, that appropriate risk management must be in place as these transitions occur.

HOW DOES ONE DEAL WITH THE ISSUE OF CONFIDENTIALITY WHEN WORKING WITH A PERSON WHO HAS SEXUALLY OFFENDED AND WHO MAY BE LIVING IN THE COMMUNITY OR WHEN ATTEMPTING TO MOVE THE PERSON INTO A LESS RESTRICTIVE ENVIRONMENT?

The question of confidentiality is one that causes great concern for all clinicians and service providers. Glaser (2009) has suggested that although models of treatment for sexual offending have incorporated mandatory limitations on confidentiality to protect the public, the dilemma continues to pervade practice as to when and under what conditions should confidentiality be breached. As Glaser (2009) suggests, "[e]thics is very much about making appropriate decisions in certain contexts" (p. 254).

If the person who offended is being treated outside of a closed facility, such as in their community home or in a group home, the person will inevitably be in contact with the public. As well, to build an enriching lifestyle for the person to increase the potential of nonoffending, it is therapeutically valuable to ensure that the person is engaged in the community as much as possible and with appropriate risk management strategies in place. But, is there an obligation for a service provider to inform the public? If the person is working in a store, attending school or just living in a neighborhood, should those who are engaging with the person know that the person has a history of a sexual offense? Public notification of persons who have sexually offended occurs in different variations in Canada, the United States, and elsewhere. In some jurisdictions, individuals who have sexually offended have their addresses made public, and in some US states, mandatory signs may be erected on their lawns identifying them as a "sex offender" or "predator" (see discussion of public notification processes in Wilson & Sandler, in press). Many parents and community members argue that it is their right to know if someone in their community poses a danger to their family. However, on the other end of the spectrum, the individual who offended has a right to community re-integration and the chance to be a functioning member of society, albeit offense free. Moreover, from a treatment and risk perspective, community disclosures of persons who have sexually offended typically result in hostile communities, which is not conducive to treatment or rehabilitation and, consequently, may increase the risk of re-offending.

In terms of confidentiality and disclosure, a more urgent decision arises if the person discloses an interest in re-offending and whether they disclose a plan to do so. This represents the limits to confidentiality and when there is a duty to report.

Section 2 of the Code (BACB, 2014), 2.0 – *Behavior Analysts Responsibility to Clients,* addresses confidentiality in detail and 2.08 below is particularly relevant to disclosures:

2.06 Maintaining Confidentiality.

(a) Behavior analysts have a primary obligation and take reasonable precautions to protect the confidentiality of those with whom they work or consult, recognizing that confidentiality may be established by law, organizational rules, or professional or scientific relationships. (b) Behavior analysts discuss confidentiality at the outset of the relationship and thereafter as new circumstances may warrant. (c) In order to minimize intrusions on privacy, behavior analysts include only information germane to the purpose for which the communication is made in written, oral, and electronic reports, consultations, and other avenues. (d) Behavior analysts discuss confidential information obtained in clinical or consulting relationships, or evaluative data concerning clients, students, research participants, supervisees, and employees, only for appropriate scientific or professional purposes and only with persons clearly concerned with such matters. (e) Behavior analysts must not share or create situations likely to result in the sharing of any identifying information (written, photographic, or video) about current clients and supervisees within social media contexts.

2.07 Maintaining Records. (a) Behavior analysts maintain appropriate confidentiality in creating, storing, accessing, transferring, and disposing of records under their control, whether these are written, automated, electronic, or in any other medium. (b) Behavior analysts maintain and dispose of records in accordance with applicable laws, regulations, corporate policies, and organizational policies, and in a manner that permits compliance with the requirements of this Code.

2.08 Disclosures. Behavior analysts never disclose confidential information without the consent of the client, except as mandated by law, or where permitted by law for a valid purpose, such as (1) to provide needed professional services to the client, (2) to obtain appropriate professional consultations, (3) to protect the client or others from harm, or (4) to obtain payment for services, in which instance disclosure is limited to the minimum that is necessary to achieve the purpose. Behavior analysts recognize that parameters of consent for disclosure should be acquired at the outset of any defined relationship and is an ongoing procedure throughout the duration of the professional relationship.

One last comment on confidentiality and working with persons with intellectual disabilities who have committed a sexual offense relates to sharing with other professionals in regard to multidisciplinary collaboration. Best practice in the field of dual diagnosis suggests that treatment and intervention should be multidisciplinary. Although traditional therapy commonly includes a perspective that all information shared in treatment is to remain confidential, in order to work in a multidisciplinary fashion where the person's needs are examined holistically, open discussion with other professionals is important. In such cases, information that is pertinent to treatment across professionals is important to share with persons who *need to know,* but only if the individual provides consent to do so (Fletcher, 2017).

GIVEN THE RISKY NATURE OF THE BEHAVIORS, HOW DOES A PRACTITIONER DEAL WITH AN INDIVIDUAL OR AN AGENCY THAT IS NOT TREATMENT COMPLIANT?

At an individual level, treatment noncompliance for a person with an intellectual disability who has sexually offended can occur both passively and actively. At a passive level, the person may show a lack of motivation to engage in treatment. At an active level, the person may be vigorously resisting change and engaging in behaviors that are known to be counterproductive to treatment, such as use of drugs or alcohol or seeking locations that are known to present stimuli that precede offending behavior.

At a systems or agency level the issue of a lack of adherence to treatment protocols and the resultant impact on treatment fidelity can present a significant ethical challenge for the practitioner overseeing the treatment plan. Hingsburger, Lee, and Salonia (2014) adopted the concept of deliberate indifference to describe some agency support, or lack thereof, of persons with intellectual disabilities in community settings. They suggested deliberate indifference in a community care setting can occur when three elements are present. First, a person or agency must be entrusted with the care of a person; second, the person or agency must be aware that there is an imminent risk associated with the behaviors of the person; and third, the person or agency must deliberately fail to put in place strategies or actions that could prevent that risk. Let us take an example of a person with an intellectual disability who has a history of sexual offending against children and who decides he wants to move from his current group home into group home that is located next to a school yard. He tells his support staff that he wants to move there and that it is his right. Despite the staff members' knowledge of his situation, they agree to move him because they say it is his right to live where he chooses. However, this move would constitute deliberate indifference. Yes, he has rights; however, fulfilling this right may potentially put others at risk and, given his personal advocacy to move to that setting, risk is likely imminent. In fact, it is likely also a case of negligence. As Ward (2011, p. 112) noted, "[r]ights imply duties, and while entitlements and other human rights are extended to offenders, these should always be balanced against the core interests and basic human rights of others and the safety of the country at large."

Often, indifference on the part of an agency or staff can be subtler, such as failure to observe people in situations that should be supervised or lax adherence to protocols, policies, or consistent consequences. Nonetheless, appropriate risk management is a critical issue in supporting persons with intellectual disabilities and histories of sexual offending when they live in community settings. Respecting the rights of the individual cannot undermine responsibility to protect both the person and others.

Hingsburger and colleagues (2014) suggested that risk reduction strategies occur at four levels, which we have adapted for this population. The first level is environmental. An agency supporting an individual who offended must provide a safe environment for that individual and others, which may involve strategically locating the person in a special setting within the community. Second, staff must be fully aware of the risk factors and precursor behaviors associated with the person's challenges, be trained in risk identification and management, and receive ongoing support in implementing the strategies necessary to prevent the behavior. Third, if at high risk, the person will likely require eyes-on supervision at all times, while providing as much autonomy as is responsibly possible. This may also include avoidance of high-risk situations and places and supervised exposure. Lastly, staff members have a responsibility to consistently take opportunities to remind and reinforce the individual of the necessary boundaries to keep both the person and the community safe. In this, the role of the behavior therapist is to ensure that ongoing training and consultation is provided to ensure that therapeutic drift over time is avoided. This can occur when a program has been ongoing and imminent danger does not appear to loom; potentially leading to complacency, which creates perfect environmental cues for inconsistent messages to occur increasing the potential for re-offense.

HOW DOES DIGNITY OF RISK FIT INTO THE TREATMENT OF PERSONS WITH INTELLECTUAL DISABILITIES WHO HAVE COMMITTED A SEXUAL OFFENSE?

Dignity of risk is a concept in working with persons with intellectual disabilities that implies that, although a person may have limitations in their abilities, the person should not be denied the opportunity to try something that they may wish to do but at which they may fail by virtue of their disability. This does not mean, however, that persons who are in a position to care for the person should turn their backs on a situation that would cause potential harm to the person or others just because the person wants to do it. In the case of a person who sexually offended against children and who is now choosing to engage in a risky behavior, such as going for a walk in a park where there are children, the person is not only putting himself at risk, but is risking the welfare of potentially vulnerable children. This discussion involves a greater dilemma that involves duty of care versus autonomy. The debate over autonomy and duty of care is ongoing in both practice and in the literature (Hawkins et al. 2011). Autonomy implies that the person, on his own, is able to make an independent decision. However, according to the ethics of care, there is a reliance on meeting the needs of those for whom care is being provided and, as such, decisions are relational (interdependent) rather than based on absolute autonomy (Held, 1996). Nonetheless, underlying this relationship is responsiveness, sensitivity, and empathy. As such, "[t]he ethics of care addresses rather than neglects moral issues arising in relationships among the unequal and dependent, relations that are often laden with emotion and involuntary" (Held, 2006, p. 10).

The ethical and moral dilemmas clinicians and support workers face must involve careful analysis of many day-to-day issues. At the heart of these issues are some basic values that hold primacy. The first is consideration of promoting beneficence (do good) while avoiding maleficence (do no harm). When considering a person's goals and individual autonomy, we must always ask: Is the individual's decision one that has potential to improve the person's life or does it pose an imminent and reasonable risk of harm to himself or others?

SUMMARY

> *There is little doubt that ethical considerations are of paramount importance in dealing with individuals with intellectual and developmental disabilities (IDD). This is no less important for those individuals entangled in the criminal justice system and the subsequent ethical aspects of working with people with IDD who have been labelled as an offender* (Griffiths, et al., 2018, p. 105).

The BACB® Code of Ethics is foundational for all assessment and treatment procedures in ABA. The challenges for this population of persons with intellectual disabilities who have sexually offended can be significant. There are often seemingly competing priorities, such as balancing risk and rights with responsibility, or treatment and management, that will create ethical dilemmas requiring the vigilance of ethical practice. Further discussion and research on this topic in the field is highly warranted.

REFERENCES

APA Presidential Task Force (2006). Evidence based practice in psychology. *American Psychologist, 61,* 271-285. Retrieved from http://www.apa.org/pubs/journals/features/evidence-based-statement.pdfn psychology

Aunos, M. & Feldman, M. A. (2002). Attitudes towards sexuality, sterilization and parenting rights of persons with intellectual disabilities. *Journal of Applied Research in Intellectual Disabilities, 15,* 285-296.

Baumeister, A. A. (1997). Behavioral research: Boon or bust? In W. E. McLean (Ed.), *Ellis' handbook of mental deficiency, psychological theory, and research.* Mahwah, NJ: Erlbaum.

Beech, A. R. & Ward, T. (2004). (2004). The integration of etiology and risk in sex offenders: A theoretical model. *Aggression and Violent Behavior, 10,* 31-63.

Behavior Analyst Certification Board (BACB) (2014). *Behavior analyst certification board professional and ethical compliance code for behavior analysts.* Retrieved from http://bacb.com/ethics-code/

Bergman, L. R., & Magnusson, D. (1997). A person-oriented approach in research on developmental psychopathy. *Development and Psychopathology, 9,* 291-319.

Birgden, A. (2009). Therapeutic jurisprudence and offender rights: a normative stance is required. *University of Puerto Rico Revista Juridica, 78,* 43–60. Retrieved from http://www.antoniocasella.eu/archipsy/birgden_2009.pdf

Birgden, A., & Cucolo, H. (2011). The treatment of sex offenders: Evidence, ethics, and human rights. *Sexual Abuse: A Journal of Research and Treatment, 23,* 295–313.

Blasingame, G. D., Boer, D. P., Guidry, L., Haaven, J., & Wilson, R. J. (2014). *Assessment, treatment, and supervision of individuals with intellectual disabilities and problematic sexual behaviors: Informational packet.* [Education & Training Committee Report] Beaverton, OR: Association for the Treatment of Sexual Abusers.

Bonta, J. & Andrews, D.A. (2017). *The psychology of criminal conduct* (6th ed.). Cincinnati, OH: Anderson.

Brown, H. & Thompson, D. (1997). The ethics of research with men who have learning disabilities and abusive sexual behavior: a minefield in a vacuum. *Disability & Society, 12*(5), 695-707.

Chamless, D. L., Baker, M., Baucom, D. H. Beutler, L. E., Calhoun, K. S., Critz-Christoph, P. M., ... McCurry, S. (1988). Update on empirically validated therapies, II. *The Clinical Psychologist, 51,* 3-16.

Coleman, E. (2002). Sexuality and developmental disabilities: rights for sexual health. In D. M. Griffiths, D. Richards, P. Fedoroff, & S. Watson (Eds.), *Ethical dilemmas: sexuality and developmental* disabilities (pp. 5-9). Kingston, NY: NADD Press.

Cullen, F. T. & Gendreau, P. (2000). Assessing correctional rehabilitation: Policy, practice, and prospects. *Criminal Justice, 3,* 109-175.

Dial, K. B. (1968). A report of group work to increase social skills of females in vocational rehabilitation program. *Mental Retardation, 6,* 11-14.

Feldman, M., Condillac, R., Tough, S., Hunt, S., & Griffiths, D. (2002). Effectiveness of community positive behavioral intervention for persons with developmental disabilities and severe behavior problems. *Behavior Therapy, 33,* 377-398.

Fletcher, R. (2017). *Diagnostic Manual- Intellectual Disabilities 2.* International Dual Diagnosis Certificate Program, Brock University, St. Catharines, ON.

Fredericks, B. & Nishioka-Evans, V. (1999). Functional assessment for a sex offender population. In A.C. Repp & R.H. Horner (Eds.), *Functional analysis of problem behavior: From effective assessment to effective support* (pp.279-303). Belmont CA: Wadsworth Publishing.

Glaser, R. (2009). Treaters or punishers? The ethical role of mental health clinicians in sex offender programs. *Aggression and Violent Behavior, 14,* 248-255.

Glenn, S. S., (1988). Contingencies and metacontingencies: Toward a synthesis of behavior analysis and cultural materialism. Behavior Analyst, 11(2), 161-179.

Griffiths, D. (in press). What Works: Ethical consideration when treating offenders with intellectual and developmental disabilities. In W. Lindsay, L. Craig & D. Griffiths (Eds.). *What works with offenders with intellectual disabilities: Theory, research and practice.* Wiley-Blackwell.

Griffiths, D. (2002). Sexual aggression. In Wm. I. Gardner (Ed.), *Aggression and other disruptive behavioral challenges: Biomedical and psychosocial assessment and treatment* (pp. 325-398). New York: National Association for Dual Diagnosis.

Griffiths, D., Hingsburger, D., Ioannou, S., & Hoath, J. (2018). Ethical considerations in working with people with intellectual disabilities who have offended. In W. Lindsay & J. Taylor (Eds.), *The Wiley handbook on offenders with intellectual disabilities: research, training and practice* (p-p.105.122). Chichester, UK: Wiley.

Griffiths, D. M., Richards, D., Fedoroff, P, & Watson S.L. (2002). *Ethical dilemmas: Sexuality and developmental disabilities.* Kingston, NY: NADD Press.

Griffiths, D., Watson, S., Lewis, R., & Stoner, K. (2004). Sexuality research and persons with intellectual disabilities. In E. Emerson, C. Hatton, T. Thompson & T. R. Parmenter (Eds.), *International handbook of applied research in intellectual disabilities* (pp.311-334). London: John Wiley & Sons.

Hamelin, J., Marinos, V., Robinson, J., & Griffiths, D. (2011). Rights and the justice system. In D. Griffiths, F. Owen, S. Watson (Eds.), *The rights agenda: An action plan to advance the rights of persons with intellectual disabilities* (pp. 223-254). Welland, ON: 3Rs Community University Research Alliance.

Hawkins, R., Redley, M., & Holland, A. J. (2011). Duty of care and autonomy: How support workers manage the tension between protecting service users from risk and

promoting their independence in a specialized group home. *Journal of Intellectual Disability Research, 55*, 873-884.
Held, V. (2006). *The ethic of care: Personal, political, and global.* New York, NY: Oxford University Press.
Hingsburger, D., Lee, D. & Salonia, C. (2014). *Deliberate indifference: understanding the legal implications of risk. Executive functioning - A newsletter for senior leadership in organizations providing human services.* Retrieved from http://www.vitacls.org/pdf/Executive%20Functioning%20-%20Vol%201%20Issue%202.pdf
Holburn, S. (2002). How science can evaluate and enhance person-centred planning. *Research and Practice in Persons with Severe Disabilities, 27*, 250-260.
Iacona, T. & Murray, V. (2003). Issues of informed consent in conducting medical research involving people with intellectual disability. *Journal of Applied Research in Intellectual Disability, 16*, 41-51.
Ioannou, S. (2013). *Managing risk in a culture of rights: providing support and treatment for sex offenders with intellectual disability in community-based settings.* Unpublished Master of Arts Thesis. Brock University, St. Catharines, ON.
Laws, D.R. & Marshall, W.L. (2003). Sexual Offenders: Part 1. Early Developments A Brief History of Behavioral and Cognitive Behavioral Approaches to Sexual Offenders: Part 1. Early Developments. *Sex Abuse: A Journal of Research and Treatment, 15*(2), 75-92.
Lindsay, W. R. (2005). A model underpinning treatment for sex offenders with mild intellectual disability: current theories of sex offending. *Mental Retardation, 43*, 428-441.
Lindsay, W. R. (2009). *The treatment of sex offenders with developmental disabilities.* West Sussex, UK: Wiley-Blackwell.
Lindsay, W. R. (June 2015). *Assessment and treatment of sexual offending behavior in persons with developmental disabilities and autism.* International Dual Diagnosis Certificate Program, Brock University, St. Catharines, Ontario.
Lindsay, W. R., Smith, A. H. W., Law, J., Quinn, K., Anderson, A., Smith, A., & Allan, R. (2004) Sexual and nonsexual offenders with intellectual and learning disabilities: A comparison of characteristics, referral patterns and outcome. *Journal of Interpersonal Violence, 19*, 875-890.
Lippke, R. L. (2002). Toward a theory of prisoners' rights. *Ratio Juris, 15*, 122–145.
Lorenzen, T. J. & V. L. Anderson (1993). *Design of experiments: a no-name approach.* New York, NY: Marcel Dekker, Inc.
Lund, C.A. (1992). Long-term treatment of sexual behavior problems in adolescent and adult developmentally disabled persons. *Annals of sex research, 5* (1), 5–31.
Lunsky, Y., Frijters, J., Griffiths, D. M., Watson, S. L., & Williston, S. (2007). Sexual knowledge and attitudes of men with intellectual disability who sexually offend. *Journal of Intellectual and Developmental Disability, 32*, 74-81.
Magnusson, D. (2003). The person approach: Concepts, measurement models, and research strategy. *New Directions for Child and Adolescent Development, 101*, 3-23.
Marshall, W.L. (2009). Manualization: A blessing or a curse? *Journal of Sexual Aggression, 15* (2), 109-120.
Miller, D. (2007). *National responsibilities and global justice.* Oxford UK: Oxford Press.

Montenegro, M. & Greenhill, B. (2015). Evaluating the 'Freda Challenge': a coproduced human rights game in services for persons with intellectual disabilities. *Journal of Applied Research in Intellectual Disabilities, 28*, 223-238.

Newsom, C., & *Hovanitz*, C. A. (*2005*). The nature and value of empirically validated interventions. In J. W. Jacobson, R. M. Foxx, & J. A. Mulick (Eds.), *Controversial therapies for developmental disabilities: Fad, fashion and science in professional practice* (pp. 31-44). Mahwah, NJ, US: Lawrence Erlbaum Associates Publishers.

Owen, F., Griffiths, D., Stoner, K., Gosse, L., Watson, S., Tardif, C.,...Vyrostko, B. (2003). Multi-level human rights training: The first step to changing systems. *Journal on Developmental Disabilities, 10*, 43-64.

Owen, F., & MacKinnon, G. (2012). The right to community living. In D. Griffiths, F. Owen, & S. L. Watson (Eds.), *Rights agenda: An action plan to advance the rights of persons with intellectual disabilities* (pp. 5-14). St. Catharines, ON: Community University Research Alliance.

Peel Behavioral Services & Wilson, R. J. (2017). *Passport to independence.* Holyoke, MA: NEARI Press.

Polvinale, R. A. & Lutzker, J. R. (1980). Elimination of assaultive and inappropriate behavioiur by reinforcement and social-restitution. *Mental Retardation, 18*, 27-30.

Risley, T. R. (1999). Foreword: Positive behavioral support and applied behavior analysis. In E.G. Carr, R.H. Horner, A.P. Turnbull, J.G. Marquis, D. Magito-McLaughlin, M.L.McAtee, C.E.Smith, K. Anderson-Ryan, M.B. Ruef,& A. Doolabh, *Positive behavior support for people with disabilities: A research synthesis.* Washington, D.C.: American Association on Mental Retardation.

Rosenthal, T. L. (1973). Response-contingent vs fixed punishment in aversion condition of pedophilia: a case study. *Journal of Nervous and Mental Disease, 156*, 440-443.

Schalock, R. L. (1994). The concept of quality of life and its current applications in the field of mental retardation/developmental disabilities. In D. Goode (Ed.), *Quality of life for persons with disabilities: international perspectives and issues* (pp. 266-284). Cambridge MA: Brookline.

Shaw, W. J. & Walker, C. E. (1979). Use of relaxation in the short-term treatment of fetishistic behavior: an exploratory case study. *Journal of Pediatric Psychology, 4*, 403-407.

Sidman, M. (1960). *Tactics of scientific research: Evaluating experimental data in psychology.* New York: Basic Books.

Skinner, B. F. (1953). Science and human behavior. New York: Macmillan.

Stancliffe, R. J. & Wehmeyer, M. L. (1995). Variability to the availability of choice to adults with mental retardation. *Journal of Vocational Rehabilitation, 5*, 319-328.

Steptoe. L., Lindsay, W. R., Forrest, D. & Power, M. (2008). Quality of life and relationships in sex offenders with intellectual disability. *Journal of Intellectual and Developmental Disability, 31*, 13-19.

Swanson, C. K., & Garwick, F. B. (1990). Treatment for low functioning sex offenders: group therapy and interagency cooperation. *Mental Retardation, 28*, 155-161.

Tilley, E., Walmsley, J., Earle, S., & Atkinson, D. (2012) 'The silence is roaring': Sterilization, reproductive rights and women with intellectual disabilities. *Disability and Society 27*, 413–426.

Tough, S. E. (2001, November). *Validation of two standard risk assessments (Rapid Risk Assessment for Sex Offense Recidivism, 1997; Static–99, 1999) on a sample of adult males who are developmentally disabled with significant cognitive deficits.* Paper presented at the Association for the Treatment of Sexual Abusers 20th Annual Research and Treatment Conference, San Antonio.

United Nations (2006). *Convention on the Rights of Persons with Disabilities.* Retrieved September 7, 2018 from www.un.org/development/desa/disabilities/convention-on-the-rights-of-persons-with-disabilities.html

Vollmer, T. R. (2014, June). Ethical issues for applied behavior analysts: Covert observation. *Severe and challenging behavior of persons with intellectual disabilities or autism: Supporting individuals in the community.* Dual Diagnosis Certificate Program, Brock University, St. Catharines, ON.

Ward, T. (2007). On a clear day you can see forever: Integrating values and skills in sex offender treatment. *Journal of Sexual Aggression, 13,* 187-201.

Ward, T. (2011). Human rights and dignity in offender rehabilitation. *Journal of Forensic Psychology Practice, 11,* 103-123.

Ward, T., Gannon, T. A., & Birdgen, A. (2007). Human rights and the treatment of sex offenders. *Sexual Abuse,* 19, 195-216.

Ward, T. & Salmon, K. (2011). The ethics of care and treatment of sex offenders. *Sexual Abuse, 23,* 397-413.

Ward, T., & Stewart, C. (2003). Criminogenic needs and human needs: A theoretical *model. Psychology, Crime & Law, 9,* 125-143.

Watson, S. L., Richards, D. A., Hayes, S., Lecomte, J., & Taua, C. (2012). The right to consent to treatment. In D. Griffiths, F. Owen, & S.L. Watson (Eds.), *Rights Agenda: An action plan to advance the rights of persons with intellectual disabilities* (pp. 5-14). St. Catharines, ON: Community University Research Alliance.

Wilson, R. J., Cortoni, F., Picheca, J. E., Stirpe, T. S., & Nunes, K. (2009). *Community-based sexual offender maintenance treatment programming: An evaluation.* [Research Report R-188] Ottawa, ON: Correctional Service of Canada.

Wilson, R. J. & McWhinnie, A. J. (2017). *Circles of Support & Accountability: A "how to" guide for establishing CoSA in your location.* Report compiled under contract to Counseling and Psychotherapy Center, Inc. for the United States Department of Justice, Office of Justice Programs, Office of Sex Offender Sentencing, Monitoring, Apprehending, Registration, and Tracking.

Wilson, R. J. & Sandler, J. C. (in press). What works (or does not) in community risk management for persons convicted of sexual offenses? A contemporary perspective. *International Journal of Offender Therapy and Comparative Criminology.*

Wong, S. E., Gaydos, G. R., & Fuqua, R. W. (1982). Operant control of pedophilia: reducing approaches to children. *Behavior Modification, 6,* 73-84.

Wulfert, E., Greenway, D., & Dougher, M. J. (1996). A logical functional analysis of reinforcement-based disorders: Alcoholism and pedophilia. *Journal of Consulting and Clinical Psychology, 64*(6), 1140-1151.